OPTUM360°

DESK REFERENCE

2018

Clinical Documentation Improvement Desk Reference for ICD-10-CM and Procedure Coding

The Clinician's Checklist for ICD-10-CM
Your copy of this manual includes *The Clinician's Checklist for ICD-10-CM*, a trifold card with documentation tips for the most common chronic and acute medical conditions. Use this card to help clinicians understand the documentation needed for accurate ICD-10-CM coding.

Optum360 Notice

Optum360
2525 Lake Park Blvd
Salt Lake City, UT 84120

Our Commitment to Accuracy

Optum360 is committed to producing accurate and reliable materials.

To report corrections, please visit www.optum360coding.com/accuracy or email accuracy@optum.com. You can also reach customer service by calling 1.800.464.3649.

American Medical Association Notice

Copyright

Made in the USA
ISBN 978-1-62254-341-0

Acknowledgments

Gregory A. Kemp, MA, *Product Manager*
Karen Schmidt, BSN, *Technical Director*
Stacy Perry, *Manager, Desktop Publishing*
Lisa Singley, *Project Manager*
Leanne Patterson, CPC, *Clinical/Technical Editor*
Deborah C. Hall, *Clinical/Technical Editor*
Tom Darr, *MD*
Tracy Betzler, *Senior Desktop Publishing Specialist*
Hope M. Dunn, *Senior Desktop Publishing Specialist*
Katie Russell, *Desktop Publishing Specialist*
Jean Parkinson, *Editor*

About the Technical Editors

Leanne Patterson, CPC

Ms. Patterson has more than 10 years of experience in the health care profession. She has an extensive background in professional component coding, with expertise in E/M coding and auditing, and HIPAA compliance. Her experience includes general surgery coding, serving as Director of Compliance, and conducting chart-to-claim audits and physician education. She has been responsible for coding and denial management in large multi-specialty physician practices and most recently served as a practice manager where she supervised implementation of a new EHR system. Ms. Patterson is credentialed by the American Academy of Professional Coders (AAPC) as a Certified Professional Coder (CPC).

Deborah C. Hall

Ms. Hall is a new product subject matter expert for Optum360. She has more than 35 years of experience in the health care field. Ms. Hall's experience includes 10 years as practice administrator for large multi-specialty medical practices. She has written several multi-specialty newsletters and coding and reimbursement manuals, and served as a health care consultant. She has taught seminars on CPT/HCPCS and ICD-9-CM coding and physician fee schedules.

Tom Darr, MD

Tom Darr, MD, is the VP of Clinical Solutions for Optum360. Through his clinical expertise and 20 years of business experience related to the revenue cycle, Dr. Darr brings a patient focus to Optum360's technology solutions and services, designed to simplify and improve the patient experience so patients and health care providers can focus their attention on treatment, healing, and care. He is certified by the American Board of Emergency Medicine and is a practicing emergency medicine physician with more than 30 years' experience.

Contents

Section 1: Introduction

Medical record documentation, whether paper or electronic, is one of the cornerstones of our health system today. Only accurate, consistent, and complete documentation can translate into the data and information necessary to ensure clinical quality, substantiate medical necessity, and determine the most appropriate reimbursement. No matter the setting, the health record documentation, as designated by the physician provider, remains the foundation upon which many decisions are based. As a result, efforts to improve the quality of that documentation have been on-going for many years.

Origins of Clinical Documentation Improvement (CDI) Efforts

Providers' focus on clinical documentation has its beginnings in the administration of President Ronald W. Reagan in the early 1980s. Ironically, President Reagan's initial opposition to government intervention in private industry gave way to the heavily regulated payment systems that characterize Medicare today. Following the creation of the Medicare program in the 1960s, Medicare costs increased rapidly. By the late 1970s, it was a "runaway" program that had thwarted all voluntary efforts by hospitals to slow costs.

However, as voluntary restraints proved to be ineffective at controlling the costs of the Medicare program, President Reagan and Congress pragmatically turned to prospective payment. The resulting diagnosis related group (DRG) system pays hospitals on the basis of a patient's medical condition and other factors, including procedures provided. Clinical documentation is a fundamental element in securing appropriate provider payment under the DRG payment system. Under DRGs, poor documentation results in lower payments.

Since its inception, Medicare's DRG payment system has saved the government hundreds of billions of dollars. Due to its success, the Centers for Medicare and Medicaid Services (CMS) has expanded its use of prospective payment systems (PPS) and introduced other payment methodologies to control Medicare program costs. In each instance, provider reimbursement hinges on documentation. CMS's intent to move to "value-based payments" is the latest example. Demonstrating value means showing how a patient's medical condition has improved or has been addressed by specific care, as found in the Quality Payment Program. Communicating a patient's improved condition relies upon clinical documentation.

The Clinician's View of CDI

There has been a long battle between administrative staff and clinicians over clinical documentation. Too often, clinical detail is lacking in clinical documentation, which makes it difficult to code claims and answer auditor's questions. There are two issues that contribute to a misalignment of physician and facility interests:

- Physicians have traditionally been paid based on procedures performed, with the patient diagnosis considered secondary. The procedure was either performed, or not performed. It is a simple matter in the mind of the physician and does not require detailed documentation. Today, however, diagnosis documentation has become more important in order to confirm medical necessity for procedures and to accurately identify the patient's medical condition. Additionally, the lack of detail of the service or procedure performed often leads to a less complex procedure or service being reported on the claim and, therefore, reimbursement is at a lower rate.
- Clinical detail required for billing is not usually an independent clinician's first concern. Extra work or effort from clinicians to help billing does not reward physicians.

Several factors, however, are now working to enhance clinician motivation toward improving documentation, including audits of professional claims by payers, such as Medicare's recovery audit contractors (RAC), and concerted efforts by billing personnel and auditors to gain clinician cooperation with documentation through CDI programs. Both internal and payer auditors find that lack of documentation is the most common reason for claim denials. But in a broader way, clinicians are now more aware of documentation issues as a result of the change from ICD-9 to ICD-10 coding systems and CMS's intention to shift payments in a way that requires more clinical detail for demonstrating value-based care.

Gain Share is Encouraging Documentation Improvement

The health plans participating in CMS's Medicare Advantage program now have nearly a third of all Medicare beneficiaries enrolled, with a significant number of the nation's physicians serving these beneficiaries. Payments to the health plans are made on a capitated, per-member, per-month basis, with rates adjusted by the patient's medical condition. Medicare Advantage plans are allowed to keep the portion of premiums not spent for care, and increasingly, physicians serving these beneficiaries are invited to participate in gain sharing. In these arrangements, physicians receive some part of the health plan revenues. Physicians contribute to health plan revenue largely by providing complete and accurate clinical documentation that earns higher capitated payments for individual patients. Involvement with gain sharing arrangements has elevated some physicians' attention to clinical documentation improvement.

In the physician office/clinic setting, reimbursement has been tied directly to diagnosis codes by substantiating the medical necessity of the service or procedure performed. Additionally, for Medicare Advantage or Part C claims, diagnosis coding can affect reimbursement under the Medicare Hierarchical Condition Category (HCC) regulations. The latest regulatory initiative that increased these efforts was the move from the ICD-9-CM coding system to ICD-10-CM for diagnoses.

Because of the increased number of codes available and their corresponding level of detail, the documentation driving that code assignment must be just as detailed and provide the additional information. Additional regulatory efforts to prevent health care fraud and abuse also require concise, complete, and accurate medical record documentation that supports the procedures or services reported.

Optum360's *Guide to Clinical Validation, Documentation and Coding* is a suggested companion to this desk reference. Visit www.Optum360Coding.com for more details.

Reasons to Implement Clinical Documentation Improvement

Clinical documentation improvement provides a number of benefits and the reasons to implement are far reaching. Some of the reasons to implement a CDI program are the following:

- To identify and clarify any confusing, incomplete, conflicting, or missing information in the physician-documented portion of the health record that is related to diagnoses or procedures
- To foster and enhance communication between members of the CDI team (such as CDI staff and coders) and the medical staff
- To provide education to medical staff members on the increased granularity inherent in ICD-10-CM and how it necessitates more detailed documentation in the medical record
- To provide continuity of care for the patient, between members of the health care team that rely on documentation in the health record for determining ongoing treatment decisions
- To provide a more robust and accurate depiction of patient severity
- To provide education to coding staff members to increase their clinical knowledge, particularly as it relates to the increased specificity in conditions, diseases, procedures, and services
- To support clinical quality initiatives, including those related to outcome scores and pay-for-performance programs
- To provide more robust clinical data to the clinical community to assist in data-driven decisions
- To decrease the provider's compliance risk as it relates to medical necessity and coverage, coding and billing, and other issues related to regulatory compliance
- To provide a defense for regulatory compliance reviews, such as those by RACs, zone program integrity contractors (ZPIC) and Medicaid integrity contractors programs
- To decrease the number of delayed or denied claims due to insufficient documentation

- To promote the goal of the hospital medical record being as complete as possible during an acute care admission
- To ensure appropriate reimbursement for the medically necessary services provided, regardless of the reimbursement mechanism

Hierarchical Condition Categories and CDI

As mentioned previously, CDI is important to ensure appropriate ICD-10-CM code assignment is supported. Clinical documentation is also important to support that Hierarchical Condition Category (HCC) assignment is correct, confirming correct code assignment and appropriate reimbursement.

Medicare is one of the world's largest health insurance programs, and about one-third of the beneficiaries on Medicare are enrolled in a Medicare Advantage (MA) private health care plan. Due to the great variance in the health status of Medicare beneficiaries, risk adjustment provides a means of adequately compensating those plans with large numbers of seriously ill patients while not overburdening other plans that have healthier individuals. Medicare Advantage plans have been using the Hierarchical Condition Category/risk adjustment model since 2004. Simplistically, based on the patient's condition and assignment of the correct ICD-10-CM code, the patient is classified to an HCC that has been determined to affect the cost of health care. Currently the following HCC models are in use:

- CMS-HCC (Medicare Advantage)
- Rx-HCC (Drugs)
- PACE/ESRD

The term "risk adjustment" is often used to describe what HCCs do. HCCs predict health care resource consumption of individuals. HCC scores are used to "risk adjust" payments to a health plan based on the level of risk the beneficiary presents to the plan. HCCs adjust payments so that there is a higher reimbursement for sicker patients.

Under the current CMS-HCC model, MA organizations collect risk adjustment (RA) data, including beneficiary diagnoses from hospital inpatient facilities, hospital outpatient facilities, and physicians during a data-collection period. MA organizations identify the diagnoses relevant to the CMS model and submit them to CMS. CMS categorizes the diagnoses into groups of clinically related diseases called HCCs and uses the HCC category, disease interactions, as well as demographic characteristics to calculate a Risk Adjustment Factor (RAF) score for each beneficiary. CMS then uses the RAF scores to adjust the monthly capitated payments to MA organizations for the next payment period.

Risk adjustment is a process of adjusting capitation payments to health plans either higher or lower to account for the differences in expected health costs of individuals. Risk adjustment is required for managed care programs that monitor changes in disease progression and population mix, set performance targets to generate outcome data, and identify patients for population health initiatives (disease or case management). RA is used by the government as well as private and commercial insurance entities, and is needed in any value-based purchasing program.

The ICD-10-CM codes that are associated with an HCC will be identified by the icon HCC next to the code. Note, in some instances, where a range of codes are identified under the topic, not all codes may be associated with an HCC. Please refer to appendix B for the specific codes within that range that are associated with an HCC.

IMPORTANT

When the HCC icon appears with a range of codes, please refer to appendix B as not all codes within the range may be associated with an HCC. Note, in some instances, where a range of codes is identified under the topic, not all codes may be associated with an HCC.

Supporting Documentation for Reporting Procedures and Services

Medical record documentation is also essential for determining the most appropriate CPT® code. The CPT code book contains many code for procedures which, while very similar, have distinct components that differentiate them. This could be something as easily identifiable as the morphology of a lesion, or something more difficult, such as specific instrumentation. The difficulty lies in educating clinicians on the exact information needed for documentation as well as the coder or CDI experts understanding the key terms that identify these components.

Failing to adequately document medical services and procedures can lead to inaccurately reported services, claim delays, claim denials or even, after postpayment review by an insurer, recoupment of payments, or allegations of fraud and abuse.

How to Use This Book

The Optum360 *Clinical Documentation Improvement Desk Reference for ICD-10-CM and Procedure Coding* is designed for use by providers and all others who are involved in the documentation and coding processes in any setting. It is organized in an easy-to-use alphabetic format, focusing on those diagnoses, services, and procedures with significant differences in the type and specificity required for accurate code assignment. This allows greater ease in providing very specific and focused information for physicians in certain specialties who provide documentation.

For example, a pulmonologist may want to review the differences in documentation requirements between ICD-9-CM and ICD-10-CM codes for a condition such as asthma. The chapter related to Diseases of the Respiratory System contains a section for asthma, and at first glance, it is apparent that the code axes, or the major way in which the codes are arranged and classified, have changed. Instead of the "extrinsic" and "intrinsic" categories in ICD-9-CM, the asthma codes in ICD-10-CM fall into the following major categories:

- Mild intermittent asthma
- Mild persistent asthma
- Moderate persistent asthma
- Severe persistent asthma
- Other and unspecified asthma

The second code axis is related to presentation of disease: Is the patient suffering from an acute exacerbation, is status asthmaticus present, or is this a chronic and uncomplicated case? The answers to these questions relate to the fifth-digit subclassification under each of the major categories listed above.

The Clinical Documentation Improvement Desk Reference for ICD-10-CM and Procedure Coding manual provides definitions for each of the major types of asthma, so that the pulmonologist may share the information with the office staff, residents, interns, and any others that may be reviewing the healthrecord documentation. These differentiating factors (mild versus moderate, intermittent versus persistent) should be clearly documented, according to the definitions provided. Obviously, the severity level determination is affected by whether any of the secondary axis items (acute exacerbation, status asthmaticus) are also documented.

In addition to conditions, *The Clinical Documentation Improvement Desk Reference for ICD-10-CM and Procedure Coding* also provides key documentation requirements that differentiate between select procedures. For example, the topic Abortion illustrates the differences between the treatment of different types of abortions and the differences in the documentation requirements for each.

There are several new features for the 2018 edition. First, there is the addition of condition-related medication lists. For most diagnosis entries, when applicable, lists of common medications used to treat a condition have been provided. The lists identify generic names along with common brand names.

There are also two new icons for 2018. The icon **HCC** identifies those ICD-10-CM codes that are associated with an HCC. A second icon, **QPP**, may appear next to a diagnosis or procedure code and indicates it is associated with a quality measure included in the Medicare Quality Payment Program (QPP).

Finally the third new feature is appendix B, "HCC and QPP Associated Codes." This table will list the codes discussed in this product that are associated with either an HCC, a Quality measure or both as shown below.

Code	Description	Associated HCC	Associated Quality Measure
I48.2	Chronic atrial fibrillation	HCC 96	Measure 326

Note: The codes identified in the table are only those codes specifically addressed in this publication; not all codes associated with an HCC or Quality measure are included. For a complete list of HCC-related diagnosis codes refer to the CMS website at:
https://www.cms.gov/Medicare/Health-Plans/MedicareAdvtgSpecRateStats/Risk-Adjustors.html.
For more information on QPP and the official list of quality measures refer to the CMS website at: https://qpp.cms.gov/.

For most entries, diagnosis or procedure, this manual provides a listing of clinical issues that need to be addressed in clinical documentation in order to help coders assign appropriate codes and distinguish a medical condition from similar but different conditions. In the example below for Crohn's disease, the clinician is prompted to identify evidence of the medical condition, and distinguish the manifestation from among the alternatives. Finally, the checklist asks about associated conditions.

Clinician Documentation Checklist

Clinician documentation should indicate the following:

- Includes
  - granulomatous enteritis
- Identify
  - manifestations such as pyoderma gangrenosum
  - part of intestinal tract involved
    - small intestine
      - Crohn's disease of duodenum
      - Crohn's disease of ileum
      - Crohn's disease of jejunum
      - regional ileitis
      - terminal ileitis
    - large intestine
      - Crohn's disease of colon
      - Crohn's disease of large bowel
      - Crohn's disease of rectum
      - granulomatous colitis
      - regional colitis
    - both small and large intestine
    - unspecified part
      - Crohn's disease
      - regional enteritis
  - associated
    - without complications
    - with complications
      - rectal bleeding
      - intestinal obstruction
      - fistula
      - abscess
      - other complication
      - unspecified complications

Another helpful tool incorporated into *The Clinical Documentation Improvement Desk Reference for ICD-10-CM and Procedure Coding* manual is "Key Terms." Under each section or condition, alternate terminology is provided that may be found in the medical record documentation. These alternative clinical descriptions ensure that all involved in the documentation and coding processes are clear concerning which conditions or services may have the same meaning and be classified together, and which conditions or services may be slightly different and should be classified elsewhere.

For example, a medical record may be documented with "idiosyncratic asthma," which is found on the list of conditions in the "Key Terms" section related to asthma. This means that the terminology is one of the inclusion conditions found under the J45 Asthma section of ICD-10-CM. Conversely, if "wood asthma" is documented, it is not on this list of conditions. While the list itself is not all-inclusive, the condition should be reviewed more closely; the ICD-10-CM index indicates that the condition wood asthma should be classified to another code under category J67.

The Clinical Documentation Improvement Desk Reference for ICD-10-CM and Procedure Coding manual also provides, where appropriate, clinical tips. For example, the topic Nerve Blocks contains a clinical tip that identifies the components of the somatic nerves and the required documentation elements that should be included when performing nerve blocks on one of these nerves.

Clinical Tip

Somatic nerves are a part of the peripheral nervous system and are associated with the voluntary control of body movements through the skeletal muscles.

Documentation should also include the reason for the nerve block and the response of prior treatment if any.

Although this manual is not considered a coding instructional manual, coding instructional notes that affect documentation are also included. For instance, under the main category for asthma (J45), an instructional note appears:

Use additional code to identify:

> *exposure to environmental tobacco smoke (Z77.22)*
> *exposure to tobacco smoke in the perinatal period (P96.81)*
> *history of nicotine dependence (Z87.891)*
> *occupational exposure to environmental tobacco smoke (Z57.31)*
> *nicotine dependence (F17.-)*
> *tobacco use (Z72.Ø)*

Because clinical researchers have identified links between use or exposure to tobacco smoke and asthma, the instructional note indicates that these conditions should be coded in addition to the code for asthma. References within the *Clinical Documentation Improvement Desk Reference for ICD-10-CM and Procedure Coding* manual prompt the physician to provide documentation for related conditions such as these, that provide detail and a more complete clinical picture.

The Clinical Documentation Improvement Desk Reference for ICD-10-CM and Procedure Coding manual also provides, in appendix 1, templates and instructions for accurately and compliantly developing physician query documents. The physician query, particularly those that seek to clarify certain conflicting or missing information, is one of the most commonly used tools to improve physician documentation. These queries must be constructed in a correct and nonleading manner in order to be compliant.

Appendix B contains a list of HCC and QPP associated codes. This table contains the ICD-10-CM and CPT® codes discussed in this product in code order, as well as the HCC and/or Quality measure associated with that code.

The process of clinical documentation improvement should be a collaborative one, involving those who provide the documentation and those who interpret it and translate the verbiage to the most appropriate numeric code. Being proactive in assisting the physician provider with the detailed information that will be necessary under the ICD-10-CM coding system can only enhance that collaboration.

Section 2: Clinical Documentation Improvement Processes—Best Practices

As mentioned earlier, the clinical documentation improvement process should be a collaborative one in order to be successful. The health care setting and whether the clinical conditions treated involve only a few, such as in a specialty clinic, or encompass the entire spectrum of diseases and disorders, such as in a full-service acute care hospital, will determine the scope and breadth of the program. However, there are many attributes that are commonly seen in successful programs of any size. Many physicians have found that participating in a CDI program at their local hospital also improves documentation in the office setting as well.

There are three main components to a successful clinical documentation improvement program: assessment, implementation, and sustainability.

Assessment

The first step in any CDI program must be an assessment. The assessment will identify those areas that are compliant as well as areas where improvement is needed.

There are several steps involved in performing the CDI assessment:

- Develop a CDI team
- Develop a review process
- Identify areas of risk
- Identify the root cause

Staffing

Before an assessment can take place, a clinical documentation improvement team must be established. This team should include members from all groups involved (e.g., clinicians, coders, information technology, etc.). Each team member can provide particular insight into what is needed for his or her particular responsibilities.

Staff members who will work on the CDI program can come from a variety of different backgrounds. Typically they include health information management (HIM) coding professionals, compliance officers, physicians, nursing staff, and other professionals with either a coding or clinical background. Some programs involve a variety of the above-mentioned individuals and job titles are not as important as specific attributes and skills, such as: clinical knowledge of the individual code sets and the reporting guidelines associated with that code set; understanding health care compliance as it relates to documentation, coding, and billing; and strong written and verbal communication skills. The importance of strong verbal skills cannot be overemphasized; these staff members will be communicating with physicians on a daily basis and must convey professionalism and significant clinical and coding knowledge. Many successful programs have one or more physician "champions," who act both as advisors to the other staff members in the program and are liaisons with the medical staff providing the documentation.

Physician Advisor or Liaison

Many CDI professionals believe that a major component of a successful program is a strong physician advisor. This major role is to act as a liaison between the CDI staff members, HIM coding, and the medical staff and to facilitate accurate coding and representation of acuity and severity. As a result, the corresponding reimbursement should also be enhanced, regardless of the setting.

Just as importantly, the physician advisor is responsible for communicating with and educating the medical staff in both the general concepts of severity and acuity as they relate to documentation and coding, and in encouraging and recommending specific documentation enhancements. To accomplish these goals, the physician advisor should have knowledge related to physician performance profiling, physician E/M payment and pay for performance, and appropriate documentation for hospital reimbursement and profiling (if working in that setting). Publicly available data tools are available that can be incorporated in the CDI strategy, including the Surgical Care Improvement Project (SCIP) outcomes, risk of mortality (ROM), and severity-of-illness (SOI) data instruments. Helping other physicians become more aware of outcomes data and the documentation and coding effect on them is a very successful way of reaching those most responsible for providing the documentation upon which these data instruments are based.

Physician advisors can also emphasize the continuity of care approach to other physicians on the medical staff. This approach reinforces the fact that what is documented accurately represents not only the patient conditions, but what was done for the patient. Other physicians participating in the care of the patient need to ensure that what they review in the medical record is accurate and complete to provide additional input and/or services. Continuity of care is an essential goal of any CDI program and should be the number one reason that conflicting information in the medical record is addressed quickly and thoroughly via the CDI process.

In addition, the physician advisor should meet on a regular basis with the CDI professionals to review selected medical records, particularly those involving traditionally confusing conditions or those with a somewhat varied set of clinical definitions. Examples of these conditions include those with respiratory failure, acute blood loss anemia, renal insufficiency versus chronic kidney disease, acute kidney injury, and urosepsis. In some cases, internal definitions of these conditions can be formulated through a collaborative process. Taking a proactive stance in handling these cases that can cause confusion on the part of both CDI/coding and the medical staff can alleviate future problems and can significantly decrease the number of physician queries required.

When physician queries are necessary, the physician advisor can provide assistance in several ways. First, the physician advisor can determine whether a query is necessary based on the initial documentation in the medical record. Secondly, he or she can help formulate physician queries that are not leading in nature, but that provide enough clinical information to make the query relevant and compliant. If queries on a particular condition become repetitive over time, the physician advisor can assist in the development of a query template, which makes further questions on the topic easier to initiate and can develop and facilitate provider education.

Another important aspect of the physician advisor role involves providing feedback to medical staff physicians on the effect of their documentation on some of the patient severity and acuity data instruments mentioned above. Providing this last link between the documentation and the resulting movement in acuity or other scores is extremely valuable, can add legitimacy, and reinforce the importance of accurate and complete documentation.

Review Process

After the team has been established, a review process should be developed. The process should be customizable depending on the particular type of review being performed. For example, a review may be to determine the completeness of the clinicians' documentation of conditions, procedures, or services or a review may be performed to determine if other clinicians can determine the patient's medical status based on the documentation in the medical record.

When developing the process, it should also be determined if the process will take place concurrently (while the patient is being treated) or retrospectively (after the patient has received treatment). In most instances, in a physician practice, concurrent review occurs prior to the submission of the claim. It may also occur at the time care is being provided. A clinician reviewer (e.g., another physician or a medical assistant trained to recognize the necessary data points) can review the medical record before the patient leaves the office.

Retrospective review usually occurs once the claim has been processed. Both types of review have benefits and it may be that each would be performed depending on the type of documentation that will be reviewed.

Regardless of the type of review selected, both can result in more detailed, accurate, and complete documentation that improves code assignment and reduces liability risk.

Implementation

Policies and procedures must be implemented for each CDI program, depending upon the size of the program, whether records consist of paper or are electronic, and staffing. The example below is a procedure for a hospital program that uses paper records:

1. After midnight, generate and obtain a hospital census report, which includes admissions. The report should, at a minimum, include the following information:
   - Patient name
   - Admission date

- Insurance information
- Attending physician name
- Admitting diagnosis

2. Each CDI staff member reviews each admission to his or her assigned floor or location in the facility. The frequency of reviews depends upon program guidelines and policies, but is typically every one to two days. Some facilities target high potential cases according to admitting diagnosis.
3. CDI staff produces an initial new admission worksheet for all new cases and the worksheet is placed in the specified location in the patient's medical record on the hospital floor. The worksheet should, at a minimum, include the following information:
   - Patient name
   - Medical record or encounter number
   - Admission date
   - Attending physician
   - Principal diagnosis
   - Secondary diagnoses
   - Principal procedure (if applicable)
   - Secondary procedures (if applicable)
4. If no query opportunity is identified, the CDI staff member reviews the case records periodically, according to facility policies. If a query opportunity is identified, the CDI staff member initiates it according to the most appropriate method (i.e., verbal, written, or electronic), detailing its existence, reason, and date on the CDI worksheet.
5. CDI physician queries are followed concurrently. If there is no response to the query within a predetermined amount of time, the physician advisor is contacted to review the current documentation and query. If appropriate, the physician advisor contacts the physician responsible for the missing or conflicting documentation.
6. After patient discharge, the coder assigns codes based on the final documentation in the medical record and any answered queries. Cases with no discrepancies are final billed. Cases with discrepancies are routed to the CDI staff member for an additional review and a physician query may be initiated after this review.
7. All cases are tracked and trended, particularly those with physician queries. The facility has a policy on the retention of queries, whether in the medical record itself or elsewhere.
8. CDI staff members meet monthly (or at other designated intervals) with the physician advisor to discuss trends in the program and any issue related to queries or documentation.
9. Quarterly meetings are scheduled between the CDI team and physician leadership and administration. Metrics and benchmarks for measuring success are reviewed, along with discussions of recently identified successes or potential problems.

Generally speaking, many of the same procedures listed above can be used in a physician practice.

1. The practice runs reports at the beginning of a month to determine possible areas where clinical documentation improvement may be needed. For example, a report may be run to determine the number of "unspecified" or "other specified" codes where assigned or the practice may wish to run a report indicating those claims that were denied because of medical necessity issues.
2. A CDI staff member reviews the reports to determine if there are patterns. For example, a report indicates that 86 percent of Dr. Smith's claims for patients with complete blood counts are performed for unspecified anemia or 62 percent of all flexible sigmoidoscopy claims are unpaid because of medical necessity issues.
3. CDI staff produces an initial CDI review worksheet for all new cases and the worksheet is placed in the specified location in the patient's medical record. The worksheet should, at a minimum, include the following information:
   - Patient name
   - Medical record or encounter number
   - Admission date
   - Attending physician
   - Principal diagnosis
   - Secondary diagnoses
   - Principal procedure (if applicable)
   - Secondary procedures (if applicable)
   - Claim denial codes (if applicable)
4. The medical record is reviewed to determine if further clinical documentation could have resulted in a better understanding of what was performed during the encounter and the reason for the service. If a query opportunity is identified, the CDI staff member initiates it according to the most appropriate method (i.e., verbal, written, or electronic), detailing its existence, reason, and date on the CDI worksheet.
5. CDI physician queries are followed concurrently. If there is no response to the query within a predetermined amount of time, the physician advisor is contacted to review the current documentation and query. If appropriate, the physician advisor contacts the physician responsible for the missing or conflicting documentation.
6. After including any additional information to the medical record that may potentially affect code assignment, the CDI staff member updates the CDI worksheet. **Note:** Caution should be used so that any additions/addenda to the medical record are made in accordance with standard clinical documentation guidelines.
7. The case is circulated back to the coder who assigns codes based on the final documentation and submits or resubmits the claim as necessary. When a claim is resubmitted, payer guidelines are carefully followed.
8. All cases are tracked and trended, particularly those with physician queries. The practice has a policy on the retention of queries, whether in the medical record itself, or elsewhere.
9. CDI staff members meet monthly (or at other designated intervals) with the physician advisor to discuss trends in the program and any issue related to queries or documentation. It is determined during these

meetings if formal education is necessary and if the education is to be provided to a specific clinician or to the entire clinical staff.

10. Quarterly meetings are scheduled between the CDI team and physician leadership and administration. Metrics and benchmarks for measuring success are reviewed along with discussions of recently identified successes or potential problems.

The Query Process

Because the physician query process is a major component of a CDI program, each facility or practice should have a policy related to query development, format, and management. The policy should specify when to query, how to format the query appropriately, and the retention policy of the query. Some programs rely heavily on one type of query, such as the written query, while others use a combination of approaches, including verbal and electronic methods. Queries may be used to request further specificity or to clarify the severity of a documented condition, to clarify a cause-and-effect relationship, or to present clinical indicators of an undocumented condition.

Appendix 1, "Physician Query Samples" in this manual, provides numerous examples of physician queries.

The following six criteria should be used when reviewing documentation and in determining whether a query is necessary:

Legibility: Poor penmanship, improper use of photocopies, poor document scans, "cut-and-paste" errors, use of templates, or improperly correcting an error in a medical record can cause problems with legibility, omissions, or additions in text that can result in errors of documentation and code assignment: does a condition warrant reporting that is a result of "cut and paste" documentation from a previous encounter problem list which was not addressed on the current encounter?

Consistency: Documentation that is conflicting, inadequate, incomplete, ambiguous, or inconsistent: is the condition exacerbated or is it stable; was the suspected condition ruled out; what is the clinical significance of the abnormal test results; or, does the provider confirm the consultant's diagnosis?

Relationships: Clinical indicators noted without a stated related diagnosis, diagnostic work-up without stated reason, treatment without identified indication or manifestations not linked to an underlying cause: does the notation ↑ Na represent a clinically significant diagnosis; what is the reason for the need of continuous O2; what was the indication and final conclusion for the performance of a glucose test; is the ulcer due to a complication of the underlying diabetes?

Specificity: Clinical results, including pathology reports, response to treatment, and/or the patient's clinical condition suggest a more specific diagnosis or level of severity than is documented: based on culture and sensitivity and patient response to treatment, can the condition be further specified as to a causative organism; can the post-op/final diagnosis be further specified due to the pathology report findings; based on the pathology report findings, which additional sites of metastasis are clinically significant?

Clinical validation: When there is a lack of clinical data or insufficient indicator(s)needed to determine a diagnosis or the necessary level of specificity necessary for reporting the most appropriate ICD-10-CM code, the decision to query a clinician may be required. For example, the PACU note stating "post-op respiratory failure" during the routine post-op intubation period without correlating clinical indicators represent a complication due to surgery, other condition, or an expected outcome immediately postsurgery; is the diagnosis of acute exacerbation supported by clinical findings, adjustment of regimen/treatment or clinical manifestation?

Other issues related to queries include the following:

When not to query: In some instances, physicians must make clinical diagnostic decisions that may not appear to agree with test results or other findings. Queries should not be formulated that question a provider's clinical judgment, but only to clarify documentation when it fails to meet one of the six criteria listed above. To help avoid clinical validation issues, the physician should indicate why a critical clinical indicator is not met for the patient when stating his or her diagnostic statement; for example, pneumonia ruled in based on clinical scenario with negative chest x-ray due to severe dehydration. Also, queries are not necessary for every unaddressed issue or discrepancy in the medical record. Insignificant or irrelevant findings typically do not warrant a query.

Clinical validation escalation policy: All entities and physician practices should have a written policy and procedure that identifies what constitutes the need for a clinical validation query, those who are part of the escalation team, and that outlines their role and the chain of responsibility.

How to notify the physician that a query has been placed in the medical record: Because a variety of members of the health care team has access to and may frequently be reviewing the medical record, it may be a challenge to ensure that the appropriate physician sees the query. Some organizations handle the issue by electronically notifying the physician when a query is placed in the record.

Ensuring that the resulting answer to a query is documented appropriately in the medical record: This issue relates to query retention. Many organizations do not consider the query form itself a part of the medical record. In that case, the physician must document the answer to the query elsewhere in the medical record, typically in the progress notes or discharge summary. The other issue related to the timing of unanswered queries involves how to track the unanswered queries. Each organization should have a policy regarding this process, including how to address a lack of response, and strategies for record completion.

Query timing for resolved conditions: Some physicians may be reluctant to document a condition, particularly an acute condition, if it has resolved by the time of the query. In this instance, it is helpful to provide information regarding patient severity. Regardless of the timing of the treatment, if the patient was treated for the condition, it should be documented and coded for appropriate acuity.

Queries for conditions not documented in the record: Queries must be based on physician documentation within the medical record and the link between the data and the condition must be made in order to support the query. For example, the routine lab test performed after a minor surgery shows slightly below normal H/H levels and the provider simply notes the lab results in a progress note; the patient's pre-op baseline is unknown and there is no mention of a condition in the progress notes nor is there any documentation of the need for monitoring or treatment of a condition. This scenario would not warrant a query: the labs were routine and not specifically ordered to monitor or evaluate for a condition and although the provider noted the results, there was no mention of their clinical significance and in fact there is no indication they were significant as there is no documentation the patient was symptomatic or required treatment.

Verbal queries: This is more commonplace when used in concurrent programs and CDI staff members are interacting with physicians on a real-time basis. These must follow the same format as written queries but in condensed form including the question and its clinical support. Each program should have a policy regarding documentation of verbal queries.

Query documentation: The use of queries on easily removable and discardable notes (such as sticky notes or scratch paper) is disallowed regardless of whether or not the query form becomes a part of the final medical record. Preferred documentation includes the CDI program-approved query template or general query form, secure email electronic form, or approved form on an IT messaging system.

Leading queries: Queries should include clinical indications and information and should ask the physician to make a clinical interpretation of these facts based on professional judgment. Queries that clearly ask the physician to document a specific condition or that illicit a specific response are inappropriate and could lead to allegations of upcoding. Queries should also never indicate that any particular response would impact reimbursement or any other measurable instrument (such as a quality reporting system).

Query formats:

Narrative: Clinical scenario is succinctly noted, followed by clinical data citing document and date, summary of clinical judgment, diagnostic statement, note of decision making including treatment plan, and patient response to therapy. The query must include relevant points and identify the need for further clarification (etiology, specificity, link, severity, clinical validation, etc.). The question must not be worded for a yes or no answer nor should it indicate a specified diagnosis or procedure. Anticipate possible answers and word the query in such a way to include them; this may prompt the need for an additional or follow-up question for an anticipated answer.

Query templates should not be titled with a diagnosis that has not already been documented in the record, as this may be considered leading. If a diagnosis of pneumonia is not already documented in the record then the written query should not be titled "pneumonia." However, if a diagnosis of pneumonia is already documented and the query is to further specify the pneumonia, then the query may be titled "pneumonia" and request further specificity/type.

Multiple choice: Clinical scenario is succinctly noted, followed by clinical data citing document and date, summary of clinical judgment, diagnostic statement, note of decision making including treatment plan and patient response to therapy. The query must include relevant points and identify the need for further clarification (etiology, specificity, link, severity, etc.). The question must not be worded for a yes or no answer. Clinically possible diagnostic choices are presented in a bulleted list along with choices of "other," "undetermined," "clinically insignificant," "integral" or "unspecified." This format allows a new diagnosis as an option, as long as it meets the clinical scenario and data from the record.

Yes/no/other choice: Clinical scenario is succinctly noted, followed by clinical data citing document and date, summary of clinical judgment, diagnostic statement, and, as appropriate, note of decision making including treatment plan and patient response to therapy. The query must include relevant points and identify the need for further clarification after review of pathology, consult, or other report findings. This format involves confirmation of an existing diagnosis from the report either as an additional or a more specified diagnosis or to resolve conflicting documentation. The list of answer choices are yes, no, other, clinically undetermined, integral, or clinically insignificant.

Multiple query questions: Multiple questions may be formulated on one physician query as long as they are distinct and none are leading. For example, in a patient with diabetes mellitus and chronic kidney failure, one query question may involve the type of diabetes (type 1, 2, drug-induced, etc.), one may involve the relationship between the diabetes and the kidney failure, and one may involve the specific renal manifestation.

Post-bill queries: Most queries of this type are a result of an internal or external audit and refer to the fact that the claim has been submitted or the remittance advice or EOB indicates the claim was paid. Most organizations have policies to help determine whether to generate physician queries at this point in time. Issues to consider include payer-specific rebilling time frames and determining the reliability of the query response given the time frame.

Query Program Sustainability

Each CDI program management should establish an auditing and monitoring program related to physician queries. Not only will this policy make queries more consistent across the organization, but it will also identify areas that require additional education and training. Three major questions should be answered after review of any query:

- Was the query necessary?
- Was the language in the query leading or in any way inappropriate?
- Did the query introduce any new diagnostic information that was not previously in the medical record?

Based on the findings from that audit, educational activities can be scheduled to ensure accurate and appropriate queries are formulated in the future.

Additional auditing activities related to queries can take the following forms:

Sampling: At regular intervals, random or targeted sampling should be done for each staff member that is formulating queries. The review should include not only the content of the query but the format as well. This auditing activity will also target areas for further education.

Tracking query response results: The response to a query can have varying effects on code assignments. A tracking form should categorize the various types of results in order to identify query effectiveness. The topic (e.g., sepsis, acute respiratory failure, excisional debridement, etc.) should also be noted to identify and quantify which issues are queried and the frequency.

Individual physician provider tracking: The total number of queries per provider should decrease over time, indicating an improvement in documentation patterns. This is also a success metric for the clinical documentation improvement program. The response time for a physician should also be tracked to identify those who fail to respond or who habitually respond beyond the specified period resulting in billing delays.

High risk, historically problematic, or confusing conditions: It is especially instructive to measure queries for problematic diagnoses before and after educational sessions, to determine educational program success.

CDI Success Metrics

One of the most important aspects of a clinical documentation improvement program is the establishment and performance of a success metrics system. Some of the data elements to consider tracking include the following:

- Risk of mortality (ROM) and severity of illness (SOI)
- Total volume of queries formulated and released per month
- Diagnoses with high volume of queries
- Physicians most often queried
- Proportion of successful versus unsuccessful queries
- Clinical or patient care area which originates highest volume of queries
- Trended elements, including query, condition, physician, CDI staff member, case-mix-index (CMI) data (if hospital-based program)
- Case-mix-index (CMI) movement as a result of the CDI program (for hospital-based programs)
- Documentation habit changes as a result of the CDI program

Most organizations have an internal average measurement of coded data that is tracked over time. In the physician office/clinic setting it may track the hierarchical condition category (HCC) conditions; in the hospital setting it typically involves the case-mix index, which can be tracked in several different ways (e.g., by coder, by physician, by clinical service area, etc.). Any unexpected change in one of these metrics may represent a potential problem with clinical documentation. It is important to be able to isolate the factor causing the metric movement in order to address it appropriately.

Using Technology for Clinical Documentation Improvement

There are a number of electronic solutions that are currently in use in the health care arena today that can and will affect clinical documentation improvement. Although the reasons for a CDI program and the benefits of a program will not change, the use of some of these automated tools can alter the day-to-day activities, scope, roles, and duties for many of the staff members in a CDI program. Several of these tools and their resulting effects and benefits are listed below.

Electronic Health Record

A significant proportion of hospitals and physician practices have transitioned to electronic health records (EHR) and, even if not in a completely paper-free environment, they use a hybrid medical record with a sizable amount of information collected and stored electronically. While this can eliminate issues related to legibility and entirely missing documentation, it may also potentially produce other problems such as overwhelming staff with the sheer amount of required documentation or the tendency to "overcode." Written policies should be in place that address the copy, paste, and clone functions in the EHR. Specific documentation should be provided for each and every patient, and each should consist of "stand-alone" information that does not rely on data from other sources that may not be present at the time of a CDI process or coding.

The EHR can be a useful tool in providing feedback and prompts to physicians for more specific documentation, if structured in a thoughtful and consistent way. The goal is not to overwhelm the providers with too many prompts and requests for further information, but to provide very specific pointers, some in template fashion that will remind the physician that more specificity is required. This will be particularly crucial after the transition to ICD-10-CM. For example, in a pulmonology practice, the EHR template should prompt the physician for more information when "asthma" is documented. In ICD-10-CM there are 18 different codes in category J45 that represent asthma. Code subcategories related to "mild intermittent," "mild persistent," "moderate persistent," and "severe persistent" are available, along with combination code components related to the presence of status asthmaticus or an acute exacerbation. Similarly, a diagnostic statement of "acute respiratory failure" is no longer sufficient. An additional piece of information related to whether coexisting hypoxia or hypercapnia is present is also required. Any CDI program must be integrated with the facility or practice EHR in order to be most efficient and effective.

Computer-assisted Coding

Computer-assisted coding (CAC) is a method of providing coded information for a variety of purposes. Its use has grown exponentially during the last several years as facilities and physicians are asked to do more with less, coupled with a need for increased coding productivity and consistency. CAC uses natural language processing (NLP) technology, which generates structured data from unstructured text. As the health care community implements ICD-10-CM and CPT coding with its greater need for specificity, the CAC tool provides a method for positively affecting both coder productivity and documentation specificity. Some CAC programs are run concurrently, along with the CDI process, in order to address documentation deficiencies immediately, at the point of care.

Most CAC systems are able to "read" input documentation and generate a list of "initial" or working ICD-10-CM, CPT, or HCPCS codes. The coding professional is then required to review the list of codes and determine whether the codes are accurate and complete and ready to be billed. The process changes the role of the coder from one that reads documentation and assigns codes to that of an auditor, which in most cases does not require as much time, thus improving productivity. However, this does require a change in the "thought" process and, therefore, additional instruction and training should be provided to the coder to ensure accuracy and efficiencies. In addition, some CAC systems can review patient documentation in real time and target cases that require CDI review and intervention. In this way, a higher proportion of the total patient population is evaluated, leading to overall consistency throughout the facility or practice.

As technology progresses, it appears that many of the electronic solutions will be integrated and provide more than one function. For example, an EHR and a computer-assisted CDI program, perhaps with CAC, may be integrated and provide several solutions concurrently. While it may be only one automated system, a need will still exist for staffing related to a coding professional, a clinical documentation specialist, a case manager, and a physician liaison; each role is distinct.

CDI Brings Many Improvements

CDI programs have become more essential under ICD-10-CM, as the increased specificity and granularity require a correspondingly higher specificity in the clinical documentation provided in the health record.

The overriding goal of clinical documentation improvement should be to ethically improve the accuracy, completeness, and specificity of clinical documentation through assessment, education, review, communication, clarification, querying, and analysis of clinical documentation patterns. Additionally, all of this must be accomplished without overburdening the clinician, confusing the clinician regarding what does or does not need to be documented as well as avoiding the tendency to "overcode" because of the additional documentation that was previously unclear or unavailable. If successful, improvements will be seen in programs related to care coordination, quality and severity of illness reporting, meaningful use initiatives, pay-for-performance programs, bundled payments of various types, RAC and other fraud and abuse auditing, and code-based reimbursement.

Section 3: Documentation Issues

This section is organized in an easy-to-use alphabetic format according to the condition or procedure addressed.

For ICD-10-CM codes the, focus is on those diagnoses with significant differences in the type and specificity required for accurate code assignment. The code axes are listed, which may include the component subcategories or each code in the section to be discussed. Information related to the entire section of codes appears next, whether related to the ICD-10-CM classification itself or to the CDI process.

The procedures included are those that have documentation issues as well as those for which multiple coding options are available.

Each topic includes clinical definitions that indicate differentiating factors that can affect code assignment. Clinical data such as physical examination findings, laboratory tests commonly ordered, and/or abnormal laboratory findings, ancillary testing provided, therapeutic procedures performed, common medications, and other significant information that may support reporting the condition are also included. A Clinician Documentation Checklist that displays the clinical factors that the clinician should document is also provided.

In addition to the elements listed above, within each of the topics covered the following components may also appear:

Clinical Tip: Provides the clinical definitions and information that must be documented in order to classify the condition, service, or procedure to this particular code or ICD-10-CM subcategory.

Documentation Tip: Provides information regarding specific elements that are needed in the documentation to differentiate the condition or procedure from other similar conditions or procedures.

CPT Alert: Identifies information that may be found in the documentation that could possibly affect procedure code assignment.

CDI Alert: Contains helpful tips for the CDI professional or other staff member who may be reviewing the physician documentation. Suggestions for ensuring the most appropriate and complete documentation appear here.

I-10 Alert: Provides information that, when found in the clinical documentation, could affect ICD-10-CM code assignment.

Key Terms: Lists synonyms or other clinical terms that may be documented in the medical record that are also classified to the code.

Clinician Note: Shares tips related to documentation for the physician practice setting, which may impact professional component reimbursement and quality initiatives.

⇨ I-10 ALERT

The *ICD-10-CM Official Guidelines for Coding and Reporting* provides useful information regarding documentation requirements, as well as reporting guidelines for the ICD-10-CM classification system. The official guidelines may be accessed at: https://www.cms.gov/Medicare/Coding/ICD10/Downloads/2017-ICD-10-CM-Guidelines.pdf.

CDI ALERT

Contains helpful tips for the CDI professional or other staff member who may be reviewing the physician documentation. Suggestions for ensuring the most appropriate and complete documentation appear here.

⇨ I-10 ALERT

Alerts the user to classification concepts unique to this code subcategory or code section along with assignment tips and/or differentiating factors. Instructions for additional coding requirements may also appear here.

Abnormal Auditory Perceptions and Acoustic (Auditory) Nerve Disorders

Code Axes

Other abnormal auditory perceptions	**H93.2**
Auditory recruitment	**H93.21-**
Diplacusis	**H93.22-**
Hyperacusis	**H93.23-**
Temporary auditory threshold shift	**H93.24-**
Central auditory processing disorder	**H93.25**
Other abnormal auditory perceptions	**H93.29-**
Disorders of acoustic nerve	**H93.3X-**

Description of Condition

Abnormal auditory perceptions and acoustic (auditory) nerve disorders

Clinical Tip

In auditory perception disorders, the patient is unable to process auditory sounds or objects, but the function of the auditory nerve is intact. The origin of dysfunction is postulated to occur in the central nervous system, not the ear or auditory nerve, and is not associated with peripheral hearing loss.

In auditory nerve disorder, there is a malfunction or compromise of the acoustic (eighth cranial) nerve which may be associated with or caused by congenital anomaly, tumor, infection or other etiology.

Auditory perception disorder is an umbrella term that encompasses a wide range of disorders, which affect the processing (or translation) of auditory information.

Auditory processing disorder may be acquired by neurological problems including tumor, injury, stroke, neurological disorders, infection, or oxygen deficiency.

Temporary auditory threshold shift is a temporary hearing loss when the sensory structures of the cochlea (inner ear) have been overstimulated or fatigued; often due to exposure to loud noise. The threshold of hearing shifts in which the lowest (softest) decibel level is higher than usual.

Diplacusis is a cochlear dysfunction causing the patient to hear single auditory stimulus as two sounds (e.g., echo), whereas hyperacusis is an acute, though usually nonpainful, hearing sensitivity.

Key Terms

Key terms found in the documentation for auditory processing disorder may include:

Central auditory processing disorder (CAPD)

Congenital auditory imperception

Word deafness

Key terms found in the documentation may include:

Acoustic neuritis

Auditory neuropathy

Auditory or acoustic neuralgia

Eighth cranial nerve disorder

Documentation Tip

Ensure that all related conditions are coded appropriately, particularly if the condition is related to other underlying diseases or disorders (e.g., vascular disease, metabolic disturbances, congenital anomalies, infection, history of trauma).

> **⇨ I-10 ALERT**
>
> ICD-10-CM classifies disorders of the acoustic (auditory) nerve (H93.3X) separately from disorders of auditory perception (H93.2). In auditory perception disorders, the patient is unable to process auditory sounds or objects, but the function of the auditory nerve is intact. In auditory nerve disorder, there is a malfunction or compromise of the auditory (eighth cranial) nerve.
>
> Auditory perception disorder is an umbrella term that encompasses a wide range of disorders, which affect the processing (or translation) of auditory information.
>
> **Note:** Conditions classified to chapter 8 include laterality (right, left, bilateral) within the code structure. All conditions should specify the affected ear(s).

Disorders of acoustic nerve (H93.3X-)

The acoustic nerve or sometimes documented as the eighth cranial nerve or vestibulocochlear nerve controls balance. Documentation will indicate that the patient complains of dizziness or feeling that he, she, or the environment, or both are spinning. Acoustic nerve disorders may also result in facial or head pain as well as tinnitus and hearing loss. Cranial nerve disorders can also cause various kinds of facial or head pain or a feeling of fullness in the ear.

> **CDI ALERT**
>
> When documentation indicates an acoustic neuroma or benign neoplasm of the acoustic nerve, ICD-10-CM code D33.3 is assigned.

Key Terms

Key terms found in the documentation may include:

Acoustic nerve compression

Cochleovestibular nerve compression syndrome

Microvascular compression syndrome

Clinical Findings

Physical Examination

History and review of systems may include:

- Visualization of the inner ear (otoscope)
- Basic hearing test
  - Weber's test
  - Rinne's test
  - free field test (whispering test)

Diagnostic Procedures and Services

- Laboratory
  - complete blood count
  - chemistry blood profile
- Imaging
  - MRI
  - CT
- Other
  - auditory brainstem response testing (ABR)
  - audiometry (hearing test)
  - tilt table test

Therapeutic Procedures and Services

- Microvascular decompression (MVD), if failure of medical (nonsurgical) therapy

Clinician Note

Documentation should list all symptoms including any circumstances that exacerbate the condition. Results of the physical examination, including normal findings should be recorded. Testing results should be included and any final diagnosis, including other conditions such as an acoustic neuroma, Meniere's disease or labyrinthitis, which are coded to other ICD-10-CM codes, should be identified.

Clinician Documentation Checklist

Clinician documentation should indicate the following:

- Symptoms
- Hearing loss
  - conversational hearing
  - percentage hearing loss
  - unilateral or bilateral
- Paroxysmal positional vertigo, if present
  - vestibulo-ocular reflex (Dix-Hallpike test)
- Procedures performed
  - MRI
  - CT
  - laboratory studies
  - auditory brainstem response testing (ABR)
  - audiometry (hearing test)
  - tilt table test
- Treatment
  - Medical intervention including medications prescribed
  - Neurology consult

Clinician Note

Specify the type of abnormal auditory perception. Differentiate between auditory recruitment, diplacusis, hyperacusis, auditory threshold shift, and auditory processing disorders.

Document whether these conditions exist in combination with other systemic disease or auditory disorder. Specify any contributory history of trauma, infection or other related condition or status (e.g., congenital anomaly, family history).

Document the laterality of the affected site (i.e., left, right, bilateral).

CDI Alert

Documentation must include the type of abnormal auditory perception to avoid reporting nonspecific diagnoses. The provider should qualify the disorder as:

- Auditory recruitment
- Diplacusis
- Hyperacusis
- Temporary auditory threshold shift
- Central auditory processing disorder
- Other (specify)

Documentation of laterality (i.e., right, left, bilateral) of affected ear or nerve should be thorough and specific to avoid reporting unspecified codes.

Abortion

Code Axes

Surgical treatment of incomplete abortion	**59812**
Surgical treatment of missed abortion	**59820–59821**
Surgical treatment of septic abortion	**59830**
Induced abortion	**59840–59857**

Description of Procedure

An abortion is the expulsion or extraction of the products of conception. Carefully review the medical record documentation to determine if the abortion is spontaneous, induced, complete, incomplete or induced as well as what type of surgical intervention was required.

Treatment of incomplete abortion, any trimester, completed surgically (59812)

An incomplete abortion occurs when some but not all of the products of conception are expelled. This code is most commonly used when reporting the surgical treatment after a woman spontaneously aborts part of the products of conception. Usually, the treatment requires dilation and curettage but, depending upon the gestation age, it may be necessary to perform dilation and vacuum extraction.

CPT Alert

This code should not be reported when documentation indicates that the dilation and curettage or evacuation was performed to terminate a viable pregnancy. In these instances, see codes 59840–59841, 59851, 59856.

Key Terms

Key terms found in the documentation may include:

- Ab with retained products of conception with D&C
- D&C for retained products of conception
- Miscarriage with D&C
- Partial ab with D&C
- Partial ab with D&E

CDI Alert

When documentation indicates that there was early fetal death, but the products of conception were retained, it is inappropriate to report 59812 for this procedure. In these instances, the service is considered the treatment of a missed abortion.

Clinician Note

Documentation should include the gestational age of the fetus as well as the specific type of surgical intervention required (dilation and curettage or dilation and evacuation) and any complicating factors such as infection or excessive bleeding.

Treatment of missed abortion, completed surgically, first trimester (59820)

Treatment of missed abortion, completed surgically, second trimester (59821)

A missed abortion is the death of the fetus before the completion of 22 weeks; however, the products of conception are retained and must be surgically extracted. In missed abortion, the fetus remains in the uterus four to eight weeks following its death. Code 59820 describes the treatment of a missed abortion in the first trimester and is usually accomplished by suction curettage. Code 59821 is used to report the surgical treatment of a missed abortion during the second trimester and may include dilation and vacuum extraction. Documentation will indicate that the provider dilated the cervical canal and then inserted a cannula into the uterus after which time the uterine contents are evacuated by rotation of the cannula. After suction curettage, a sharp curette may be used to gently scrape the uterus to ensure that the uterus is empty.

Clinical Tip

Ultrasonography may be needed to determine the size of the fetus to determine the type of procedures required prior to the procedure and is reported separately.

Key Terms

Key terms found in the documentation may include:

D&C for missed ab

Treatment missed miscarriage

Treatment of missed ab

Clinician Note

Because appropriate code selection is dependent upon the gestation age of the fetus, it is imperative that the gestation age be recorded.

CDI ALERT

Gestational age is often recorded by the number of weeks gestation completed. The chart below can be used to convert the gestation age to the trimester.

Weeks Completed	Trimester
1–13	First
14–27	Second
28–42	Third

Treatment of septic abortion, completed surgically (59830)

A septic abortion is one complicated by generalized fever and infection. Documentation will also indicate inflammation and infection of the endometrium and in the cellular tissue around the uterus. The infection is treated with intravenous antibiotics and blood transfusions as necessary and, when treated surgically, will indicate that the provider performed a dilation and curettage or vacuum extraction of the products of conception.

Key Terms

Key terms found in the documentation may include:

D&C for septic abortion

Septic abortion treated surgically

Clinician Note

When known, the specific infectious agent should be recorded in the medical record documentation.

Induced abortion, by dilation and curettage (59840)

Induced abortion, by dilation and evacuation (59841)

Induced abortion, by 1 or more intra-amniotic injections (59850–59852)

Induced abortion, by 1 or more vaginal suppositories (59855–59857)

Code 59840 is used to report the termination by dilation and curettage (D&C). Code 59841 describes the termination by dilation and evacuation (D&E). Because D&E requires wider cervical dilation than curettage, the physician may dilate the cervix with a laminaria several hours to several days before the procedure. For pregnancies through 16 weeks, the cannula will usually evacuate the pregnancy. For later pregnancies, the cannula is used to drain amniotic fluid and to draw tissue into the lower uterus for extraction by forceps. In either case, a sharp curette may be used to gently scrape the uterus to ensure that it is empty. These types of induced abortions are commonly performed for the legal termination of the pregnancy.

Examination of the documentation may also indicate that the termination of a pregnancy was performed by inducing labor with amniocentesis and intra-amniotic injections (59850–59852). This method is usually used after the first trimester (13 weeks or more). Documentation will indicate that the physician inserts an amniocentesis needle into the abdomen to obtain a free flow of clear amniotic fluid. A hypertonic solution is then administered by gravity drip. The hypertonic solution results in fetal death and labor usually results. Code 59851 is used when this method fails to expel all products of conception, and documentation supporting the assignment of this code includes indications that a dilation and curettage and/or evacuation were used to remove the remaining tissue. Code 59852 is used when documentation indicates that an incision in the abdominal wall and uterus was made in order to remove the remaining tissue.

CPT ALERT

When medical record documentation indicates that the abortive service was performed to reduce the number of fetuses, otherwise known as multifetal pregnancy reduction or MPR, see CPT code 59866.

Termination can also be by means of vaginal suppositories. In this method labor is induced with vaginal suppositories. Before using the suppositories, documentation may indicate that a laminaria, which is an applicator made of kelp or synthetic material, was inserted in the cervix to soften and expand the cervical canal. Once the cervix is ready, the physician inserts the vaginal suppositories and labor usually results. The fetus and placenta are delivered through the vagina (59855). Code 59856 is used when this method fails to expel all products of conception, and a dilation and curettage and/or evacuation is used to remove the remaining tissue. Code 59857 is used when this method fails to expel all products of conception, and a hysterotomy, through an incision in the abdominal wall and uterus, is used to remove the remaining tissue.

Key Terms

Key terms found in the documentation may include:

Induced abortion

Legal abortion

Termination of pregnancy

Clinical Findings

Physical Examination

History and review of systems may include:

- Review of GU and GI symptoms including vaginal bleeding and urinary tract infection.
- Determine if vaginal bleeding is present for an inevitable, incomplete, or complete abortion.
- Determine if dilation is present in cervical os. Cervical os may be closed in spontaneous, threatened, inevitable, incomplete, or missed abortion.
- Determine if fever, chills, constant abdominal or pelvic pain and/or purulent vaginal discharge is present in septic abortion. Cervical os is opened in septic abortion.
- Palpate abdomen for tenderness, rebound, rigidity, and guarding.
- Perform fetal Doppler for fetal heart sounds.

Diagnostic Procedures and Services

- Laboratory studies
  - β-hCG

Gestation weeks	Whole HCG units
<1	5–50
2	50–500
3	100–10,000
4	1,000–30,000
5	3,500–115,000
6–8	12,000–270,000
12	15,000–270,000

Note: HCG units may indicate a dropping level when the pregnancy is no longer viable.

  - CBC
  - blood type with Rh typing
- Imaging
  - ultrasound for fetal viability in cases of suspected inevitable, incomplete, or complete abortion

Therapeutic Procedures and Services

- Surgical intervention including dilation and curettage, dilation and evacuation or intra-amniotic injections

Clinician Documentation Checklist

Clinician documentation should indicate the following:

- Type of abortion
  - spontaneous
  - induced
  - complete
  - incomplete
- Surgical intervention
  - D&C
  - D&E
- Gestation age of fetus (weeks)
- Septic abortion

Acute Myocardial Infarction (AMI)

Code Axes

ST elevation (STEMI) myocardial infarction of anterior wall	**I21.Ø1, I21.Ø2, I21.Ø9** HCC QPP
ST elevation (STEMI) myocardial infarction of inferior wall	**I21.11, I21.19** HCC QPP
ST elevation (STEMI) myocardial infarction of other and unspecified sites	**I21.21, I21.29, I21.3** HCC QPP
Non-ST elevation (NSTEMI) myocardial infarction	**I21.4** HCC QPP
Acute myocardial infarction, unspecified	**I21.9**
Myocardial infarction type 2	**I21.A1**
Other myocardial infarction type	**I21.A9**
Subsequent ST elevation (STEMI) myocardial infarction of anterior/inferior walls	**I22.Ø, I22.1** HCC
Subsequent non-ST elevation (NSTEMI) myocardial infarction	**I22.2** HCC
Subsequent ST elevation (STEMI) myocardial infarction of other/unspecified site	**I22.8, I22.9** HCC
Old myocardial infarction	**I25.2** HCC
Intraoperative acute myocardial infarction, during cardiac surgery	**I97.79Ø**
Intraoperative acute myocardial infarction, during other surgery	**I97.791**
Postprocedural acute myocardial infarction, following cardiac surgery	**I97.19Ø**
Postprocedural acute myocardial infarction, following other surgery	**I97.191**

Description of Condition

Acute myocardial infarction (MI) is a leading cause of morbidity and death worldwide. Myocardial infarction occurs when reduced blood supply to the heart (myocardial ischemia) results in irreversible myocardial heart damage. Myocardial can be categorized as:

Common Clinical Diagnosis

STEMI ST elevation myocardial infarction

NSTEMI No ST elevation myocardial infarction

⇨ I-10 ALERT

The ICD-10-CM definition of initial acute myocardial infarction (category I21) is that with a stated duration of four weeks (28 days) or less from onset. A subsequent AMI is defined as one occurring within four weeks (28 days) of a previous AMI. If a patient is still receiving treatment for the myocardial infarction after the four week time frame, an appropriate aftercare code should be reported.

Classified by Clinical Scenario

Type 1 Spontaneous MI related to ischemia

Type 2 Secondary to Ischemia from supply and demand mismatch

Type 3 MI resulting in sudden cardiac death

Type 4a MI associated with percutaneous coronary intervention

Type 4b MI associated with in-stent thrombosis

Type 4c MI associated with a rise and/or fall of cTn values in patients with ≥50% stenosis

Type 5MI associated with coronary artery bypass

ST elevation (STEMI) myocardial infarction (I21.Ø-, I21.1-, I21.2-, I21.3)

An ST elevation myocardial infarction (STEMI) involves electrocardiogram (ECG) evidence of the ST-segment elevation, meaning that there is active and ongoing transmural myocardial damage due to the coronary artery being totally blocked. Patients with STEMI can develop Q-waves, which indicate an area of dead myocardium and irreversible damage. STEMI AMIs reflect a higher severity level than non-STEMI AMIs.

Clinical Tip

AMIs may affect the anterior wall, which includes the following:

- Left main coronary artery
- Left anterior descending coronary artery
- Diagonal coronary artery
- Anteroapical, anterolateral, or anteroseptal AMIs

The inferior wall AMIs include the following:

- Right coronary artery
- Inferolateral AMI

Other areas where AMIs may occur include:

- Left circumflex coronary artery
- Apical-lateral, basal-lateral, high lateral, posterobasal, posterolateral, posteroseptal

Key Terms

Key terms found in the documentation may include:

AMI with ST elevation

Coronary artery embolism, occlusion, rupture, or thrombosis

Infarction of heart, myocardium, or ventricle

ST AMI

Transmural Q-wave infarction

CDI ALERT

If a STEMI AMI converts to an NSTEMI due to thrombolytic therapy, it is still classified as a STEMI, due to the higher severity level of the STEMI and the fact that the patient was treated for the condition. If an NSTEMI evolves into a STEMI, then it is classified as a STEMI AMI. Review documentation carefully if both STEMI and NSTEMI appear in the medical record.

Clinician Note
Clinician documentation should also include information indicating tPA status and tobacco exposure, use, or dependence since these should be coded additionally. Similarly, when the body mass index (BMI) is documented, the appropriate code should be reported additionally.

Non-ST elevation (NSTEMI) myocardial infarction (I21.4)

A non-STEMI acute myocardial infarction results from a partially blocked coronary artery and is diagnosed on ECG, which indicates no ST-elevation. In a non-STEMI AMI there is less permanent damage to the myocardium. The non-STEMI is also known as a non-transmural AMI because the damage does not involve the entire thickness of the ventricular wall.

Key Terms
Key terms found in the documentation may include:

Acute subendocardial myocardial infarction
Coronary artery embolism, occlusion, rupture, or thrombosis
Non-Q wave myocardial infarction
Nontransmural myocardial infarction

CDI ALERT

Review documentation carefully for AMI cases, particularly as it involves time frames and patients who have been readmitted. An acute MI is defined in ICD-10-CM terms as that occurring within the last 28 days. In ICD-10-CM terms, a "subsequent" AMI is defined as an additional AMI that has occurred within 28 days of another previous AMI. Documentation should also be reviewed carefully to ensure that there is no confusion between a non-STEMI AMI and acute coronary syndrome, with symptoms of unstable angina. If an acute MI is more than 28 days old, it should be classified as an old myocardial infarction (I25.2).

Myocardial infarction type 2 (I21.A1)

Key Terms
Key terms found in the documentation may include:

Myocardial infarction due to demand ischemia
Myocardial infarction secondary to ischemic imbalance

Other myocardial infarction type (I21.A9)

Key Terms
Key terms found in the documentation may include:

Myocardial infarction associated with revascularization procedure
Myocardial infarction type 3
Myocardial infarction type 4a
Myocardial infarction type 4b
Myocardial infarction type 4c
Myocardial infarction type 5

Subsequent ST elevation (STEMI) and non-ST elevation myocardial infarction (I22.Ø–I22.9)

The definitions related to STEMI versus NSTEMI and locations of AMI for subsequent AMIs are the same as those for initial AMIs. The differentiating factor involves the timing of the AMI, and whether multiple AMIs have occurred.

Documentation Tip

Heart auscultation for timing and ST heart sound and second heart sound: documentation indicates a click or snap for valve murmurs and gallops or rubs.

Documentation indicating possible myocardial infarction include tachycardia, bradycardia, tachypnea, hypotension, shortness of breath, asymmetric breath sounds or pulses, new heart murmurs and pulses paradoxus.

Clinical Findings

Physical Examination

History and review of systems may include:

- Other cardiac conditions
  - myocardial ischemia
  - unstable angina
  - myocardial infarctions
  - coronary artery bypass graft
- Past medical conditions
  - hypertension
  - diabetes
  - risk of bleed
  - other
- Patient's complaints
  - chest discomfort
  - other associated symptoms
- Heart rate and blood pressure
- A brief, focused and limited neurological examination to determine cognitive deficits
- An inspection of the neck for venous distention and hepatojugular reflux
- An examination of lungs for presence of symmetry of breath sounds and signs of congestion such as dry or wet rales, pleural friction rubs or decreased breath sounds
- Examination of lower extremity to determine presence or absence of edema and arterial pulses.

Diagnostic Procedures and Services

- Laboratory
  - CBC
  - cardiac biomarkers/enzymes
  - myoglobin levels
  - chemistry panel
  - creatinine kinase MB
  - cardiac troponins (cTnI, cTnT, troponin C, troponin I troponin T)

Note: Increased cardiac enzymes support myocardial infarction.

- Imaging
  - cardiac MRI
  - echocardiography
- Other
  - EKG/ECG
    - findings that support a STEMI diagnosis:
      - new ST elevation at the J point in two contiguous leads of >0.1 mV in all leads other than leads V2–V3
      - for leads V2–V3, the following cut points apply: ≥0.2 mV in men ≥40 years, ≥0.25 mV in men <40 years, or ≥0.15 mV in women
      - the presence of reciprocal ST depression helps confirm the diagnosis
      - no Q-wave EKG findings support a non-STEMI diagnosis

Medication List

- Anticoagulants
  - apixaban (Eliquis)
  - dabigatran (Pradaxa)
  - heparin
  - rivaroxaban (Xarelto)
  - warfarin (Coumadin)
- Antiplatelet agents and antiplatelet therapy
  - aspirin
  - clopidogrel (Plavix)
  - dipyridamole
  - prasugrel (Effient)
- Angiotensin-converting enzyme (ACE) inhibitors
  - benazepril (Lotensin)
  - captopril (Capoten)
  - enalapril (Vasotec)
  - fosinopril (Monopril)
  - lisinopril (Prinivil, Zestril)
  - quinapril (Accupril)
  - ramipril (Altace)
- Beta blockers
  - acebutolol (Sectral)
  - atenolol (Tenormin)
  - betaxolol (Kerlone)
  - bisoprolol (Zebeta)
  - metoprolol (Lopressor, Toprol XL)
  - propranolol (Inderal)

- Vasodilators
  - nitroglycerin (Nitrostat)
  - nesiritide (Natrecor)
  - hydralazine (Apresoline)
  - nitrates
  - minoxidil

Clinician Note

When ischemic dilated cardiomyopathy (IDCM) is documented prior to the MI, the medical necessity of an implantable cardioverter-defibrillator is supported.

Intraoperative acute myocardial infarction, during cardiac or other surgery (I97.79Ø, I97.791)

Postprocedural acute myocardial infarction, following cardiac or other surgery (I97.19Ø, I97.191)

Patients at increased risk of intraoperative or postprocedural acute myocardial infarction include those with a diagnosis of decompensated congestive heart failure, severe cardiac valvular diseases, significant arrhythmias, and unstable or severe angina. The vast majority of these cases develops by postoperative day two and can significantly affect clinical progress.

Clinician Note

If the cause-and-effect relationship between the medical intervention and the acute MI is not clearly documented in the medical record, however the relationship is suspected, the Clinician should be queried for additional information clarifying the relationship if present.

⇨ I-10 ALERT

Work-up is the same as for myocardial infarction; however, EKG findings are negative and chest discomfort subsides with rest and medications.

Other ischemic heart diseases: angina pectoris (I2Ø.-)

Some patients may experience acute ischemic cardiac conditions without progression to acute myocardial infarction. Documentation should be reviewed in order to appropriately classify these patients and ensure consistency. Documentation for angina must be specific; there are four ICD-10-CM codes for the condition, ranging from unstable angina to angina pectoris with documented spasm, to other and unspecified forms of the disease.

Documentation Tip

Documentation for the cardiac work-up is the same as for myocardial infarction; however, EKG findings are negative and chest discomfort subsides with rest and medications.

Key Terms

Key terms found in the documentation for angina may include:

- Accelerated or crescendo angina
- Angina equivalent
- Angiospastic or Prinzmetal angina
- Cardiac angina
- Coronary slow flow syndrome
- De novo effort angina
- Intermediate coronary syndrome
- Ischemic chest pain
- Preinfarction syndrome
- Spasm-induced or variant angina

Clinician Note

Documentation should include information regarding use, exposure to, history of, or dependence to tobacco products. Additionally, documentation should be reviewed to determine if the coronary atherosclerosis is due to lipid rich plaque. Look for terms such as fibrous atherosclerosis or coronary plaque.

⇨ I-10 ALERT

For codes in the angina category, only two codes (I20.0 and I20.1), representing unstable angina and angina pectoris with documented spasm, are designated as CC (complication/comorbidity) conditions. Ensure that documentation is clear to support these codes.

Other acute ischemic heart diseases (I24.-)

Patients may experience acute ischemic conditions that do not progress to acute myocardial infarction; it is essential that documentation be clear and accurate, particularly in cases in which the patient had a coronary embolism, occlusion, or thromboembolism not related to AMI.

Dressler's syndrome, or postmyocardial infarction syndrome, involves a persistent low-grade fever, pleuritic chest pain, a pericardial friction rub, and/or a pericardial effusion. Most patients develop the condition three to six weeks following an acute MI. It is usually a self-limiting condition and is thought to be due to an autoimmune response.

Key Terms

Key terms found in the documentation for Dressler's syndrome may include:

- Postcardiac injury syndrome
- Postmyocardial infarction syndrome
- Postpericardiotomy syndrome

Clinician Note

When documentation contains terms such as acute coronary embolism, occlusion, or thromboembolism but does not mention myocardial infarction, a code from category I24 may be supported.

Clinician Documentation Checklist

Clinician documentation should indicate the following:

- Episode of care
  - initial: initial infarction
  - subsequent: the second MI within the acute phase
- Time frame for acute phase of myocardial infarction (MI) is four weeks
- Document the site of the myocardial infarction
  - anterolateral
  - posterior
  - anterior wall
  - inferior wall
- Document the type of MI
  - non-STEMI
  - STEMI
- Document the involved vessel
  - left anterior descending
  - left main
  - right coronary artery
  - left circumflex
  - other coronary artery
    - if non-STEMI evolves into a STEMI, document STEMI only
    - if STEMI converts to non-STEMI due to thrombolytic therapy, document STEMI
- Sequencing of initial and subsequent MI
  - Depends on the circumstances of admission
  - If patient is admitted for AMI and has subsequent AMI during hospitalization, the first MI is sequenced first with the subsequent MI sequenced second
  - If patient is discharged following treatment for an initial AMI, then has subsequent AMI that requires readmission within the four-week acute phase of the initial AMI, the subsequent AMI is sequenced first followed by the initial AMI
- Types of subsequent MI
  - transmural MI of anterior wall
  - transmural (Q wave) MI of anterior wall NOS
  - anteroapical transmural (Q wave)
  - anterolateral transmural (Q wave)
  - anteroseptal transmural (Q wave)
  - transmural infarction (Q wave) diaphragmatic wall
  - transmural infarction (Q wave) inferior wall
  - inferolateral transmural (Q wave)
  - inferoposterior transmural (Q wave)
  - subendocardial MI

  - non-Q wave
  - nontransmural
  - apical-lateral transmural
  - basal-lateral transmural
  - high lateral transmural
  - transmural lateral wall NOS
  - posterior true transmural
  - posterobasal transmural
  - posterolateral transmural
  - posteroseptal transmural
  - septal NOS transmural
  - subsequent acute MI of unspecified site
  - subsequent MI (acute) NOS
- Complications of MI
  - hemopericardium
  - atrial septal defect
  - ventricular septal defect
  - rupture of cardiac wall
  - rupture of chordae tendineae
  - rupture of papillary muscle
  - thrombosis:
    - atrium
    - auricular appendage
    - ventricle
  - sequencing of myocardial infarction and complications is dependent on when the MI and complications occurred
- Old myocardial infarction should be documented, if applicable
- Use of TPA should be documented
  - previous facility
  - current facility

Alcohol Abuse

Code Axes

Alcohol abuse, uncomplicated	**F1Ø.1Ø**
Alcohol abuse, in remission	**F1Ø.11**
Alcohol abuse with intoxication, uncomplicated	**F1Ø.12Ø** HCC
Alcohol abuse with intoxication delirium	**F1Ø.121** HCC
Alcohol abuse with intoxication, unspecified	**F1Ø.129** HCC
Alcohol abuse with alcohol-induced mood disorder	**F1Ø.14** HCC
Alcohol abuse with alcohol-induced psychotic disorder with delusions	**F1Ø.15Ø** HCC
Alcohol abuse with alcohol-induced psychotic disorder with hallucinations	**F1Ø.151** HCC
Alcohol abuse with alcohol-induced psychotic disorder, unspecified	**F1Ø.159** HCC
Alcohol abuse with alcohol-induced anxiety disorder	**F1Ø.18Ø** HCC
Alcohol abuse with alcohol-induced sexual dysfunction	**F1Ø.181** HCC
Alcohol abuse with alcohol-induced sleep disorder	**F1Ø.182** HCC
Alcohol abuse with other alcohol-induced disorder To use this code, the other alcohol-related disorder must be specified and not found in any other subcategory.	**F1Ø.188** HCC
Alcohol abuse with unspecified alcohol-induced disorder	**F1Ø.19** HCC

⇨ I-10 ALERT

Report blood alcohol level (BAC), when available and clinically relevant.

Description of Condition

Alcohol abuse (F1Ø.1-)

Alcohol abuse is characterized by recurring misuse of alcohol in excess with identifiable harmful and dysfunctional behaviors and negative consequences for health, psychosocial state, and employment. It lacks the criteria of dependency. Time frame for consideration of abuse would be persisting for at least one month or has occurred repeatedly within a 12-month period.

Key Terms

Key terms found in the documentation may include:

- Alcohol abuse
- Dipsomania (without documentation of addiction)
- ETHO abuse

Clinician Note

The provider must state the pattern of harmful usage (dependence, abuse or use) and its current clinical state (uncomplicated, intoxication, remission, etc.) and indicate the relationship to any identified mental, behavioral, or physical disorder or its relevance to the patient's status or encounter including its clinical significance.

First Listed Diagnosis Note

Admit for acute alcohol intoxication with alcohol abuse: The appropriate code from category F1Ø.1- will be the first listed diagnosis, followed by all reported alcohol-induced complications and comorbidities.

Admit for toxicity due to alcohol abuse and cocaine use with aspiration pneumonia: The appropriate code from the Table of Drugs and Chemicals for poisoning will be the first listed diagnosis (either alcohol (absolute, beverage) or cocaine), followed by all documented manifestations, complications, and comorbidities.

Admit for encephalopathy due to alcohol abuse: The appropriate code from the Table of Drugs and Chemicals for poisoning will be the first listed diagnosis (alcohol, absolute, beverage), followed by the code for alcohol abuse with other alcohol-related disorder, then toxic encephalopathy. Follow with all documented manifestations, complications, and comorbidities.

Clinical Findings

Physical Examination

Patient's history may indicate that there are findings of a failure to fulfill obligations, drinking in physically hazardous situations (such as driving or boating), legal issues arising from alcohol use or that there are social and/or interpersonal problems without the evidence of dependence.

Physical examination may indicate health issues such as:

- cardiac arrhythmia
- dyspepsia
- liver disease
- depression
- anxiety
- insomnia
- trauma related to alcohol use

The following screening questions may be asked when determining the level of alcohol-related problems:

- On any single occasion during the past three months have you had greater than five drinks containing alcohol?
- On a typical day when you drink, how many drinks do you have?
- What is the maximum number of drinks you had on any given day in the past month?

Clinician Documentation Checklist

Clinician documentation should indicate the following:

- Name of substance
  - alcohol
    - identify blood alcohol level
  - polysubstance
- Level of substance use
  - use
  - abuse
  - dependence
- Any additional description of use
  - intoxication
  - remission
  - withdrawal
- Associated psychoactive-induced disorders
  - anxiety
  - delirium
  - delusions
  - hallucinations
  - mood disorder
  - perception disturbance
  - persisting amnestic disorder
  - persisting dementia
  - psychotic disorder
  - sexual dysfunction
  - sleep disorder

Alcohol Dependence

Code Axes

Alcohol dependence, uncomplicated	**F1Ø.2Ø** HCC
Alcohol dependence, in remission	**F1Ø.21** HCC
Alcohol dependence with intoxication, uncomplicated	**F1Ø.22Ø** HCC
Alcohol dependence with intoxication delirium	**F1Ø.221** HCC
Alcohol dependence with intoxication, unspecified	**F1Ø.229** HCC
Alcohol dependence with withdrawal, uncomplicated	**F1Ø.23Ø** HCC
Alcohol dependence with withdrawal delirium	**F1Ø.231** HCC
Alcohol dependence with withdrawal with perceptual disturbance	**F1Ø.232** HCC
Alcohol dependence with withdrawal, unspecified	**F1Ø.239** HCC
Alcohol dependence with alcohol-induced mood disorder	**F1Ø.24** HCC
Alcohol dependence with alcohol-induced psychotic disorder with delusions	**F1Ø.25Ø** HCC
Alcohol dependence with alcohol-induced psychotic disorder with hallucinations	**F1Ø.251** HCC
Alcohol dependence with alcohol-induced psychotic disorder, unspecified	**F1Ø.259** HCC
Alcohol dependence with alcohol-induced persisting amnestic disorder	**F1Ø.26** HCC
Alcohol dependence with alcohol-induced persisting dementia	**F1Ø.27** HCC
Alcohol dependence with other alcohol-induced disorders, anxiety	**F1Ø.28Ø** HCC
Alcohol dependence with other alcohol-induced disorders, sexual dysfunction	**F1Ø.281** HCC
Alcohol dependence with other alcohol-induced disorders, sleep disorder	**F1Ø.282** HCC
Alcohol dependence with other alcohol-related disorder To use this code, the other alcohol-related disorder must be specified and not found in any other subcategory.	**F1Ø.288** HCC
Alcohol dependence with unspecified alcohol-induced disorder	**F1Ø.29** HCC

⇨ I-10 ALERT

Delirium tremens (DT) is reported in subcategories of F1Ø that identify "delirium."

Description of Condition

Alcohol dependence (F1Ø.2-)

Alcohol dependence (i.e., alcoholism) is a chronic disorder characterized by large or frequent consumption of ethanol in which the individual becomes physically and mentally dependent upon to function. Long-term consequences are physical, psychological, and behavioral, some of which are liver disease, undernutrition with electrolyte disorders and vitamin deficiencies, coagulopathy, depression, dementia, psychosis, heart disease, and violent behavior. Criterion denoting dependence is increased tolerance and continued use despite impairment of health, social life, and job performance. Cessation results in withdrawal symptoms, including early seizures.

⇨ I-10 ALERT

Report the blood alcohol level (BAC), when available and clinically relevant.

Clinical Tip

Beer potomania is severe hyponatremia accompanied by mental status changes occurring as a rare syndrome associated with binge beer ingestion and inadequate dietary intake.

Key Terms

Key terms found in the documentation may include:

Alcohol addiction

Alcohol dependence

Chronic alcoholism

CDI ALERT

Alcohol taken in conjunction with other drugs, prescribed or nonprescribed, which results in toxicity or other reaction as a consequence of the interaction between the alcohol and drug, is classified as a poisoning. All manifestations (e.g., coma, seizure, respiratory failure, etc.) should be documented. If aspiration occurs, it should be specified as to the site of the aspiration (e.g., esophagus, trachea, bronchus, lung, etc.) and its clinical significance.

Documentation Tip

Detoxification treatment should be documented in orders and in the progress notes, including the drugs or substances used and their administration. Medication administration records completed by nursing staff should include date, start and end time, route, and substance.

First Listed Diagnosis Note

Admit for detoxification or rehab: The appropriate code from category F1Ø.2- will be the first listed diagnosis, followed by all reported alcohol-induced complications and comorbidities.

Admit for acute alcohol intoxication in alcoholism: The appropriate code from category F1Ø.2- will be the first listed diagnosis, followed by all reported alcohol-induced complications and comorbidities. Document and report any associated alcohol and drug dependence, abuse or use. Include the reason for the type of service-complexity (observation, outpatient, inpatient).

⇨ I-10 ALERT

Personal history of alcohol dependence is reported as alcohol dependence in remission.

Admit for toxicity due to alcohol and cocaine use with aspiration pneumonia: The appropriate code from the Table of Drugs and Chemicals for poisoning will be the first listed diagnosis (either alcohol (absolute, beverage) or cocaine), followed by all documented manifestations, complications, and comorbidities. Document and report any associated alcohol and drug dependence, abuse or use.

Admit for alcohol withdrawal with seizure: The code for alcohol dependence with withdrawal will be reported as the first listed diagnosis, followed by alcohol dependence with other alcohol-induced disorder, then seizure (other) code. Follow with all documented manifestations, complications and comorbidities.

Clinician Note

The provider must state the pattern of harmful usage (dependence, abuse, or use) and its current clinical state (uncomplicated, intoxication, remission, etc.) and indicate the relationship to any identified mental, behavioral, or physical disorder or its relevance to the patient's status or encounter including its clinical significance.

Medication List

- Acamprosate (Campral)
- Disulfiram (Antabuse)
- Fluoxetine (Prozac)
- Naltrexone (ReVia, Vivitrol)
- Ondansetron (Zofran)
- Topiramate (Topamax)

Clinician Documentation Checklist

Clinician documentation should indicate the following:

- Name of substance
  - alcohol
    - identify blood alcohol level
  - polysubstance
- Level of substance use
  - use
  - abuse
  - dependence
- Any additional description of use
  - intoxication
  - remission
  - withdrawal
- Associated psychoactive-induced disorders
  - anxiety
  - delirium
  - delusions
  - hallucinations
  - mood disorder
  - perception disturbance
  - persisting amnestic disorder
  - persisting dementia
  - psychotic disorder
  - sexual dysfunction
  - sleep disorder

CDI ALERT

Documentation will indicate the consumption of large amounts of alcohol with ≥3 of the following:

- Tolerance
- Withdrawal symptoms
- Drinking larger amounts than intended
- Persistent decisions to reduce use without success
- Substantial time spent obtaining, drinking, or recovering from alcohol
- Sacrifice of other life events for drinking
- Continued use despite physical or psychological problems

Alcohol Use

Code Axes

Alcohol use, unspecified with intoxication, uncomplicated	**F1Ø.92Ø** HCC
Alcohol use, unspecified with intoxication delirium	**F1Ø.921** HCC
Alcohol use, unspecified with intoxication, unspecified	**F1Ø.929** HCC
Alcohol use, unspecified with alcohol-induced mood disorder	**F1Ø.94** HCC
Alcohol use, unspecified with alcohol-induced psychotic disorder with delusions	**F1Ø.95Ø** HCC
Alcohol use, unspecified with alcohol-induced psychotic disorder with hallucinations	**F1Ø.951** HCC
Alcohol use, unspecified with alcohol-induced psychotic disorder, unspecified	**F1Ø.959** HCC
Alcohol use, unspecified with alcohol-induced persisting amnesia disorder	**F1Ø.96** HCC
Alcohol use, unspecified with other alcohol-induced persisting dementia	**F1Ø.97** HCC
Alcohol use, unspecified with alcohol-induced anxiety disorder	**F1Ø.98Ø** HCC
Alcohol use, unspecified with alcohol-induced sexual dysfunction	**F1Ø.981** HCC
Alcohol use, unspecified with alcohol-induced sleep disorder	**F1Ø.982** HCC
Alcohol use, unspecified with other alcohol-induced disorder	**F1Ø.988** HCC
Alcohol use, unspecified with unspecified alcohol-induced disorder	**F1Ø.99** HCC

Description of Condition

Alcohol use (F1Ø.9-)

Harmful alcohol use is characterized by mental, behavioral and physical disorders due to alcohol use when dependency or abuse is not documented. Alcohol use without negative consequences documented, e.g., mere usage, is not reported with category F1Ø. Provider documented BAC levels should be reported when the clinical significance is stated and has relevance to the encounter (Y9Ø.-).

Key Terms
Key terms found in the documentation may include:

Alcohol intoxication

Alcohol intoxication, unknown usage

Alcohol use with clinical manifestation/state

Drunkenness

ETHO intoxication

Clinician Note
The provider must state the pattern of harmful usage (dependence, abuse or use) and its current clinical state (uncomplicated, intoxication, remission, etc.) and indicate the relationship to any identified mental, behavioral or physical disorder or its relevance to the patient's status or encounter including its clinical significance.

First Listed Diagnosis Note
Admission for acute alcohol poisoning with coma, teen with history of infrequent recreational use: The appropriate code from the Table of Drugs and Chemicals for poisoning will be the first listed diagnosis (alcohol, absolute, beverage), followed by the code for coma and alcohol use, unspecified with other alcohol-induced disorder.

Clinician Documentation Checklist
Clinician documentation should indicate the following:

- Name of substance
  - alcohol
    - identify blood alcohol level
  - polysubstance
- Level of substance use
  - use
  - abuse
  - dependence
- Any additional description of use
  - intoxication
  - remission
  - withdrawal
- Associated psychoactive-induced disorders
  - anxiety
  - delirium
  - delusions
  - hallucinations
  - mood disorder
  - perception disturbance
  - persisting amnestic disorder

- persisting dementia
- psychotic disorder
- sexual dysfunction
- sleep disorder

Amyloidosis

Code Axes

Non-neuropathic heredofamilial amyloidosis	**E85.Ø**
Neuropathic heredofamilial amyloidosis	**E85.1**
Heredofamilial amyloidosis, unspecified	**E85.2**
Secondary systemic amyloidosis	**E85.3**
Organ-limited amyloidosis	**E85.4**
Other amyloidosis	**E85.8-**
Amyloidosis, unspecified	**E85.9**

Description of Condition

Amyloidosis is a potentially fatal condition in which insoluble, fibril-like proteins (amyloid) build up in one or more organs and tissues within the body such as the heart, kidneys, liver, spleen, nervous system, or digestive tract. The material cannot be broken down and interferes with the normal function of the organ. The disease may be inflammatory, hereditary, or neoplastic in nature.

Heredofamilial amyloidosis (E85.Ø, E85.1, E85.2)

This is an inherited disorder caused by an abnormal recessive gene. This type of amyloidosis is most common in ethnic groups from the eastern Mediterranean region.

Key Terms

Key terms found in the documentation may include:

Hereditary amyloid nephropathy

Amyloid polyneuropathy (Portuguese)

Familial

Genetic

Secondary systemic amyloidosis (E85.3)

When another disease leads to amyloidosis, the disorder is considered secondary. Secondary amyloidosis can occur as a result of several infectious, inflammatory, and malignant conditions. Common causative conditions include tuberculosis, osteomyelitis, rheumatoid arthritis, Crohn's disease, and Castleman disease.

Key Terms
Key terms found in the documentation may include:

Secondary amyloidosis

Hemodialysis-associated amyloidosis

Familial Mediterranean fever

Organ-limited amyloidosis (E85.4)

Also known as localized amyloidosis, organ-limited amyloidosis appears to be caused by local deposits of amyloid proteins within an organ. These localized deposits typically involve the upper and lower airways, lung tissue, liver, skin, breasts, and eyes. These amyloid protein deposits in the brain can contribute to Alzheimer's disease.

Light Chain (AL) and Wild-type transthyretin-related (ATTR) amyloidosis (E85.81, E85.82)

AL is caused by overproduction of an amyloidogenic immunoglobulin light chain in patients with a B cell lymphoproliferative disorder.

ATTR is caused by misfolding and deposition of wild-type TTR. This type of amyloidosis targets the heart and has been linked as a cause for infiltrative cardiomyopathy in older male patients.

Clinical Tip
Wild-type ATTR and AL amyloidosis can both cause cardiomyopathy. It is essential to identify the correct type of amyloid to ensure appropriate treatment.

Amyloidosis, unspecified (E85.9)

If no other underlying disease is present and the main symptoms stem from amyloidosis, the amyloidosis is considered primary.

Clinical Tip
Common areas for amyloid deposits include the kidneys, GI tract, liver, spleen, heart, nerves, blood vessels, and skin.

Key Terms
Key terms found in the documentation may include:

Primary amyloidosis

Clinical Findings

Physical Examination

Signs and symptoms of systemic amyloidosis may be nonspecific but history, review of systems, and examination may include:

- Abnormal heart rhythm
- Chronic diarrhea or constipation

- Shortness of breath
- Difficulty swallowing or chewing
- Enlarged liver or spleen
- Enlarged tongue
- Fatigue
- Joint pain
- Joint swelling
- Memory problems
- Nerve pain
- Numbness or tingling
- Skin changes
- Vomiting
- Weakness
- Weight loss

Diagnostic Procedures and Services

- Laboratory
  - blood tests for abnormal proteins
  - urine tests for abnormal proteins
  - liver function tests
- Imaging
  - abdominal ultrasound
  - echocardiogram
  - chest CT
- Other
  - pulmonary function tests
  - abdominal fat pad biopsy
  - bone marrow biopsy
  - skin biopsy

Therapeutic Procedures and Services

For secondary disease, the underlying condition is treated. For primary amyloidosis, treatment may include:

- Chemotherapy
- Organ transplant
- Stem cell transplant

Medication List

- Chemotherapy using an alkylating agent
- Colchicine (Colcrys)

Clinician Documentation Checklist

Clinician documentation should indicate the following:

- Identification of
  - primary or secondary disease
  - genetic disease
  - familial disease
  - hereditary disease
    - neuropathic
    - non-neuropathic
  - hemodialysis associated disease
  - localized disease
    - organ involved

Anemia — Acquired Hemolytic

Code Axes

Drug-induced autoimmune hemolytic anemia	**D59.Ø** HCC
Other autoimmune hemolytic anemias	**D59.1** HCC
Drug-induced nonautoimmune hemolytic anemia	**D59.2** HCC
Hemolytic-uremic syndrome	**D59.3** HCC
Other nonautoimmune hemolytic anemias	**D59.4** HCC
Paroxysmal nocturnal hemoglobinuria (Marchiafava-Micheli)	**D59.5** HCC
Hemoglobinuria due to hemolysis from other external causes	**D59.6** HCC
Other acquired hemolytic anemias	**D59.8** HCC
Acquired hemolytic anemia, unspecified	**D59.9** HCC

I-10 Alert

The ICD-10-CM subcategories for acquired hemolytic anemia now include classifications for drug-induced conditions, whether autoimmune or nonautoimmune. When the condition is drug-induced, an additional adverse effect ICD-10-CM code should be assigned from categories T36–T5Ø, with fifth or sixth character 5, indicating a therapeutic use adverse effect.

Description of Condition

Drug-induced autoimmune hemolytic anemia (D59.Ø)

Some therapeutic drugs may cause the patient's immune system to inappropriately target its own red blood cells for destruction through development of antibodies. These antibodies attach themselves to the red blood cells and cause early destruction. Cephalosporins are a class of antibiotics most commonly associated with the condition, but others are listed below:

- Cephalosporins
- Dapsone
- Levodopa
- Levofloxacin
- Methyldopa
- Nitrofurantoin
- Nonsteroidal anti-inflammatory drugs (NSAIDs)
- Penicillin and its derivatives
- Phenazopyridine (Pyridium)
- Quinidine

CDI Alert

Ensure that the documentation specifies that the condition is determined to be drug-induced. Initial symptoms include dark urine, jaundice, tachycardia, shortness of breath, and weakness.

Key Terms

Key terms found in the documentation may include:

Acquired hemolytic anemia, chemical induced

Other autoimmune hemolytic anemias (D59.1)

There are two major types of disorders in this classification: cold antibody hemolytic anemia and warm antibody hemolytic anemia. In the cold antibody type, the autoantibodies become most active and attack red blood cells only at temperatures well below normal body temperature, whereas in the warm antibody type, the autoantibodies attach to and destroy red blood cells at temperatures equal to or higher than normal body temperature.

CDI ALERT

Diagnosis is typically made on the initial blood test, with an increase in the number of red blood cells that are immature (reticulocytes). Also, tests indicate increased amounts of certain antibodies, either attached to red blood cells (direct antiglobulin or direct Coombs' test) or in the liquid portion of the blood (indirect antiglobulin or indirect Coombs' test). Initial symptoms include dark urine, jaundice, tachycardia, shortness of breath, and weakness and may progress to splenomegaly.

Key Terms

Key terms found in the documentation may include:

Autoimmune hemolytic disease
Chronic cold hemagglutinin disease
Cold agglutinin disease
Cold agglutinin hemoglobinuria
Immune complex hemolytic anemia
Immunohemolytic anemia
Secondary cold type hemolytic anemia
Secondary warm type hemolytic anemia

Drug-induced nonautoimmune hemolytic anemia (D59.2)

This condition is similar to that listed above for code D59.Ø, except that the drug's adverse reaction is not associated with the body's autoimmune response. Instead, an oxidative mechanism occurs, where a component of the therapeutic drug binds to the red blood cells, resulting in oxygen deprivation and oxygen delivery to the tissues is impaired. This resulting condition is called methemoglobinemia.

CDI ALERT

Ensure that the documentation specifies that the condition is determined to be drug-induced. Initial symptoms include dark urine, jaundice, tachycardia, shortness of breath, and weakness.

Several of the drugs most commonly associated with the condition are listed below:

Dapsone
Phenazopyridine
Primaquine
Ribavirin

Key Terms

Key terms found in the documentation may include:

Drug-induced enzyme deficiency anemia

I-10 ALERT

ICD-10-CM Instructional note: Use additional code for any associated: *E. coli* infection (B96.2-), pneumococcal pneumonia (J13), or *Shigella dysenteriae* (AØ3.9).

Hemolytic-uremic syndrome (D59.3)

Hemolytic-uremic syndrome (HUS) is a combination of three major components: hemolytic anemia (destruction of red blood cells), acute kidney failure, and a low platelet count (thrombocytopenia). The condition most commonly affects children and very often is preceded by an episode of infectious, sometimes bloody, diarrhea caused by *E. coli* O157:H7, which is acquired as a foodborne illness.

Clinical Tip
Acquired hemolytic anemias are uninherited disorders involving premature destruction of erythrocytes (red blood cells). Causes may include injury, infection, drugs, or blood transfusions (autoimmune). The condition is also classified as either intrinsic, where the cause is related to the red blood cell (RBC) itself, or extrinsic, where outside factors are believed to cause the disorder.

Key Terms
Key terms found in the documentation may include:

Drug-induced enzyme deficiency anemia
HUS

CDI ALERT

Review documentation carefully. Initially, HUS can be very hard to distinguish from thrombotic thrombocytopenic purpura, so documentation may appear in the medical record related to ruling out either condition.

Clinical Findings

Physical Examination

A complete physical examination with particular attention to pallor, abdominal distention, petechiae, and heart murmur. Hypoxia may also be indicated.

Diagnostic Procedures and Services

- Laboratory
  - CBC: Findings may indicate normochromic-monocystic, reticulocytosis or marrow erythroid hyperplasia
  - chemistry panel may indicate elevated serum bilirubin and LDH
  - stool guaiac: negative as anemia is not due to blood loss
  - ferritin
  - total iron binding capacity
  - serum iron
  - iron saturation

Note: Hemolytic anemia results usually note that a ferritin serum iron and iron saturation levels are normal and a TIBC are normal or low.

Therapeutic Procedures and Services

Type of treatment is dependent upon the severity and cause and may include the following:

- Blood transfusions
- Plasmapheresis
- Treatment with intravenous immune globulin (to strengthen the immune system)

Medication List
- Corticosteroids (Prednisone)
- Cyclosporine
- Rituximab

Clinician Documentation Checklist

Clinician documentation should indicate the following:

- Type of acquired hemolytic anemia:
  - autoimmune or nonautoimmune
  - drug-induced autoimmune or nonautoimmune:
    - specify drug and any adverse effect
  - hemolytic-uremic syndrome
    - specify associated disorder
      - *Escherichia coli*
      - pneumococcal pneumonia
      - *Shigella dysenteriae*
  - paroxysmal nocturnal hemoglobinuria (Marchiafava-Micheli)
  - hemoglobinuria due to hemolysis from other external cause
    - Specify the external cause
      - from exertion
      - march hemoglobinuria
      - paroxysmal cold hemoglobinuria
- Other autoimmune types
  - autoimmune hemolytic disease (cold, warm)
  - chronic cold hemagglutinin disease
  - cold agglutinin disease
  - cold agglutinin hemoglobinuria
  - cold hemolytic anemia (secondary, symptomatic)
  - warm hemolytic anemia (secondary, symptomatic
- Other nonautoimmune types
  - mechanical hemolytic anemia
  - microangiopathic hemolytic anemia
  - toxic hemolytic anemia

Anemia — Iron-Deficiency

Code Axes

Iron deficiency anemia secondary to blood loss (chronic)	**D5Ø.Ø**
Other and unspecified iron deficiency anemias	**D5Ø.8, D5Ø.9**

Description of Condition

Iron deficiency anemia secondary to blood loss (chronic) (D5Ø.Ø)

Iron deficiency anemia due to chronic blood loss most commonly results from a recurrent bleeding lesion in the gastrointestinal tract, such as a gastric ulcer or diverticulitis. Note that acute posthemorrhagic anemia is excluded from this category. The two conditions are clinically very dissimilar and have different causes.

Key Terms

Key terms found in the documentation may include:

- Asiderotic anemia
- Chlorosis
- Chronic blood loss anemia
- Chronic posthemorrhagic anemia (D5Ø.Ø)
- Hypoferric anemia
- Hypochromic or microcytic anemia
- IDA due to inadequate nutrition
- Idiopathic hypochromic anemia

Other and unspecified iron deficiency anemias (D5Ø.8, D5Ø.9)

These classifications are available when the documentation indicates conditions that either have no specific code assignment, or there is no specific documentation for the condition. Iron deficiency anemia secondary to inadequate dietary iron intake is indexed to code D5Ø.8.

Key Terms

Key terms found in the documentation may include:

- IDA due to inadequate nutrition
- Iron deficiency anemia due to inadequate dietary iron intake
- Refractory sideropenic anemia

CDI ALERT

Ensure that the anemia is specified as chronic (and not acute posthemorrhagic) to assign codes from this category.

CDI ALERT

Laboratory work-up typically reveals depleted iron stores and small, pale red blood cells (RBC), erythrocyte count less reduced than hemoglobin, serum ferritin below 12 ng/mL, low serum iron, and increased total iron-binding capacity. The physician must document the underlying cause of the anemia; no cause and effect may be assumed.

Clinical Findings

Physical Examination

History and review of systems may include:

- Signs and symptoms
  - fatigue
  - loss of stamina
  - shortness of breath
  - weakness and pallor

Diagnostic Procedures and Services

- Laboratory
  - CBC: low hemoglobin and hematocrit are below normal levels (In early stages, the hemoglobin may be normal.)
  - serum iron
  - total iron binding
  - iron saturation
  - serum ferritin
  - bone marrow evaluation

Note: In uncomplicated iron deficiency anemia the ferritin and serum iron levels are below normal while the TIBC may be elevated. Iron saturation results are either normal or low.

Therapeutic Procedures and Services

In most instances iron supplements are provided either in the oral or intramuscular method.

In severe cases a blood transfusion may be performed.

Medication List

- Carbonyl iron (Feosol)
- Ferrous sulfate (Feratab, Fer-Iron, Slow-FE)
- Iron sucrose (Venofer)

Clinician Documentation Checklist

Clinician documentation should indicate the following:

- Type of iron deficient anemia
  - secondary to blood loss
  - due to inadequate dietary iron intake
  - due to inadequate nutrition
  - asiderotic
  - chlorosis
  - hypoferric
  - idiopathic hypochromic
  - refractory sideropenic

Anemia — Postoperative

Code Axes

Postoperative (postprocedural) anemia due to (acute) blood loss	**D62**
Postoperative (postprocedural) anemia, due to chronic blood loss	**D5Ø.Ø**
Postoperative (postprocedural) anemia, specified NEC	**D64.9**

Description of Condition

Postoperative (postprocedural) anemia due to (acute) blood loss (D62)

Anemia due to blood loss that is acute is the result of rapid, sudden loss of blood following trauma, a hemorrhagic condition, hemophilia, acute leukemia or loss during surgery. Postoperative anemia due to blood loss (posthemorrhagic) must be evidenced by clinically significant lab values that are indicative of the diagnosis. The diagnosis of anemia must be documented by the provider; the code cannot be reported based on lab values alone. The term 'acute' is not required to report postoperative blood loss anemia as D62, but the anemia *must* be described as "[due to] blood loss" *and* a stated link to the surgery/procedure would verify the cause/effect relationship with terms/phrases such as "postoperative," "due to," as "a result of" the surgery or procedure. It should be noted that this code is not a "complication" code but is identifying a condition that is occurring postoperatively or acutely due to bleeding/hemorrhage as "acute hemorrhagic anemia."

Clinical Tip

If a diagnosis of anemia is specified in the absence of documentation of significant surgical blood loss, review operative records for documentation of administration of excessive fluids (e.g., colloids, crystalloids, plasma, etc.) intraoperatively which could result in iatrogenic dilutional anemia. An immediate drop in hemoglobin in the absence of significant blood loss during surgery may be indicative of a dilutional anemia rather than anemia due to acute blood loss. Any multiple choice clinician query for acute blood loss during surgery should also include the clinically reasonable choice of dilutional anemia along with any clinical indicators.

Key Terms

Key terms found in the documentation may include:

Acute blood loss anemia

Acute posthemorrhagic anemia

Acute post-op anemia due to blood loss

Acute post-op anemia due to blood loss as a result of surgery

P/O blood loss anemia

CDI ALERT

When the clinical scenario and clinical indicators are suggestive of anemia due to blood loss after a procedure or surgery, and only the diagnosis of anemia is made, a query would be appropriate to clarify the link and nature for specificity.

CDI ALERT

Arrows: up and down arrows do not indicate a diagnosis. Query the provider as to the meaning of the symbols and request the information be fully stated including the clinical significance.

Post-op anemia due to blood loss

Postprocedure blood loss anemia

Documentation Tip

The baseline or preoperative H/H should be documented in order to qualify the type of anemia. Note that treatment is not required in order to report D62.

Arthroscopies

Code Axes

Arthroscopy, temporomandibular joint	**29800–29804**
Arthroscopy, shoulder	**29805–29828**
Arthroscopy, elbow	**29830–29838**
Arthroscopy, wrist	**29840–29848**
Arthroscopy, hip	**29860–29863, 29914–29916**
Arthroscopy, knee	**29866–29887**
Arthroscopy, ankle	**29891, 29894–29899**
Arthroscopy, metacarpophalangeal joint	**29900–29902**
Arthroscopy, subtalar joint	**29904–29907**

Description of Procedure

An arthroscopy is the visualization of a joint using a fiberoptic scope and may be performed as a diagnostic tool or as a surgical intervention. It requires two or more small surgical incisions and the scope and surgical instrumentation, often referred to as trocars, are inserted into the joint space. A number of surgical procedures may be performed through the scope, including but not limited to the removal of loose bodies (bone and/or cartilage), debridement, partial or complete synovectomy, or meniscus repairs.

CDI ALERT

The documentation should be carefully reviewed to determine what exact procedures were performed. There are times when the procedure performed and listed at the beginning of the operative report will not be the actual procedure described in the body of the report.

When reviewing documentation to ascertain correct code selection, it is important to note the anatomical location (joint) but also additional terms such as medial, lateral, and the specific ligament being treated. The instrumentation used can also help to determine the exact type of surgical intervention being performed.

Key Terms

Key terms found in the documentation may include:

Arthroscopy with _____________

Debridement (debride): The smoothing of rough or torn cartilage as well as osteophytes and loose body removal that interfere with the motion of the joint Documentation may indicate the use of a shaver as well as other instruments such as rasps, curettes, spoons, and awls.

Meniscectomy (meni): The removal of the meniscus, a fibrocartilaginous structure that divides a joint space in half Meniscectomies are commonly performed knee arthroscopic procedures and physicians often use specialized instruments called meniscectomies when performing this service.

Synovectomy (syno): The partial removal of all or part of the synovium of a joint and documentation will often refer to motorized shaver.

Clinician Note

Documentation should clearly indicate any services or procedures performed at the time of arthroscopic examination and should clearly identify the location within the joint that the procedure is performed.

Clinician Documentation Checklist

Clinician documentation should indicate the following:

- Indicate the medical condition being treated
- Anatomical location
- Instrumentation
- Surgical procedures performed
  - removal of loose material
  - debridement
  - synovectomy
  - meniscus repair
  - other

Asthma

Code Axes

Note: All asthma codes (with the exception of subcategory J45.99) have fifth or sixth characters that represent the following three classification axes: uncomplicated, with (acute) exacerbation, with status asthmaticus: defined as an acute exacerbation of asthma that does not respond to standard treatments of bronchodilators and steroids.

Mild intermittent asthma	**J45.2-** HCC
Mild persistent asthma	**J45.3-** HCC
Moderate persistent asthma	**J45.4-** HCC
Severe persistent asthma	**J45.5-** HCC
Other and unspecified asthma	**J45.9-** HCC
Other asthma (exercise induced bronchospasm, cough variant asthma, other)	**J45.99-** HCC

Description of Condition

Clinical Tip

Respiratory insufficiency is integral to asthma. Hypoxemias are reported separately as it is not inherent.

Key Terms

Key terms found in the documentation may include:

- Allergic asthma
- Allergic bronchitis
- Allergic rhinitis with asthma
- Atopic asthma
- Extrinsic allergic asthma
- Hay fever with asthma
- Idiosyncratic asthma
- Intrinsic nonallergic asthma
- Nonallergic asthma
- Reactive airway disease

I-10 ALERT

Classification axes for extrinsic and intrinsic asthma have been eliminated in ICD-10-CM. Instead, asthma severity levels, as have been defined by pulmonologists, have been introduced.

CDI ALERT

If there is an obstructive component to the patient's asthma, ensure that it is documented appropriately. These cases are coded and classified differently and require two codes, one from category J44 and one from category J45.

Asthma Severity Levels

Mild intermittent asthma (J45.2-)

Mild intermittent asthma is the least severe of all types, involves a frequency of symptoms no more than two days a week, and nighttime symptoms no more than two times a month. This type of asthma typically does not interfere at all with daily activities.

Mild persistent asthma (J45.3-)

Patients with mild persistent asthma may have symptoms more than twice weekly, but not daily, and the condition can typically be controlled with one controller medication. A rescue inhaler may be used on a regular basis, but not daily. This type of asthma may interfere with daily activities in a minor way.

Moderate persistent asthma (J45.4-)

A classification of moderate persistent asthma requires that the patient have asthma symptoms daily that are controlled with two medications. A rescue inhaler may be used daily, and the patient may wake with asthma symptoms more than once a week, but not daily. The effect on daily activities is moderate.

Severe persistent asthma (J45.5-)

This is the most severe asthma classification and these patients have asthma symptoms daily. In some cases symptoms are experienced throughout the day, regardless of the use of two or more medications. The patient wakes from asthma symptoms nightly and must use a rescue inhaler multiple times a day. The effect on daily activities is extreme.

Exercise induced bronchospasm (J45.990)

This condition is defined as a reversible transient bronchoconstriction that affects patients both with and without a history of asthma. The symptoms of shortness of breath, wheezing, cough, or chest tightness occurs during strenuous exercise and may peak at five to ten minutes after exercising. Spirometry is commonly used to rule out underlying asthma.

Cough variant asthma (J45.991)

The major symptom of cough variant asthma is a dry non-productive cough that has persisted for six to eight weeks. There are no other more typical asthma symptoms, such as wheezing, or shortness of breath. The condition may be triggered by cold air or environmental allergens and is treated with a rescue inhaler.

Clinical Findings

Physical Examination

History and review of systems may indicate:

- Coughing
- Wheezing
- Chest tightness
- Shortness of breath

Diagnostic Procedures and Services

- Imaging
  - pulmonary function tests (PFT)
  - chest x-ray
  - electrocardiogram
  - allergy testing

Medication List

- Bronchodilator
  - long-acting beta agonists (LABAs)
    - — formoterol (Foradil, Perforomist)
    - — salmeterol (Serevent)
  - short-acting beta agonists
    - — albuterol (Proventil, Ventolin)
    - — ipratropium (Atrovent)
    - — levalbuterol (Xopenex)
  - theophylline (Theo-24, Uniphyl)
- Inhaled corticosteroids
  - beclomethasone (QVAR)
  - budesonide (Pulmicort)
  - ciclesonide (Alvesco)
  - flunisolide (Aerospan HFA)
  - fluticasone (Flovent HFA)
  - mometasone (Asmanex Twisthaler)
- Leukotriene modifiers
  - montelukast (Singulair)
  - zafirlukast (Accolate)
  - zileuton (Zyflo)
- Combination inhalers: Corticosteroids and long-acting beta agonists
  - fluticasone and salmeterol (Advair Diskus)
  - budesonide and formoterol (Symbicort)
  - mometasone and formoterol (Dulera)
- Oral or intravenous corticosteroids

Clinician Documentation Checklist

Clinician documentation should indicate the following:

- Identify any triggers
- Exposure to environmental tobacco smoke
- Exposure to tobacco smoke in the perinatal period
- History of tobacco use
- Occupational exposure to environmental tobacco smoke
- Tobacco dependence
- Tobacco use
- Include additional conditions
  - allergic (predominantly) asthma
  - allergic bronchitis
  - allergic rhinitis with asthma
  - atopic asthma
  - extrinsic allergic asthma
  - fever with asthma
  - idiosyncratic asthma
  - intrinsic nonallergic asthma
  - nonallergic asthma
- Type
  - mild intermittent
  - mild persistent
  - moderate persistent
  - severe persistent
  - other
    - exercise-induced bronchospasm
    - cough variant asthma
  - unspecified
    - asthmatic bronchitis
    - childhood asthma
    - late onset asthma
  - document if any of the above type is:
    - uncomplicated
    - with (acute) exacerbation
    - with status asthmaticus

Atelectasis

Code Axes

Atelectasis	**J98.11**
Postprocedural atelectasis	**J95.89** **J98.11**

Description of Condition

Atelectasis (J98.11)

Atelectasis is an incomplete expansion of lung segments that may result in partial or complete lung collapse. It occurs to some degree in many patients undergoing upper abdominal or thoracic surgery. Prognosis depends on prompt removal of any airway obstruction, relief of hypoxia, and re-expansion of the collapsed lung. Prolonged immobility, anesthesia, mechanical ventilation, prolonged bed rest with few changes in position, underlying lung diseases, or any condition that inhibits full lung expansion or makes deep breathing painful, with shallow breathing are risk factors.

Postprocedural atelectasis (J95.89, J98.11)

Atelectasis is an expected condition within the first 48 hours postoperatively when the patient has undergone a general anesthetic with moderately high oxygen concentrations. It is often an incidental x-ray/physical finding that is frequently self-limiting. It will usually resolve spontaneously without treatment. When it becomes symptomatic and requires work-up or additional monitoring or treatment, and it is documented as a complication of a procedure, it will be reported as a postprocedure complication.

CDI Alert

When atelectasis is associated with significant findings, such as fever, or requires further diagnostic or therapeutic work up, such as chest x-ray (as part of work-up, not routinely/incidentally), urinalysis/blood culture, or respiratory therapy, or is linked to an extended hospital stay, then it is reportable.

Clinical Findings

Physical Examination

History and review of systems may include:

- Coarse lung sound and/or decreased lung sound
- Cough
- Dyspnea
- Shortness of breath
- Chest pain
- Transudate pleural effusion

Diagnostic Procedures and Services

- Imaging
  - chest x-ray
- Other
  - spirometry

Therapeutic Procedures and Services

- Chest physiotherapy
- Deep breathing
- Directed cough
- Nebulizer

Clinician Documentation Checklist

Clinician documentation should indicate the following:

- Recent procedures requiring general anesthesia
- Complications that occurred were
  - during procedure (intraoperative)
  - after procedure (postprocedural)
- Significant symptoms
  - shortness of breath
  - dyspnea
  - respiratory failure
  - decreased breath sounds
  - dullness to percussion
  - chest pain
  - transudate pleural effusion
  - fever
- Additional diagnostic or therapeutic workup
  - chest x-ray
  - blood culture
  - respiratory therapy
- Reason for an extended hospital stay

Body Mass Index

Code Axes

Body mass index (BMI) 25.Ø-29.9, adult	**Z68.25–Z68.29**
Body mass index (BMI) 3Ø.Ø-39.9, adult	**Z68.3Ø–Z68.39**
Body mass Index (BMI) ≥4Ø.Ø, adult	**Z68.41–Z68.45** HCC

⇨ I-10 ALERT

Codes Z68.25–Z68.45 are unacceptable as principal diagnoses for facility billing.

Description of Condition

Overweight = Body Mass Index (BMI) 25.Ø–29.9, adult (Z68.25–Z68.29)

Key Terms

Key terms found in the documentation may include:

Dietary counseling

Overweight

Obesity = Body Mass Index (BMI) 3Ø.Ø–39.9, adult (Z68.3Ø–Z68.39)

Morbid Obesity = Body Mass Index (BMI) ≥4Ø.Ø, adult (Z68.41–Z68.45)

This disorder is defined as excess body weight. Causes are typically multifactorial and may include side effects of prescription medication, a hormone imbalance, or genetic predisposition.

Clinical Tip

Untreated obesity tends to progress and can lead to many common health problems. Common complications include diabetes, cardiovascular disorders, metabolic syndrome, many cancers, osteoarthritis, fatty liver, depression, and obstructive sleep apnea.

Key Terms

Key terms found in the documentation may include:

BMI >30

BMI >40

Dietary management

Excess abdominal fat

Excessively overweight

Lose 5 to 10 percent of body weight

Morbid obesity

Obesity

Severe obesity

CDI ALERT

BMI can be reported based on documentation by a nurse, dietitian, etc. However, a diagnosis of obesity must be based on physician documentation.

Clinician Documentation Checklist

Clinician documentation should indicate the following:

- Obesity
  - morbid or severe
    - drug induced (document drug)
    - due to excess calories
    - familial
    - glandular
- Body mass index (BMI) = weight (kg) divided by the square of the height
- Document associated conditions or resources used
  - dietary consult
  - dietary plan
  - increase in OR time
  - special equipment

Bronchoscopy

Code Axes

Bronchoscopy, rigid or flexible **31622–31654**

Description of Procedure

A bronchoscopy is the examination of the bronchi by means of a fiberoptic scope that can be either flexible or rigid. Rigid bronchoscopies are performed less frequently and are usually used when a wider aperture or channels are required for diagnosing and treating such conditions as:

- Large pulmonary hemorrhages
- Some types of foreign bodies
- Some types of obstructive endobronchial lesions that may require laser debulking and/or stent placement

Flexible fiberoptic scopes are used in most other scenarios.

Like other endoscopic procedures, bronchoscopies can be diagnostic in nature, or when medically indicated, can be therapeutic. Appropriate code selection is dependent upon what, if any, additional procedures or services are documented in the medical record.

Endobronchial ultrasound (sometimes recorded as EBUS in the medical record) is performed to determine the presence of peripheral lesions. Documentation often indicates that a transducer was passed through the bronchoscope to better visualize vascular and nonvascular structures. When documentation indicates that this service was performed, code 31654 is reported additionally.

CDI ALERT

The documentation should be carefully reviewed to determine what exact procedures were performed. There are times when the procedure performed and listed at the beginning of the operative report will not be the actual procedure described in the body of the report.

Bronchoscopy, with balloon occlusion (31634)

Documentation will indicate that a balloon occlusion was performed to treat an air leak when the documentation states that the physician advanced a balloon catheter through the bronchoscope to the site of the leak and inflated the balloon until the leak is occluded. While keeping the balloon inflated, a sealant such as fibrin is injected. Once the air leak is resolved, the balloon catheter is removed.

An endobronchial valve is a device placed and subsequently removed via the bronchoscope that permits one-way air movement. The valve closes when the patient inhales preventing air flow to the diseased area of the lung. The valve opens during exhalation to allow air to escape from the diseased area of the lung. It is used to treat persistent air leak from the lung into the pleural space.

Key Terms

Balloon occlusion

Endobronchial ultrasound (EBUS)

Endobronchial valve

Transbronchial needle aspiration (TBNA)

Clinician Note

Because some codes may be reported to indicate that additional lobes were treated, the medical record documentation must clearly specify the anatomical location where the procedure or service was performed.

Clinician Documentation Checklist

Clinician documentation should indicate the following:

- Identify the medical condition being treated
- Purpose of bronchoscopy
  - diagnostic
  - therapeutic
- Includes
  - transbronchial needle aspiration (TBNA)
  - endobronchial ultrasound (EBUS)
  - balloon occlusion
  - endobronchial valve
- Anatomical location of procedure

Cataract — Age-related (Senile)

Code Axes

Age-related incipient cataract	**H25.Ø-**
Age-related nuclear cataract	**H25.1-**
Age-related cataract, Morgagnian type	**H25.2-**
Other age-related cataract	**H25.8-**
Unspecified age-related cataract	**H25.9**

Note: Conditions classified to chapter 7 include laterality (right, left, bilateral) within the code structure. All ophthalmic conditions should specify the affected eye(s).

Description of Condition

Age-related cataract (H25.--)

Clinical Tip
Cataract is the partial or total opacity of the crystalline lens or lens capsule. Age-related (senile) cataract is slowly progressive partial or total opacity of the lens due to degenerative changes in patients over 55 years of age. Clinical classification of cataract considers the zones of the lens in which the opacity appears: cortical, subcapsular (anterior and posterior poles), and nuclear. Opacities may overlap these zones, encompassing combined clinical classification types. A morgagnian cataract is a mature cataract in which the nucleus moves freely throughout a liquefied cortex. Other causes that contribute to age-related degenerative cataract formation include systemic disease (e.g., diabetes), lifestyle factors (e.g., smoking), exposures (e.g., lead, ultraviolet light), and other intraocular diseases (e.g., glaucoma, retinal defects).

Key Terms
Key terms found in the documentation may include:

- Cataracta brunescens
- Coronary cataract
- Hypermature cataract
- Immature cataract
- Incipient cataract
- Indolent cataract
- Nuclear sclerosis cataract
- Punctate cataract

⇨ I-10 ALERT

ICD-10-CM classification for cataract includes a terminology change in the tabular list from "senile" to "age-related" for cataracts attributed to the effects of the aging process. However, note that the ICD-10-CM alphabetic index refers the coder to "*see* Cataract, senile" to index specific subterm for code assignment.

⇨ I-10 ALERT

Category H25 includes valid codes that are five or six characters in length. The following axes of classification describe those characters:

- Fourth character:
  - Type of age-related cataract (incipient, nuclear, morgagnian, other)
- Fifth character:
  - Location of cataract: point of origin of lens opacification
  - Type (Other: combined forms)
  - Laterality
- Sixth character:
  - Laterality

Senile or age-related

Water clefts

Clinician Note

Specify the nature and location of age-related cataract. Differentiate between opacities originating in the lenticular cortex, lenticular nucleus, and subcapsular poles (anterior or posterior). Document the specific type, as appropriate.

State whether opacification is partial or complete. Document any complications associated with the cataract, including the degree of visual impairment or related ophthalmic (local) conditions and manifestation, such as:

- History of eye surgeries and associated complications
- Myopia
- Glaucoma
- Retinal disease, detachment or defect
- Chronic inflammation or infection (e.g., iridocyclitis, uveitis)

Document any associated or underlying chronic or systemic disease processes. If conditions are inter-related, document the cause-and-effect relationship.

Clinician Documentation Checklist

Clinician documentation should indicate the following:

- Age-related incipient cataract
  - cortical age-related cataract
  - anterior subcapsular polar age-related cataract
  - posterior subcapsular polar age-related cataract
  - other age-related incipient cataract
    - coronary age-related cataract
    - punctate age-related cataract
    - water clefts
- Age-related nuclear cataract
  - cataracta brunescens
  - nuclear sclerosis cataract
- Age-related cataract, morgagnian type
  - age-related hypermature cataract
- Other age-related cataract
  - subtype:
    - combined forms of age-related cataract
    - other age-related cataract
- Unspecified age-related cataract
  - senile cataract

- Identify laterality of eye
  - right
  - left
  - bilateral

Cataract — Complicated

⇨ I-10 ALERT

ICD-10-CM includes a specific subcategory to classify complicated cataract. Subcategory H26.2 includes cataract due to certain ocular disorders or associated with other ophthalmic complications.

Note: Conditions classified to chapter 7 include laterality (right, left, bilateral) within the code structure. All ophthalmic conditions should specify the affected eye(s).

Code Axes

Other cataract	**H26**
Complicated cataract	**H26.2-**
Unspecified complicated cataract	**H26.20**
Cataract with neovascularization	**H26.21-**
Cataract secondary to ocular disorders	**H26.22-**
Glaucomatous flecks	**H26.23-**

Description of Condition

Complicated cataract (H26.2--)

Clinical Tip

Complicated cataract in ICD-10-CM includes cataract due to other ocular disorders or cataracts occurring as complications of other certain ophthalmic disorders. Certain ophthalmic diseases have long-term effects on the physiology of the intraocular lens. Complicated cataract often originates at the posterior subcapsular area and progresses to opacify the entire lens if the underlying or precipitating ocular disease remains untreated. Neovascularization occurs when the trabecular meshwork becomes obstructed or ischemic, resulting in deposit buildup on the lens epithelium. Chronic intraocular disease commonly associated with complications of cataract includes recurrent uveitis, glaucoma, retinitis pigmentosa, and retinal detachment or defect.

Key Terms

Key terms found in the documentation for complicated cataract may include:

- Cataracta complicata
- Degenerative cataract
- Glaucomatous flecks
- Glaukomflecken
- Inflammatory cataract
- Neovascularization cataract
- Subcapsular flecks

Clinical Findings

Physical Examination

History and review of systems may include:

Ophthalmoscopy followed by slit-lamp examination. Documentation may indicate well-developed gray, white, or yellow-brown opacities in the lenses. Small cataracts may be described as a dark defect in the red reflex. Documentation indicating a larger cataract may include the obliteration of the red reflex.

Therapeutic Procedures and Services

Surgical removal of the cataract with the placement of an intraocular lens

Clinician Documentation Checklist

Clinician documentation should indicate the following:

- Specify type
  - infantile and juvenile cataract
    - subtype
      - infantile and juvenile cortical, lamellar, or zonular cataract
      - infantile and juvenile nuclear cataract
      - anterior subcapsular polar infantile and juvenile cataract
      - posterior subcapsular polar infantile and juvenile cataract
      - combined forms of infantile and juvenile cataract
      - other infantile and juvenile cataract
      - unspecified infantile and juvenile cataract
        - presenile cataract
  - traumatic cataract
    - identify the external cause
    - subtype
      - localized traumatic opacities
      - partially resolved traumatic cataract
      - total traumatic cataract
      - unspecified traumatic cataract
  - complicated cataract
    - subtype
      - cataract with neovascularization
        - identify associated, such as chronic iridocyclitis
      - cataract secondary to ocular disorders (degenerative) (inflammatory)
        - identify associated ocular disorder
      - glaucomatous flecks (subcapsular)
        - identify underlying glaucoma type

        - ♦ unspecified complicated cataract
            - ❖ cataracta complicata
    - drug-induced cataract
        - — toxic cataract
        - — identify the drug, if applicable
    - secondary cataract
        - — subtype
            - ♦ Soemmering's ring
            - ♦ other secondary cataract
            - ♦ unspecified secondary cataract
    - other specified cataract
        - — cataract due to radiation
        - — electric cataract
        - — glass-blower's cataract
        - — heat ray cataract
- Identify laterality of eye
    - right
    - left
    - bilateral

Cataract — Removal of

Code Axes

Extracapsular cataract removal	**66982, 66984**
Intracapsular	**66983**

Description of Procedure

A cataract is opacity of the lens of the eye and can be congenital or degenerative. There are two types of procedures performed to extract the lens. Intracapsular is when the lens is removed in one piece and extracapsular, the more commonly performed service, is when the hard central nucleus is removed in one piece and then the soft cortex is removed in multiple pieces.

CPT Alert

When documentation indicates that a special pupil-stretching device, rings, or hooks are used, code 66982 indicating a complex procedure is supported. Documentation may indicate the use of a device such as a Beehler pupil stretcher or Kuglen hooks.

Extracapsular cataract removal (66982, 66984)

Intracapsular cataract removal (66983)

Clinical Tip

Dropless cataract surgery: A new cataract procedure known as the dropless cataract procedure is performed when the physician injects (intravitreal) compounded medications (antibiotics and steroids) thus reducing or in some instances preventing the need of medicated eye drops postoperatively. Most payers include the injection in the service; therefore, it should not be billed separately.

Key Terms

Key terms found in the documentation may include:

Extracapsular

Extracapsular cataract extraction (ECCE)

Intracapsular

Intracapsular cataract extraction (ICCE)

Intraocular lens (IOL)

Senile or age related

Clinician Note

State whether opacification is partial or complete. Document any complications associated with the cataract, including the degree of visual impairment or related ophthalmic (local) conditions and manifestations.

Clinician Documentation Checklist

Clinician documentation should indicate the following:

- Type of cataract
  - age-related
  - congenital
  - presenile
  - secondary
  - senile
- Conditions and manifestations
  - opacity
    - partial
    - complete
  - complications
    - degree of visual impairment
    - glaucoma
    - diabetes
- Type of removal
  - intracapsular
  - extracapsular
    - pupil stretching device used
  - phacoemulsification
  - dropless procedure
- Location
  - anterior
  - posterior
- Laterality
  - left
  - right

Cellulitis and Acute Lymphangitis

Code Axes

Cellulitis and acute lymphangitis of finger and toe	**LØ3.Ø-**
Cellulitis and acute lymphangitis of other parts of limb	**LØ3.1-**
Cellulitis and acute lymphangitis of face and neck	**LØ3.2-**
Cellulitis and acute lymphangitis of trunk	**LØ3.3-**
Cellulitis and acute lymphangitis of other sites	**LØ3.8-**
Cellulitis and acute lymphangitis, unspecified	**LØ3.9-**

Description of Condition

Cellulitis and acute lymphangitis (LØ3)

Clinical Tip

Cellulitis describes an infection of the skin and subcutaneous tissues most commonly caused by bacterial infection that spreads to the deeper layers of the dermis from an opening in the skin surface (e.g., open wound or puncture, burn, foreign body penetration). The skin becomes hot, reddened, swollen and painful.

Lymphangitis is an infection of the lymph channels or vessels. In lymphangitis, infection causes the lymph vessels to become inflamed. The abrupt onset of severe swelling is often a clinical indicator of worsening infection and increased risk for septicemia or sepsis. Reddened lines (streaks) may appear, running along the course of the lymphatic vessels in the affected area.

Key terms

Key terms found in the documentation may include:

- Finger:
  - Felon
  - Whitlow
- Nail:
  - Onychia
  - Perionychia
  - Paronychia

I-10 ALERT

ICD-10-CM classifies cellulitis (LØ3) and abscess (LØ2) in separate code categories based on whether the infection is encapsulated or contained (i.e., abscess, furuncle, carbuncle) or spread throughout the skin, subcutaneous tissues (cellulitis), and lymph channels (lymphangitis).

Infection of the lymph glands or nodes (LØ4) are classified separately.

CDI ALERT

Abscess and cellulitis are classified separately in ICD-10-CM by severity, anatomic site, and laterality. Ensure documentation is specific regarding extent of infection to avoid misrepresentation of severity.

Ensure documentation of site and laterality is thorough and specific to avoid reporting unspecified codes.

Code category LØ3 may indicate a severity progression of infection from localized to adjacent tissues that increases the risk for potentially fatal serious systemic infection (sepsis) from circulating pathogens.

Clinical Findings

Physical Examination

The infected anatomical location is examined and indicates erythema and tenderness. The skin is recorded as hot and red. The borders are described as either indistinct or sharply demarcated. In cases of lymphangitis the findings indicate that there is lymph node enlargement as well as the pain and tenderness.

Diagnostic Procedures and Services

- Laboratory
  - white blood count
  - wound cultures

Therapeutic Procedures and Services

- In some instances incision and drainage may be necessary.

Medication List

- Antibiotics
  - azithromycin
  - cephalexin (Keflex)
  - clarithromycin (Biaxin)
  - clindamycin
  - dicloxacillin
  - levofloxacin (Levaquin)
  - trimethoprim (Bactrim, Septra)
- Topical antibiotics

Clinician Note

Differentiate between cellulitis and lymphangitis accurately in the diagnosis. Document the specific anatomic site. For upper limb infections, the axilla is a separately identifiable anatomic site from the upper limb. For paired anatomic sites, specify laterality (right or left).

For example:

Acute lymphangitis of right axilla (LØ3.121)

Acute lymphangitis of right upper limb (LØ3.123)

⇨ I-10 ALERT

Category LØ3 Cellulitis and lymphangitis, includes valid codes that are four to six characters in length. The following axes of classification describe:

Fourth character:
- Anatomic site or region

Fifth character:
- Type of infection: abscess furuncle or carbuncle
- Anatomic site

Sixth character:
- Anatomic site specificity (further specification of site)
- Laterality

Clinician Documentation Checklist

Clinician documentation should indicate the following:

- Identify
  - infectious organism (e.g., bacterial, viral, etc.)
- Document site of cellulitis and acute lymphangitis
  - finger
    - — felon
    - — whitlow
    - — hangnail with lymphangitis of finger

   — infection of nail
   — onychia
   — paronychia
   — perionychia
- toe
   — hangnail with lymphangitis of toe
   — infection of nail
   — onychia
   — paronychia
   — perionychia
- Other parts of limb
   — axilla
   — upper limb
   — lower limb
   — unspecified part of limb
- face
- neck
- trunk
   — abdominal wall
   — back (any part except buttock)
   — chest wall
   — groin
   — perineum
   — umbilicus
   — buttock
   — unspecified part of trunk
- other sites
   — head (any part, except face)
      ♦ scalp
   — other site
- unspecified site

Cerebrovascular Infarction and Hemorrhage

Code Axes

Nontraumatic subarachnoid hemorrhage	I6Ø.- HCC
Nontraumatic intracerebral hemorrhage	I61.- HCC
Other and unspecified nontraumatic intracranial hemorrhage	I62.- HCC I62.Ø[Ø-3] HCC I62.1 HCC
Cerebral infarction due to thrombosis of precerebral arteries	I63.Ø- HCC QPP
Cerebral infarction due to embolism of precerebral arteries	I63.1- HCC QPP
Cerebral infarction due to unspecified occlusion or stenosis of precerebral arteries	I63.2- HCC QPP
Cerebral infarction due to thrombosis of cerebral arteries	I63.3- HCC QPP
Cerebral infarction due to embolism of cerebral arteries	I63.4- HCC QPP
Cerebral infarction due to unspecified occlusion or stenosis of cerebral arteries	I63.5- HCC QPP
Cerebral infarction due to cerebral venous thrombosis, nonpyogenic	I63.6 HCC QPP
Other and unspecified cerebral infarction	I63.8, I63.9 HCC QPP

Description of Condition

A cerebral vascular accident (CVA) is a sudden, focal interruption of the blood to the brain that results in neurologic deficit. Documentation for cerebrovascular accident must identify the type and artery involved:

Type	Location
Occlusion and stenosis Thrombosis Embolism	Precerebral arteries: right, left, or bilateral vertebral artery; basilar artery; right, left, or bilateral carotid artery
Occlusion and stenosis Thrombosis Embolism	Cerebral arteries: right, left, or bilateral middle artery; right, left, or bilateral anterior; right, left, or bilateral posterior artery; right, left, or bilateral cerebellar artery

CDI Alert

Cerebral amyloid angiopathy (CAA) (E85.4/I68.Ø) refers to protein amyloid deposits in the blood vessels of the brain that can cause the blood vessels to crack, allowing blood to leak out causing hemorrhagic strokes.

Nontraumatic subarachnoid hemorrhage (I6Ø.-)

The nontraumatic hemorrhages described in category I6Ø describe bleeding into the subarachnoid space, the area between the arachnoid membrane and the pia mater surrounding the brain. The codes specify where the bleeding is **from**, which includes the following locations:

- Anterior communicating artery
- Basilar artery
- Carotid siphon and bifurcation
- Middle cerebral artery
- Posterior communicating artery
- Vertebral artery
- Other intracranial arteries
- Unspecified intracranial artery

Key Terms

Key terms found in the documentation may include:

- Meningeal hemorrhage
- Ruptured cerebral aneurysm
- Ruptured (congenital) berry aneurysm
- Ruptured (congenital) cerebral aneurysm
- Rupture of cerebral arteriovenous malformation
- Subarachnoid hemorrhage (nontraumatic) from cerebral artery
- Subarachnoid hemorrhage (nontraumatic) from communicating artery

⇨ I-10 Alert

ICD-10-CM codes for these categories contain many subcategories representing laterality (where appropriate), specific site of infarction or hemorrhage, and type of disease process, such as thrombosis or embolism.

Nontraumatic intracerebral hemorrhage (I61.-)

An intracerebral hemorrhage involves bleeding inside the brain tissue, and may be caused by a number of conditions, such as hypertension, infections, tumors, blood clotting abnormalities, or arteriovenous malformations. For conditions in this category, the code description includes the terminology of a hemorrhage in a certain location, such as the following:

- Brain stem
- Cerebellum
- Hemisphere (cortical, subcortical, or unspecified)
- Intraventricular
- Multiple localized
- Other and unspecified

CDI Alert

Refer to CT and MRI reports to help clarify the site of the hemorrhage. Physician documentation must be consistent when reporting site, laterality and type of hemorrhage.

Key Terms

Key terms found in the documentation may include:

- Cerebral lobe hemorrhage (nontraumatic)
- Deep intracerebral hemorrhage (nontraumatic)
- Superficial intracerebral hemorrhage (nontraumatic)

Other and unspecified nontraumatic intracranial hemorrhage (I62.-)

Intracranial hemorrhages involve bleeding within the skull and subdural hemorrhages are a result of vein rupture in the subdural space between the dura and arachnoid mater. Conditions in this category are classified according to severity, with designations of acute, subacute, chronic, and unspecified subdural hemorrhages.

CDI ALERT

Refer to CT and MRI reports to help clarify the site of the infarction. Physician documentation must be consistent when reporting site, laterality, and type of infarction.

The mechanism of the hemorrhage is also included in the classification of these conditions. The following diagnoses are described in the cerebral infarction categories:

- Thrombosis
- Embolism
- Unspecified occlusion or stenosis

Cerebral infarction (I63.-)

When a blood vessel that supplies a part of the brain becomes blocked or leakage occurs outside the vessel walls, the condition is known as a cerebral infarction. The loss of blood supply results in tissue death of that area. Cerebral infarctions may be classified to the following locations:

Anterior cerebral artery (right, left, unspecified)
Basilar artery
Carotid artery (right, left, unspecified)
Cerebellar artery (right, left, unspecified)
Middle cerebral artery (right, left, unspecified)
Posterior cerebral artery (right, left, unspecified)
Vertebral artery (right, left, unspecified)
Other cerebral artery
Other precerebral artery

I-10 ALERT

There is no time limit restricting the reporting of sequelae (late effect) codes. Residual conditions may occur months or years following the causal condition. When a patient has had previous cerebral infarctions and presents with a current infarction, coders should refer to medical record documentation to determine if a sequela is the result of the current or previous infarction.

Clinical Tip

Impending or threatened CVA is only reported as a CVA when confirmed, otherwise only the symptoms are reported.

Symptoms that last for one hour or less do not often result in neurologic damage and are classified as transient ischemic attacks (TIA).

Prolonged reversible ischemic neurological deficit ((P)RIND) is a cerebral infarct that lasts between 24 and 72 hours.

Key Terms

Key terms found in the documentation may include:

Cerebral Infarction due to:
- Embolism
- Hemorrhagic
- Narrowing, obstructing
- Obstruction
- Occlusion and stenosis
- Postoperative
- Thrombosis
- Vasospasm

CVA due to:

- Embolism
- Hemorrhagic
- Narrowing, obstructing
- Obstruction
- Occlusion and stenosis
- Postoperative
- Thrombosis
- Vasospasm
- Stroke

Clinical Findings

Symptoms with abrupt onset vary and some reflect infarct or hemorrhage and origin (cerebral/precerebral) or area of brain involved. Stroke severity and progression are often assessed using the standardized scoring scale such as the National Institutes of Health Stroke Scale (NIHSS), Canadian Neurological Scale (CNS), or the Mathew Stroke Scale.

Physical Examination

History and review of systems may include:

- Confusion
- Weakness/paresis
- Hemiplegia/quadriplegia
- Hemisensory loss
- Gaze preference
- Neurological neglect
- Facial droop
- Photophobia
- Stiff neck/pain/chemical meningitis
- Papilledema
- Monocular/binocular blindness
- Blurred vision or visual field defects: homonymous hemianopia
- Eye movement abnormalities (diplopia or nystagmus)
- Anisocoria
- Hyperglycemia
- Dysphagia
- Dysarthria or difficulty understanding speech
- Vertigo
- Ataxia
- Aphasia
- Headache (worst headache of my life, thunderclap)
- Nausea/vomiting
- Syncope

⇨ I-10 ALERT

When patients admitted for symptomatic cerebral hemorrhage associated with known cerebral amyloid angiopathy, code I61.9 is assigned as the first-listed diagnosis, followed by the codes for the cerebral amyloid angiopathy E85.4 and I68.0. According to the *ICD-10-CM Official Guidelines for Coding and Reporting*: "When there are two or more interrelated conditions (such as diseases in the same ICD-10-CM chapter or manifestations characteristically associated with a certain disease) potentially meeting the definition of first listed diagnosis, either condition may be sequenced first, unless the circumstances of the admission, the therapy provided, the tabular list, or the alphabetic index indicate otherwise."

- New onset seizure
- Acute neurological deficit
- Altered loss of consciousness
- Cytotoxic cerebral edema: causes deterioration during the first 48–72 hours after onset
- Hydrocephalus
- Increased intracranial pressure
- Encephalopathy
- Coma/obtunded (GCS ≤ 8)
- Hypertension (systolic BP > 220 mm Hg)
- Fever (indication of neurological deterioration)
- Brain herniation/compression/midline shift
- Decorticate/decerebrate posturing

Diagnostic Procedures and Services

- Laboratory
  - CBC
  - platelet count (<100,000/µl)
  - prothrombin time test (PT)/partial thromboplastin time test (PTT)
  - fasting blood glucose
  - lipid profile
  - homocysteine
  - erythrocyte sedimentation rate (ESR)
  - other tests as warranted for specific dx workup
- Imaging
  - CT: after 24 hours ischemic infarct visible; initial neuroimaging
  - diffusion weighted MRI: follow-up to CT, especially when initial CT is negative
  - gradient echo MRI
  - angiography
  - carotid duplex ultrasonography
- Other
  - ECG
  - swallow study for dysphagia
  - lumbar puncture for subarachnoid hemorrhage (SaH)
  - transesophageal echocardiography to evaluate cardiac etiology

CDI ALERT

Review documentation carefully to determine whether the cerebral infarction patient had tPA administered in another facility, prior to this encounter. This is important information that affects the specific case, as well as general clinical research efforts.

Clinician Note

There is no time limit restricting the reporting of sequelae (late effect) codes.

Residual conditions may occur months or years following the causal condition. When a patient has had previous cerebral infarctions and presents with a current infarction, careful attention must be paid to medical record documentation to determine if a sequela is the result of the current or previous infaction.

Clinician Documentation Checklist

Clinician documentation should indicate the following:

- Time of symptom onset
- The symptoms and associated conditions
- How long the symptoms lasted
- History including medical and family history relevant to the encounter
- Type of stroke
  - thrombosis, embolism, other occlusion/stenosis
  - hemorrhagic including site of hemorrhage/infarct, including laterality and cause of hemorrhage (aneurysm, AVM, conversion, treatment)
- Neurology consult
- Procedures performed
  - CT
  - MRI
  - laboratory
  - cardiovascular screening
  - swallow testing
- Evaluation/therapy
  - physical therapy
  - occupational therapy
  - speech
  - nutrition
- Medications provided including tPA
- Discharge summary and discharge disposition

Description of Condition

Cerebral amyloid angiopathy (E85.4/I68.Ø)

Cerebral amyloid angiopathy (CAA) refers to protein amyloid deposits in the blood vessels of the brain that can cause the blood vessels to crack, allowing blood to leak out causing hemorrhagic strokes.

First Listed Diagnosis Note

Admit for symptomatic cerebral hemorrhage associated with known cerebral amyloid angiopathy: As reason for admission was cerebral hemorrhage, code I61.9 is assigned as the first listed diagnosis, followed by the codes for the cerebral amyloid angiopathy E85.4 and I68.Ø. According to Official Coding Guidelines: "When there are two or more interrelated conditions (such as diseases in the same ICD-10-CM chapter or manifestations characteristically associated with a certain disease) potentially meeting the definition of first listed diagnosis, either condition may be sequenced first, unless the circumstances of the admission, the therapy provided, the Tabular List, or the Alphabetic Index indicate otherwise."

Chemotherapy Administration

Code Axes

Injection and intravenous infusion chemotherapy and other highly complex drug or highly complex biologic agent administration	**96401–96417**
Intra-arterial chemotherapy and other highly complex drug or highly complex biologic agent administration	**96420–96425**
Other injection and infusion services	**96440–96542**

Description of Procedure

Chemotherapy is the parenteral administration of nonradionuclide antineoplastic drugs. These drugs can be administered by either injection or infusion. Careful documentation indicating the method of administration as well as the site of the administration (venous, arterial, intrathecal) is required. Documentation must also indicate the substance administered.

Clinical Tip

The following flow chart can be used to determine if the correct code is supported by the medical record documentation.

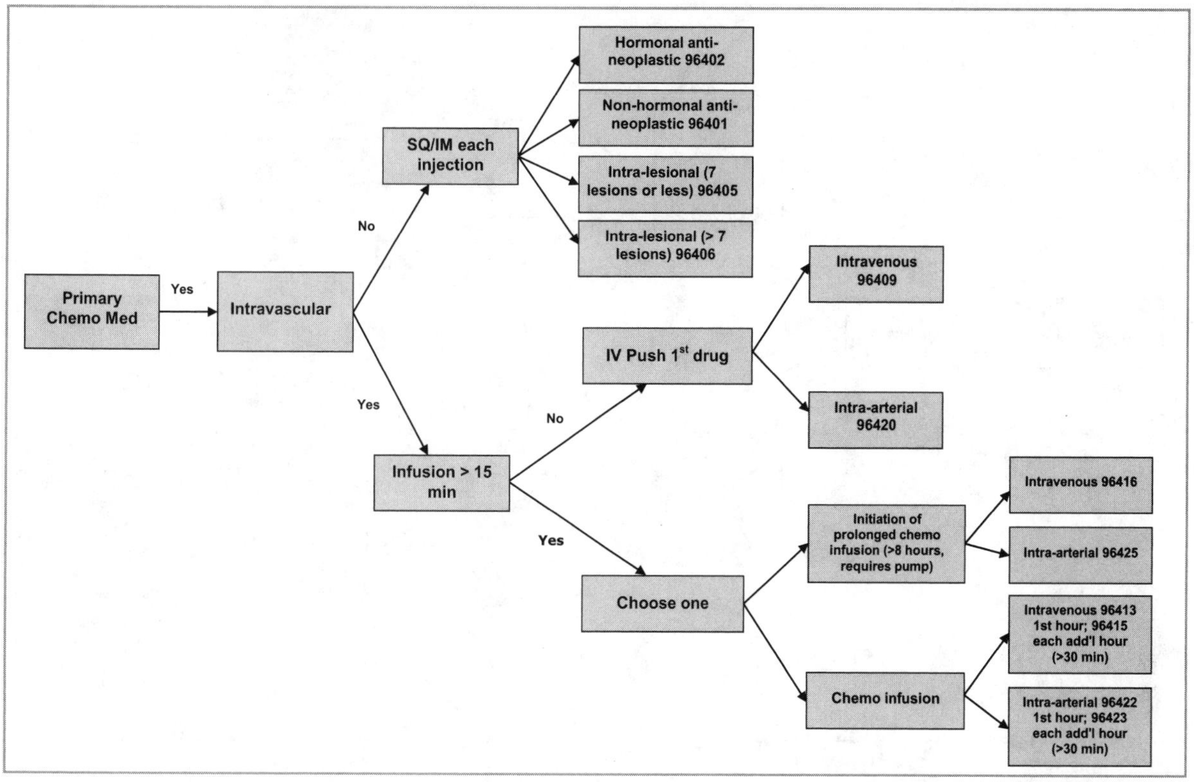
Primary Chemo Med
Yes
Intravascular
No
SQ/IM each injection
Hormonal anti-neoplastic 96402
Non-hormonal anti-neoplastic 96401
Intra-lesional (7 lesions or less) 96405
Intra-lesional (> 7 lesions) 96406
Yes
Infusion > 15 min
No
IV Push 1st drug
Intravenous 96409
Intra-arterial 96420
Yes
Choose one
Initiation of prolonged chemo infusion (>8 hours, requires pump)
Intravenous 96416
Intra-arterial 96425
Chemo infusion
Intravenous 96413 1st hour; 96415 each add'l hour (>30 min)
Intra-arterial 96422 1st hour; 96423 each add'l hour (>30 min)

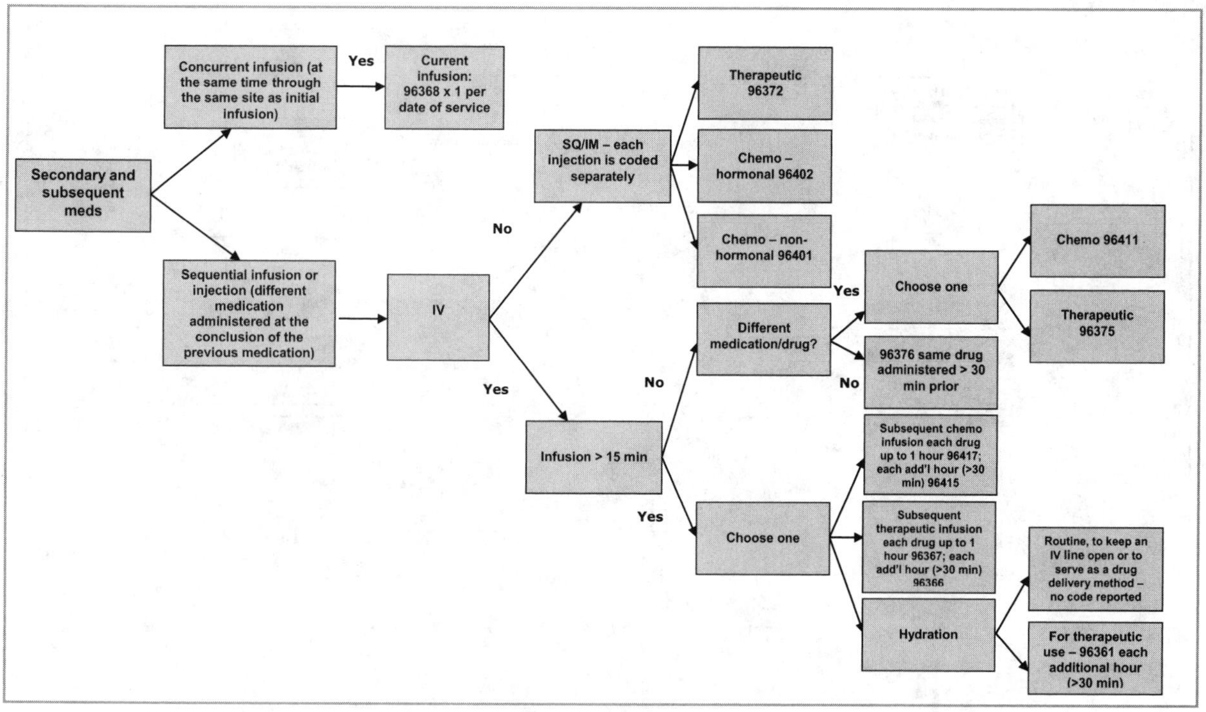
Secondary and subsequent meds
Concurrent infusion (at the same time through the same site as initial infusion)
Yes
Current infusion: 96368 x 1 per date of service
Sequential infusion or injection (different medication administered at the conclusion of the previous medication)
IV
No
SQ/IM – each injection is coded separately
Therapeutic 96372
Chemo – hormonal 96402
Chemo – non-hormonal 96401
Yes
Infusion > 15 min
No
Different medication/drug?
Yes
Choose one
Chemo 96411
Therapeutic 96375
No
96376 same drug administered > 30 min prior
Yes
Choose one
Subsequent chemo infusion each drug up to 1 hour 96417; each add'l hour (>30 min) 96415
Subsequent therapeutic infusion each drug up to 1 hour 96367; each add'l hour (>30 min) 96366
Hydration
Routine, to keep an IV line open or to serve as a drug delivery method – no code reported
For therapeutic use – 96361 each additional hour (>30 min)

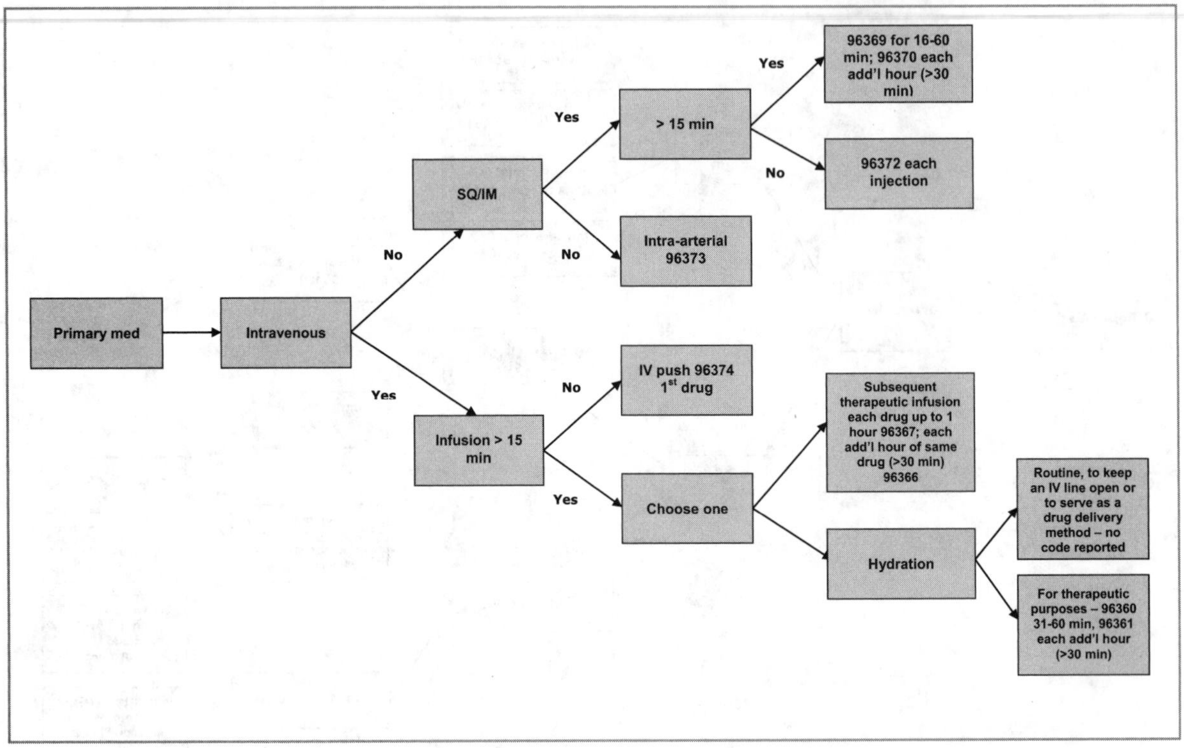
Primary med
Intravenous
No
SQ/IM
Yes
> 15 min
Yes
96369 for 16-60 min; 96370 each add'l hour (>30 min)
No
96372 each injection
No
Intra-arterial 96373
Yes
Infusion > 15 min
No
IV push 96374 1st drug
Yes
Choose one
Subsequent therapeutic infusion each drug up to 1 hour 96367; each add'l hour of same drug (>30 min) 96366
Hydration
Routine, to keep an IV line open or to serve as a drug delivery method – no code reported
For therapeutic purposes – 96360 31-60 min, 96361 each add'l hour (>30 min)

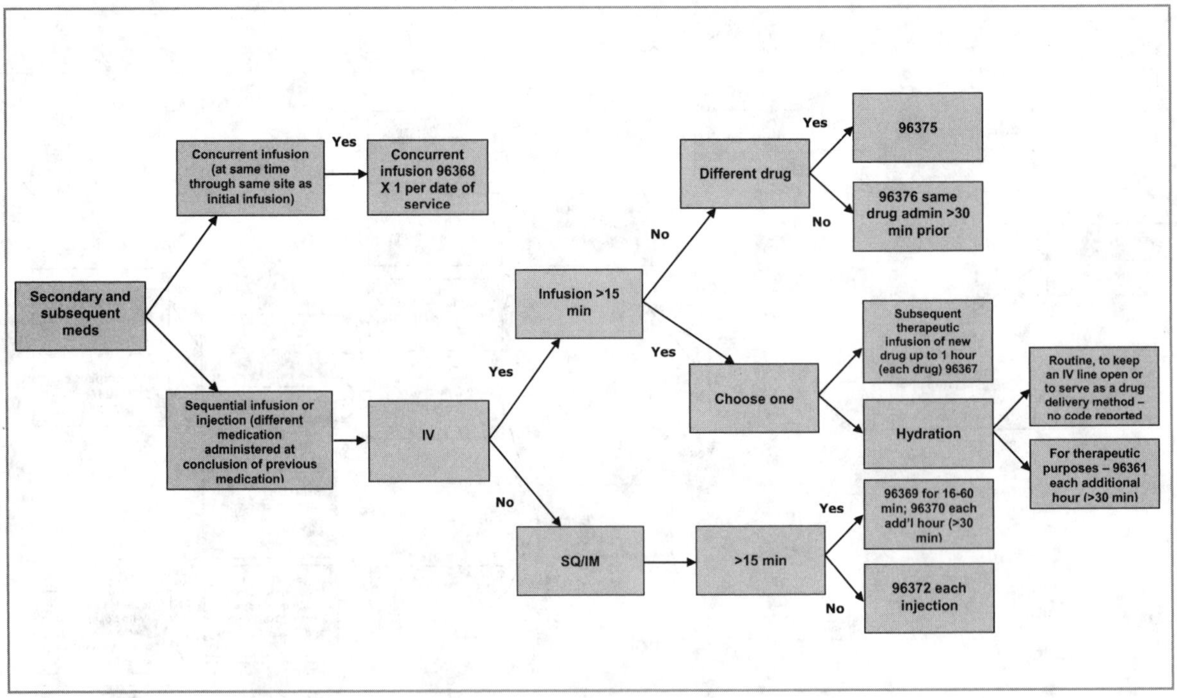
Secondary and subsequent meds
Concurrent infusion (at same time through same site as initial infusion)
Yes
Concurrent infusion 96368 X 1 per date of service
Sequential infusion or injection (different medication administered at conclusion of previous medication)
IV
Yes
Infusion >15 min
No
Different drug
Yes
96375
No
96376 same drug admin >30 min prior
Yes
Choose one
Subsequent therapeutic infusion of new drug up to 1 hour (each drug) 96367
Hydration
Routine, to keep an IV line open or to serve as a drug delivery method – no code reported
For therapeutic purposes – 96361 each additional hour (>30 min)
No
SQ/IM
>15 min
Yes
96369 for 16-60 min; 96370 each add'l hour (>30 min)
No
96372 each injection

Chemotherapy administration, subcutaneous or intramuscular (96401–96402)

Documentation will indicate that the physician or supervised assistant prepares and administers nonhormonal (96401) or hormonal (96402) medication to combat diseases such as malignant neoplasms or microorganisms. These codes apply to medication injected under the skin (subcutaneous) or into a muscle (intramuscular) often in the arm or leg.

Key Terms

Key terms found in the documentation may include:

IM (intra muscular)

Inj (injection)

Injection

Sq (subcutaneous)

SubQ (subcutaneous)

Clinician Note

Note any complications that occur during the service.

Chemotherapy administration; intravenous, push technique, single or initial substance/drug (96406)

Chemotherapy administration; intravenous, push technique, each additional substance/drug (List separately in addition to code for primary procedure) (96411)

The drug is administered through intravenous (IV) push technique in which the physician or supervised assistant is continuously present to administer the injection and observe the patient or for an infusion of less than 15 minutes.

Key Terms

Key terms found in the documentation may include:

IV

Push

Clinician Note

The medical record should include the disease being treated with the name and dosage of the drug being administered.

Chemotherapy administration, intra-arterial; push technique (96420)

Chemotherapy administration, intra-arterial; infusion technique, up to 1 hour (96422)

Chemotherapy administration, intra-arterial; infusion technique, each additional hour (list separately in addition to code for primary procedure) (96423)

Chemotherapy administration, intra-arterial; infusion technique, initiation of prolonged infusion (more than 8 hours), requiring the use of a portable or implantable pump (96245)

Documentation for these services must indicate that the infusion was intra-arterial. The medical record should identify the vessels used.

Key Terms

Key terms found in the documentation may include:

IA therapy

Clinician Note

The medical record should include the disease being treated with the name and dosage of the drug being administered.

Clinician Documentation Checklist

Clinician documentation should indicate the following:

- The disease being treated
- The treatment phase
  - induction
  - consolidation
  - maintenance
  - intensification
- Substance administered (drugs and dosage)
  - alkylating agents: mechlorethamine, chlorambucil, melphalan
  - antimetabolites: methotrexate, cytarabine
  - plant alkaloids: vincas, vinblastine, podophyllotoxins
  - antibiotics: doxorubicin, bleomycin, mitomycin
  - nitrosoureas: carmustine, lomustine
  - inorganic ions: cisplatin, carboplatin
  - biologic response modification: IFN
  - enzymes: asparaginase
  - hormones: tamoxifen, flutamide
  - high dose infusion interleukin 2

- aldesleukin
- interferon gamma
- antiemetics
  - indicate whether the medication administered is
    - initial/primary medication
    - subsequent or additional medication

- Route of administration
  - injection
  - infusion
  - IV push
- Site of administration
  - venous
  - arterial
  - intrathecal
  - subcutaneous/intramuscular
- Timing
  - concurrent infusion
  - subsequent infusion or injection
- Hydration
  - routine
  - therapeutic
- Administration time
  - start
  - stop
- Additional patient pathology
  - nausea and vomiting
  - dehydration
  - anemia
  - neutropenia
  - pancytopenia
  - fatigue
  - mood changes
  - orthostatic hypotension

Chronic Ischemic Heart Disease

I-10 ALERT

ICD-10-CM codes combine the clinical concepts of coronary atherosclerosis and several different forms of angina. A cause-and-effect relationship may be assumed when a patient has both coronary atherosclerosis and angina (Official Coding Guideline 1.C.9.b). An additional code for the angina is not necessary. Review documentation of angina carefully to ensure correct classification.

CDI ALERT

Refer to cardiac stress test reports, cardiac catheterization reports, and other cardiology results for documentation of coexisting angina. Physician documentation should be consistent throughout the record concerning which of these conditions existed at the time of the encounter.

Code Axes

Arteriosclerotic heart disease (ASHD)

ASHD of native coronary artery with and without angina pectoris	**I25.10–I25.119** HCC QPP
ASHD of coronary artery bypass graft(s) and coronary artery of transplanted heart with angina pectoris	**I25.700–I25.709** HCC QPP
ASHD of autologous vein coronary artery bypass graft(s) with angina pectoris	**I25.710–I25.719** HCC QPP
ASHD of autologous artery coronary artery bypass graft(s) with angina pectoris	**I25.720–I25.729** HCC QPP
ASHD of nonautologous biological coronary artery bypass graft(s) with angina pectoris	**I25.730–I25.739** HCC QPP
ASHD of native coronary artery of transplanted heart with angina pectoris	**I25.750–I25.759** HCC QPP
ASHD of bypass graft of coronary artery of transplanted heart with angina pectoris	**I25.760–I25.769** HCC QPP
ASHD of other coronary artery bypass graft(s) with angina pectoris	**I25.790–I25.799** HCC QPP
Other and unspecified forms of chronic ischemic heart disease	**I25.8–I25.9** HCC QPP

Clinical Tip

Many patients carry a diagnosis of chronic ischemic heart disease, or more specifically, of atherosclerotic heart disease. The key for correct classification in ICD-10-CM is determining the severity level and whether or not unstable or another form of angina is also present at the time of the encounter. The disease process is similar regardless of whether it is present in a native artery or a bypassed vessel; however, the risk and severity level is higher for bypassed vessels and, if the patient has had any bypass procedures, the status of these vessels should be clearly documented.

Key Terms

Key terms found in the documentation for coronary atherosclerosis may include:

- Atherosclerotic cardiovascular disease (ASCVD)
- Atherosclerotic heart disease (ASHD)
- Atherosclerotic heart disease with angina
- Atherosclerotic heart disease with ischemic chest pain
- Coronary (artery) atheroma
- Coronary (artery) atherosclerosis

Coronary (artery) disease (CAD)

Coronary (artery) sclerosis

Clinician Note

According to Medicare coverage guidelines, coronary artery disease with a documented prior MI, a measured left ventricular ejection fraction (LVEF) ≤ 0.35, and inducible, sustained VT or VF at EP study supports the medical necessity of an implanted cardiodefibrillator. The MI must have occurred more than 40 days prior to defibrillator insertion. The EP test must be performed more than 4 weeks after the qualifying MI.

Clinical Findings

Physical Examination

History and review of systems may include:

Patients may be asymptomatic. When present, signs and symptoms include stable exertional angina, intermittent claudication, symptoms of unstable angina or infarction, ischemic stroke, or rest pain in limbs. Palpation of extremity pulses is performed. Heart sounds are recorded and any bruits are noted.

Diagnostic Procedures and Services

- Laboratory
  - total cholesterol
  - HDL cholesterol
  - triglycerides
  - glucose
  - lipids
- Imaging
  - CT angiography
  - Ultrasonography
- Other
  - EKG
  - Doppler of extremities when decreased pulses or complaints of pain and cramping

Therapeutic Procedures and Services

Lifestyle changes including patient diet (low fat), desist tobacco use and to increase physical activity.

Medication List

- Statin use
- ACE inhibitors
- Beta blockers
- Antiplatelet drugs

Clinician Documentation Checklist

Clinician documentation should indicate the following:

- Other acute
  - acute coronary thrombosis without MI
  - Dressler's syndrome
  - other acute ischemic heart disease
  - unspecified acute ischemic heart disease
- Chronic
  - location
    - native vessels
    - bypass graft(s), unspecified
    - bypass graft(s), autologous vein
    - bypass graft(s), autologous artery
    - bypass graft(s), nonautologous biological
    - bypass graft(s) with transplanted heart
    - native vessels of transplanted heart
    - other bypass graft(s)
  - complications/symptoms
    - angina pectoris
    - unstable angina pectoris
    - documented spasm
    - other forms of angina pectoris
    - unspecified angina pectoris
  - types
    - total occlusion of coronary artery
    - due to lipid rich plaque
    - due to calcified coronary lesion
    - other ischemic heart disease
    - ischemic heart disease (chronic) NOS

Chronic Kidney Disease (CKD)

Code Axes

Chronic kidney disease, stage 1	**N18.1**
Chronic kidney disease, stage 2 (mild)	**N18.2**
Chronic kidney disease, stage 3 (moderate)	**N18.3**
Chronic kidney disease, stage 4 (severe)	**N18.4** HCC
Chronic kidney disease, stage 5	**N18.5** HCC
End stage renal disease	**N18.6** HCC
Chronic kidney disease, unspecified	**N18.9**

Description of Condition

CKD is long-standing, progressive loss of renal function. It usually develops gradually as a consequence of a wide variety of diseases such as primary and secondary glomerular disease, diabetes mellitus, hypertension, obstructive uropathy, chronic infection (pyelonephritis), interstitial nephritis, and/or congenital diseases such as polycystic kidney disease. When CKD reaches advanced stages, dangerous levels or electrolytes, fluid, and wastes can build up in the body.

Clinical Tip

CKD is defined as either kidney damage or glomerular filtration rate (GFR) < 60 mL/min/1.73 m^2 for ≥ 3 months. As kidney disease gets worse, the GFR number goes down.

Stages of Chronic Kidney Disease Defined by the National Kidney Foundation

Stage	Description	GFR, mL/min
At increased risk	Risk factors for kidney disease (e.g., diabetes, high blood pressure, family history, older age, ethnic group)	More than 90
1	Kidney damage with normal kidney function	90 or above
2	Kidney damage with mild loss of kidney function	89 to 60
3a	Mild to moderate loss of kidney function	59 to 44
3b	Moderate to severe loss of kidney function	44 to 30
4	Severe loss of kidney function	29 to 15
5	Kidney failure	Less than 15

Key Terms
Key terms found in the documentation may include:

- Chronic kidney disease
- CKD
- Glomerulopathy
- Glomerular filtration rate (GFR)
- Mild
- Moderate
- Nephropathy
- Renal insufficiency
- Severe
- Stage 1
- Stage 2
- Stage 3
- Stage 4
- Stage 5

CDI ALERT

If both a stage of CKD and ESRD are documented, assign code N18.6 for ESRD only.

End stage renal disease (N18.6)

Clinical Tip
End stage renal disease (ESRD) usually occurs when kidney function is less than 10 percent of normal, requiring chronic dialysis or kidney transplant.

Key Terms
Key terms found in the documentation may include:

- Chronic dialysis
- Complete loss of renal function
- End stage renal disease
- ESRD

Chronic kidney disease, unspecified (N18.9)

I-10 ALERT

Code associated diabetic chronic kidney disease or hypertensive chronic kidney disease first, before the code for the CKD.

Key Terms
Key terms found in the documentation may include:

- Chronic renal disease
- Chronic renal failure NOS
- Chronic renal insufficiency
- Chronic uremia

Clinical Tip
Patients with mild to moderate renal insufficiency may be asymptomatic even with an elevated BUN and creatinine.

Clinical Findings

Physical Examination

History and review of systems may include:

- Anorexia
- Changes in amount of urination
- Decreased mental awareness
- Diabetes mellitus
- Edema in feet and ankles
- Fatigue
- Hyperreflexia
- Hypertension
- Loss of appetite
- Muscle cramps
- Nausea
- Nocturia
- Persistent itching (pruritus)
- Restless leg syndrome
- Unpleasant taste in mouth
- Vomiting
- Weight loss

In advanced CKD, the following are common:

- GI ulceration and bleeding
- Hypertension
- Pericarditis

Diagnostic Procedures and Services

- Laboratory
  - albumin
  - BUN
  - CBC
  - calcium
  - creatinine
  - electrolytes
  - glomerular filtration rate
  - phosphate
  - urinary sediment
- Imaging
  - ultrasound
- Other
  - renal biopsy

Therapeutic Procedures and Services

- Possible dietary restriction of phosphate, potassium and sodium
- Vitamin D supplement
- Treatment of the underlying disorder(s)
  - anemia
  - diabetes mellitus
  - edema
  - hypertension
  - primary or secondary kidney disease
- Treatment of ESRD include:
  - creation of arteriovenous (AV) fistula
  - dialysis
    - hemodialysis
    - peritoneal dialysis
  - renal transplant

Medication List

There are no specific drugs to treat renal failure. Medications are used to treat the underlying disorder or disease manifestations as stated above.

Clinician Documentation Checklist

Clinician documentation should indicate the following:

- Identify any associated
  - Diabetic chronic kidney disease
  - Hypertensive chronic kidney disease
  - Kidney transplant status, if applicable
- Document stage of chronic kidney disease
  - Chronic kidney disease, stage 1
  - Chronic kidney disease, stage 2 (mild)
  - Chronic kidney disease, stage 3 (moderate)
  - Chronic kidney disease, stage 4 (severe)
  - Chronic kidney disease, stage 5
  - End stage renal disease
    - Chronic kidney disease requiring chronic dialysis
    - Specify dialysis status
  - Unspecified chronic kidney disease
    - Includes:
      - chronic renal disease
      - chronic renal failure
      - chronic renal insufficiency
      - chronic uremia
      - renal disease

Chronic Obstructive Pulmonary Disease (COPD)

Code Axes

Chronic obstructive pulmonary disease with acute lower respiratory infection — **J44.Ø** HCC QPP

Chronic obstructive pulmonary disease with (acute) exacerbation — **J44.1** HCC QPP

Chronic obstructive pulmonary disease, unspecified — **J44.9** HCC QPP

Clinical Tip

Chronic obstructive pulmonary disease is an umbrella term that contains other conditions, but there are two primary types of COPD: one involves chronic bronchitis, which is usually manifested with a chronic cough and mucous production. The other type of COPD is emphysema (discussed above), which involves lung destruction over time.

Key Terms

Key terms found in the documentation may include:

Asthma with chronic obstructive pulmonary disease
Chronic airflow limitation
Chronic asthmatic (obstructive) bronchitis
Chronic bronchitis with emphysema
Chronic emphysematous bronchitis
Chronic obstructive airway disease
Chronic obstructive asthma
Chronic obstructive bronchitis
Chronic obstructive lung disease
Chronic obstructive respiratory disease
Chronic obstructive tracheobronchitis
COPD

⇨ I-10 Alert

Ensure that the underlying infection is documented appropriately; an additional code is necessary for proper classification.

Description of Condition

Chronic obstructive pulmonary disease with acute lower respiratory infection (J44.Ø)

Clinical Tip

An acute exacerbation of COPD is not the same thing as a superimposed infection, although the exacerbation may be triggered by the infection. Ensure that documentation is clear concerning the infectious process.

Chronic obstructive pulmonary disease with (acute) exacerbation (J44.1)

⇨ I-10 Alert

If the COPD exacerbation is in the setting of an acute bronchitis, the Excludes 2 note under J44.1 indicates both J44.Ø and J44.1 may be reported together when appropriate.

Clinical Tip

An acute exacerbation of COPD is defined as a decompensation of the disease, with increased symptoms such as wheezing and shortness of breath. Treatment typically consists of easing symptoms and returning the patient to their baseline respiratory status.

Key Terms

Key terms found in the documentation may include:

Decompensated COPD

Decompensated COPD with acute exacerbation

Clinical Findings

Physical Examination

Indicators include dyspnea, poor exercise tolerance, chronic cough with or without sputum, wheezing, decreased breath sounds, respiratory failure, or cor pulmonale. A diagnosis is confirmed when the patient has symptoms of COPD and has a postbronchodilator FEV1/FVC ratio of less than 0.70.

Diagnostic Procedures and Services

- Imaging
  - chest x-ray
  - chest CT
- Other
  - spirometry
  - pulse oximetry

Therapeutic Procedures and Services

Treatment depends upon the severity and may include:

- Nebulizer
- Oxygen

Medication List

- Antibiotics
- Bronchodilator
  - aclidinium (Tudorza)
  - arformoterol (Brovana)
  - formoterol (Foradil, Perforomist)
  - indacaterol (Arcapta)
  - salmeterol (Serevent)
  - tiotropium (Spiriva)
  - short-acting beta agonists
    - albuterol (Proventil, Ventolin)
    - ipratropium (Atrovent)
    - levalbuterol (Xopenex)

- theophylline (Theo-24, Uniphyl)
- Inhaler
  - beclomethasone (QVAR)
  - fluticasone (Flovent)
- Leukotriene modifiers
  - montelukast (Singulair)
- Combination inhalers: Corticosteroids and long-acting beta agonists
  - budesonide and formoterol (Symbicort)
  - fluticasone and salmeterol (Advair Diskus)
  - fluticasone and vilanterol (Breo Ellipta)
  - mometasone and formoterol (Dulera)

Clinician Documentation Checklist

Clinician documentation should indicate the following:

- Identification of
  - exposure to environmental tobacco smoke
  - history of tobacco use
  - occupational exposure to environmental tobacco smoke
  - tobacco dependence
  - tobacco use
- Includes
  - asthma with chronic obstructive pulmonary disease
  - chronic asthmatic (obstructive) bronchitis
  - chronic emphysematous bronchitis
  - chronic bronchitis
    - with airway obstruction
    - with emphysema
  - chronic obstructive
    - asthma
    - bronchitis
    - tracheobronchitis
  - identify type of asthma
- Type of COPD
  - COPD with acute lower respiratory infection
    - identify the infection
  - COPD with (acute) exacerbation
    - decompensated COPD
    - decompensated COPD with (acute) exacerbation
  - unspecified
    - chronic obstructive airway disease
    - chronic obstructive lung disease

Chronic Pain

Code Axes

Chronic pain, not elsewhere classified	**G89.2-**
Neoplasm related pain (acute)(chronic)	**G89.3**
Chronic pain syndrome	**G89.4**

Description of Condition

Chronic pain is pain that persists for months or even years, persists longer than one month after resolution of an acute injury, or is associated with a nonhealing lesion. Common causes include low back injury, cancer, arthritis, nerve damage, serious infection, and diabetes.

Clinical Tip

Some patients suffer chronic pain in the absence of any past injury or disease, in these cases the cause of pain is less obvious and may be referred to as psychogenic pain. Chronic pain may also lead to or intensify psychologic issues such as depression. Differentiating psychologic cause from effect is often difficult. Even if a significant psychologic contribution to the pain is probable, a physical cause should always be sought.

Chronic pain due to trauma (G89.21)

Chronic post-thoracotomy pain (G89.22)

Other chronic and chronic post procedural pain (G89.28, G89.29)

These diagnoses are reported for pain that is not classified elsewhere and pain not associated with a documented disease process. Pain conditions in these categories are due to trauma, post-thoracotomy, or postprocedural are typically more severe and more intractable than would normally be expected.

Key Terms

Severe/intractable postoperative pain

⇨ I-10 ALERT

Normal or expected levels of pain following trauma or surgery should not be reported with codes in this category.

Neoplasm related pain (acute) (chronic) (G89.3)

Key Terms

- Cancer associated pain
- Tumor associated pain
- Pain due to malignancy

Documentation Tip

If pain is documented as being associated, related, or due to cancer or tumor, code G89.3 should be assigned regardless of whether the pain is acute or chronic. If the primary reason for the encounter is documented as pain management, G89.3 may be assigned as the principal diagnosis and the underlying neoplasm would be reported as an additional diagnosis.

Chronic pain syndrome (G89.4)

Documentation Tip

The clinician must specifically document chronic pain syndrome in order to report G89.4.

Clinical Tip

The effect of pain on the patient's life should be evaluated; evaluation by an occupational therapist may be necessary. Formal psychiatric evaluation should be considered if a coexisting psychiatric disorder (e.g., major depression) is suspected as cause or effect.

Documentation Tip

If pain is documented but not specified as acute or chronic, postprocedural, or neoplasm related; or if a definitive diagnosis is established, unless the encounter is for pain management, a code from category G89 should not be reported.

⇨ I-10 ALERT

Category G89 codes may be listed as principal diagnosis when pain management is the reason for the encounter.

Clinical Findings

Physical Examination

History and review of systems should include the location of the pain, duration of the pain, the severity of the pain, pain triggers, treatments that have alleviated the pain, past traumas, surgical procedures, or malignancies. The history may also include a detailed review of:

- Gastrointestinal system
- Musculoskeletal system
- Neuropsychological systems
- Psychosocial history
- Reproductive system
- Urologic system

Diagnostic Procedures and Services

Blood tests, urinalysis, MRI, CT scan and other diagnostic work-up may be necessary to rule out or confirm a suspected disease or disorder.

Therapeutic Procedures and Services

Nonsurgical treatment may include:

- Behavioral modifications
- Biofeedback therapy
- Local electrical stimulation
- Nerve blocks

- Physical therapy
- Psychotherapy

Surgical treatment may include:

- Implantation of spinal cord stimulators
- Insertion of morphine pumps

Clinician Note

There is no time frame that identifies when pain can be defined as chronic. It is solely at the physician's discretion to determine whether pain is chronic. Code assignment is based on the physician's documentation.

Clinician Documentation Checklist

Clinician documentation should indicate the following:

- Identify previous treatment modalities
- Identify related psychological factors associated with pain
- Type of pain
  - acute pain
  - central pain syndrome
  - chronic pain
    - due to trauma
    - postoperative pain
    - post-thoracotomy pain
  - neoplasm related pain (acute)(chronic)
    - cancer associated pain
    - pain due to malignancy
    - tumor associated pain

Colectomies and Enterectomies

Code Axes

Enterectomy, resection of small intestine	**44120–44128** QPP
Colectomy, partial	**44140–44147, 44160** QPP
Colectomy, total, abdominal, without proctectomy	**44150–44151**
Colectomy, total, abdominal, with proctectomy	**44155–44158**

Description of Procedure

An enterectomy is the removal of a portion of the small bowel. A colectomy is the removal of a portion of the large bowel. Careful documentation indicating the anatomical site and the amount of intestine removed is critical for correct code assignment.

These services can be performed as treatment for both diseases and congenital abnormalities. Additionally, it may be necessary to remove multiple segments and to anastomose the intestine multiple times.

Enterectomy, resection of small intestine; single resection and anastomosis (44120)

Enterectomy, resection of small intestine; each additional resection and anastomosis (List separately in addition to code for primary procedure) (44121)

Clinical Tip

These procedures are commonly performed for the following conditions and when documented, will support the medical necessity of the service:

- A blockage in the intestine caused by scar tissue or congenital (from birth) deformities.
- Bleeding, infection, or ulcers caused by inflammation of the small intestine. Three conditions that may cause inflammation are regional ileitis, regional enteritis, and Crohn's disease.
- Cancer
- Carcinoid tumor
- Injuries to the small intestine
- Meckel's diverticulum
- Noncancerous (benign) tumors
- Precancerous polyps (nodes)

Key Terms

Key terms found in the documentation may include:

Anastomosis

Resection

CPT ALERT

When significant additional time and effort is documented, it is appropriate to append modifier 22 and submit a cover letter along with the operative report.

Colectomy, partial (44140–44147)

Codes within this range represent the removal of a segment of the large bowel. They are differentiated by other procedures that may be performed during the same surgical session or the anatomical approach.

Key Terms

Key terms found in the documentation may include:

Cecostomy

Coloproctostomy

Colostomy

Ileostomy

Clinician Documentation Checklist

Clinician documentation should indicate the following:

- The disease or condition being treated
- Procedure
  - enterectomy
    - resection–single
    - resection–multiple
    - anastomosis
    - enterostomy
  - colectomy
    - resection–single
    - resection–multiple
    - anastomosis
    - colostomy
    - ileostomy
    - loop ileostomy
    - coloprotostomy
    - rectal mucosectomy

Coma

Code Axes

Unspecified coma	**R40.20** HCC
Coma scale, eyes open	**R40.21-** HCC
Coma scale, best verbal response	**R40.22-** HCC
Coma scale, best motor response	**R40.23-** HCC
Glasgow coma scale, total score	**R40.24-** HCC

Clinical Tip

In table format, the Glasgow coma scale appears as below:

Criteria Type & Points	1	2	3	4	5	6
Eyes Open	Never	To pain	To sound	Spontaneous	N/A	N/A
Best Verbal Response	None	Incompre-hensible words	Inappropriate words	Confused conversation	Oriented; converses normally	N/A
Best Motor Response	None	Extension to painful stimuli	Abnormal flexion to painful stimuli	Flexion withdrawal from painful stimuli	Localizes painful stimuli	Obeys com-mands

Generally, brain injury is classified according to the Glasgow coma scale (GCS) score:

- Severe, with GCS < 9
- Moderate, GCS 9–12
- Minor, GCS ≥ 13

Clinical Tip

In order to produce a valid score, one value (and code) from each subcategory (R40.21-, R40.22-, R40.23-) should be assigned. A seventh character designating when the scores were taken (e.g., in the field (EMT), at the hospital ED, at the time of hospital admission) should be assigned to each of the component Glasgow coma scale (GCS) score codes; all three should match. If only the GCS total score is documented in the medical record, a code from subcategory R40.24- may be assigned.

The GCS score codes should be reported in conjunction with traumatic brain injury (TBI) codes, or acute cerebrovascular disease or sequelae of cerebrovascular disease codes. They should never be sequenced as principal or first-listed diagnoses.

⇨ I-10 Alert

The ICD-10-CM classification for coma is vastly improved and expanded. The classification is based on the Glasgow coma scale, which provides a neurologically objective way to measure the conscious state of a person for an initial as well as a subsequent assessment. A patient is assessed against the criteria of the scale and the resulting points provide a patient score between 3 (indicating deep unconsciousness) and 15 (fully awake).

CDI Alert

The detail of the Glasgow coma scale score may be found in emergency department or trauma records. In some facilities, the ICU will track GCS over time.

Key Terms

Key terms found in the documentation for coma may include:

Comatose

Unconsciousness NOS

⇨ I-10 ALERT

New guidelines in 2017 allow the coma scale to be used to evaluate the status of the central nervous system for other nontrauma conditions, including monitoring patients in the intensive care unit regardless of medical condition. In these circumstances the coma scale code will be sequenced after the diagnosis code.

Clinical Findings

Physical Examination

History and review of systems may include:

- Neurological examination
  - decreased consciousness
  - stimuli to arouse a patient that is briefly or not at all
  - eye abnormality including dilation, pinpoint or unequal (One or both pupils may be fixed in midposition.)
  - confusion or inappropriate responses
  - limited or no response to pain
- Respiratory
  - possible abnormal breathing patterns including Cheyne-Stokes or Biot's respirations
- Cardiac
  - tachycardia
  - cardiac arrest
  - hypotension
- Other
  - nausea
  - vomiting
  - ataxia

Therapeutic Procedures and Services

- Immediate stabilization of airway and circulation
- Supportive measures including control of intracranial pressure (ICP)
- Treatment of underlying conditions

Clinician Note

Coordination of benefits is often required for payment from third-party payers so the documentation should indicate how the injury occurred (e.g., auto accident, fall from ladder at work, fall when riding a bike).

Clinician Documentation Checklist

Clinician documentation should indicate the following:

- Coma Scale
  - Coma Scale Eyes Open
    - — never
    - — to pain

- — to sound
- — spontaneous
- Coma Scale Best Verbal Response
  - — none
  - — incomprehensible words
  - — inappropriate words
  - — confused conversation
  - — oriented
- Coma Scale Best Motor Response
  - — none
  - — extension to pain
  - — abnormal flexion
  - — flexion withdrawal
  - — localizes pain
  - — obeys commands
- Glasgow Coma Scale Score
  - — specify the actual number of the score
- persistent vegetative state
- transient alteration of awareness

Congenital Malformations of Great Arteries

Code Axes

Patent ductus arterious	Q25.Ø
Coarctation of aorta	Q25.1
Atresia of aorta	Q25.2-
Supravalvular aortic stenosis	Q25.3
Other congenital malformation of aorta	Q25.4-
Atresia of pulmonary artery	Q25.5
Stenosis of pulmonary artery	Q25.6
Other congenital malformation of pulmonary artery	Q25.7-
Other congenital malformation of other great arteries	Q25.8
Congenital malformation of great arteries, unspecified	Q25.9

Description of Condition

Coarctation of aorta (Q25.1)

This condition is the narrowing of the aortic lumen resulting in upper extremity hypertension, left ventricular hypertrophy, and malperfusion of the abdominal organs and lower extremities.

Key Terms

Key terms found in the documentation may include:

Coarctation of aorta

Clinical Findings

Physical Examination

History and review of systems may include:

- Headache
- Chest pain
- Fatigue
- Intracranial hemorrhage

Diagnostic Procedures and Services

- Imaging
  - echocardiogram
  - chest x-ray

  - chest CT
  - chest MRI
  - cardiac catheterization
- Other
  - electrocardiogram
  - extremity blood pressure measurements

Therapeutic Procedures and Services

- Surgical repair

Clinician Documentation Checklist

Clinician documentation should indicate the following:

- Aorta
  - patent ductus arteriosus
    - — patent ductus botalli
    - — persistent ductus arteriosus
  - coarctation of aorta
    - — preductal
    - — postductal
  - supravalvular aortic stenosis
    - — absence of aorta
    - — aneurysm of sinus of Valsalva (ruptured)
    - — aplasia of aorta
    - — congenital aneurysm of aorta
    - — congenital malformation of aorta
    - — congenital dilatation of aorta
    - — double aortic arch (vascular ring of aorta)
    - — hypoplasia of aorta
    - — persistent convolutions of aortic arch
    - — persistent right aortic arch
- Pulmonary artery
  - atresia
  - stenosis
    - — supravalvular
  - coarctation
  - arteriovenous malformation
    - — arteriovenous aneurysm
  - other
    - — aberrant
    - — agenesis
    - — aneurysm
    - — anomaly
    - — hypoplasia

- Other congenital malformation of other great arteries
- Unspecified congenital malformation of great arteries

Great Veins

- Vena cava
  - stenosis (inferior) (superior)
  - persistent left superior vena cava
- Pulmonary
  - total anomalous pulmonary venous connection (TAPVR)
    - subdiaphragmatic
    - supradiaphragmatic
  - partial anomalous pulmonary venous connection (venous return)
  - unspecified
- Portal
  - anomalous portal venous connection
  - portal vein-hepatic artery fistula
- Other congenital malformations of great veins
  - absence of vena cava (inferior) (superior)
  - azygos continuation of inferior vena cava
  - persistent left posterior cardinal vein
  - scimitar syndrome
- Unspecified

Coumadin Toxicity

Code Axes

Poisoning, adverse effect of and underdosing of anticoagulants	**T45.51**
Poisoning by anticoagulants, accidental (unintentional)	**T45.511**
Poisoning by anticoagulants, intentional self-harm	**T45.512**
Poisoning by anticoagulants, assault	**T45.513**
Poisoning by anticoagulants, undetermined	**T45.514**
Adverse effect of anticoagulants	**T45.515**
Underdosing of anticoagulants	**T45.516**

Clinician Note
Laboratory studies to evaluate the patient's anticoagulation status are necessary for treatment and monitoring and, therefore, it is necessary to document this therapeutic treatment. Documentation should also indicate any adverse effects when present.

I-10 ALERT

ICD-10-CM has combined several different components of poisoning classifications, and has sequenced the poisoning, adverse effect, and new underdosing codes together in subcategories for each type of drug. No additional external cause code is required. The type of encounter is also classified in these codes, whether initial or subsequent encounter, or sequela.

Poisoning by anticoagulants, [all types] (T45.511–T45.514)

Clinical Tip
Although most poisonings are accidental, other examples of poisonings include errors in drug prescriptions and intentional overdoses of drugs. In addition, it is important to note that even if the drug in question was taken correctly, if it was taken in combination with another properly prescribed and administered drug, the resulting effect is classified as a poisoning. The same concept applies if the drug was taken in combination with alcohol; the resulting affect is a poisoning.

Clinician Note
Ensure that all other conditions are appropriately coded, such as specific drug reactions or complications of poisonings and adverse effects.

CDI ALERT

The documentation must clearly indicate the type of drug reaction, whether it was an adverse reaction, a poisoning, or an underdosing. If the issue involved a poisoning, the intent (e.g., accidental, self-harm, etc.) should also be documented in the medical record. It is important to determine what is meant by documentation indicating a drug "toxicity," because it could mean either a poisoning or an adverse effect.

Adverse effect of anticoagulants (T45.515)

Clinical Tip
An adverse effect of a drug is defined as an unintended consequence of a drug ingestion that was correctly prescribed and properly administered. It is important to note that the code representing the specific adverse effect (tachycardia, nausea and vomiting, etc.) should be reported first, followed by the adverse effect code.

Clinician Note
Ensure that all other conditions are appropriately coded, such as specific drug reactions or complications of poisonings and adverse effects.

Clinical Tip
An anticoagulant prevents blood from clotting; therefore, bleeding is a common adverse effect. When coagulopathy causing bleeding is due to anticoagulant therapy that is properly prescribed and administered, the nature of the adverse effect (manifestation) is reported first, followed by the code T45.515 with the appropriate seventh character to identify anticoagulation medication.

A prolonged PT/PTT or elevated INR is an expected result of anticoagulation therapy. This increases the risk for bleeding; when this level is excessive, requires treatment to lower or extends care, but has no overt bleeding condition, this is reported with R79.1 as the adverse effect manifestation, followed by T45.515 with the appropriate seventh character.

First Listed Diagnosis Note

Admit to reverse anticoagulation prior to a procedure: The reason/condition for the procedure is the first listed diagnosis, followed by Z51.81 for drug monitoring, Z79.Ø1 for long-term anticoagulant use and the code for the condition under treatment/prophylaxis by the medication.

Admit due to skin necrosis due to anticoagulation therapy: Gangrene I96 will be the first listed diagnosis as the nature of the adverse effect (manifestation) followed by T45.515 with the appropriate seventh character.

Underdosing of anticoagulants (T45.516)

CDI ALERT

Although it may appear counterintuitive to have an underdosing circumstance classified together with drug poisonings and adverse effects, the circumstances surrounding any encounter involving either prescribed or over the counter drugs must be documented clearly. Ensure that clinicians are aware that this classification axis is now available.

Clinical Tip
Underdosing is a new concept in ICD-10-CM and is defined as a circumstance in which a patient has taken less of a medication than is prescribed by a provider or a manufacturer's instruction. Taking less of a drug than prescribed can cause breakthrough symptoms of the underlying condition or may cause other problems. The clinical effects of underdosing of a drug should be classified separately.

Clinician Note
Ensure that all other conditions are appropriately coded, such as specific drug reactions or complications of poisonings, adverse effects, and underdosings.

Clinical Findings

Physical Examination

History and review of systems may include:

- Ecchymoses
- Subconjunctival hemorrhage
- Epistaxis
- Vaginal bleeding
- Bleeding gums
- Hematuria

Diagnostic Procedures and Services

- Laboratory
  - prothrombin elevated

Therapeutic Procedures and Services

- Blood transfusion may be necessary (packed red cells)
- Medication
  - vitamin K

Clinician Documentation Checklist

Clinician documentation should indicate the following:

- Identify the medical condition being treated
- Adverse effect was a result of
  - accidental poisoning
  - intentional self-harm
  - assault
  - undetermined
  - under dosing

Critical Care Services

Code Axes

Critical Care **99291–99292** OPP

Description of Procedure

These services are rendered for the care of a patient who has an illness or injury to one or more vital organ systems such that there is the high probability of imminent or life-threatening deterioration to the patient's condition. These services are based upon the time spent involved in activities directly related to the patient's care and need not be strictly spent at the bedside but rather on a patient's floor or unit.

Critical care, evaluation and management of the critically ill or critically injured patient (99291–99292)

Documentation Tip

The clinician documentation must indicate the time spent providing the critical care services, the procedures and services performed, and the nature of the condition requiring the service. Note that there are a number of procedures bundled into critical care services and, therefore, not separately reported. See the CPT® book or payer guidelines for a list of these services.

Clinician Documentation Checklist

Clinician documentation should indicate the following:

- Identify illness or injury reason for encounter
- Type of vital organ failure
  - central nervous system failure
  - circulatory failure
  - shock
  - renal
  - hepatic
  - metabolic
  - respiratory
- Start/stop time spent providing critical care services
- Procedures performed

Crohn's Disease

Code Axes

Note: Sixth characters for subcategories K5Ø.Ø1, K5Ø.11, K5Ø.81, and K5Ø.91 include that for rectal bleeding, intestinal obstruction, fistula, abscess, and other and unspecified complications.

Crohn's disease of small intestine without complications	**K5Ø.ØØ** HCC
Crohn's disease of small intestine with complications	**K5Ø.Ø1-** HCC
Crohn's disease of large intestine without complications	**K5Ø.1Ø** HCC
Crohn's disease of large intestine with complications	**K5Ø.11-** HCC
Crohn's disease of both small and large intestine without complications	**K5Ø.8Ø** HCC
Crohn's disease of both small and large intestine with complications	**K5Ø.81-** HCC
Crohn's disease, unspecified, without complications	**K5Ø.9Ø** HCC
Crohn's disease, unspecified, with complications	**K5Ø.91-** HCC

Clinical Tip

Crohn's disease is similar to other inflammatory bowel diseases including irritable bowel syndrome and ulcerative colitis and is usually differentiated by location and severity. While Crohn's disease can affect the mucus membranes of the digestive tract from the mouth to the anus, it most commonly affects the ileum (small bowel) and the cecum. Ulcerative colitis primarily affects the large bowel. Additionally, some experts use the following three endoscopic findings as evidence of Crohn's:

Aphthous ulcers: Small, discrete aphthous ulcers (canker sores) appear in the early stages of the disease and progress to involve the entire wall of the bowel; may grow to several centimeters.

Cobblestoning: Normal tissues in between the ulcers indicate the typical cobblestone appearance.

Discontinuous lesions: Areas of inflammation are scattered between normal bowel "skip areas."

Ulcerative colitis and Crohn's disease are very similar. The table below describes some of the differences.

Ulcerative Colitis	Crohn's Disease
Limited to colon	Entire GI tract (mouth to anus)
Continuous inflammation	Inflammation with intermittent inflammation
Inner most lining	All layers within bowel walls

I-10 ALERT

Combination codes include information related not only to site of the disease, but to specific complication.

CDI ALERT

Ensure that if any of the following complications are present, they are clearly documented in the medical record: rectal bleeding, intestinal obstruction, fistula, or abscess. Any other complications that are indicated as being due to Crohn's disease should also be documented.

Key Terms

Key terms found in the documentation may include:

CD

Crohn's disease

Crohn's disease of colon, large bowel, or rectum

Granulomatous colitis

Regional enteritis

Regional ileitis or colitis

Terminal ileitis

Clinical Findings

Physical Examination

- Check for bowel sounds
- Abdominal palpation for pain, tenderness, and distention

Diagnostic Procedures and Services

- Laboratory
  - stool guaiac: positive if active bleeding
  - CBC: may indicate blood loss anemia or elevated WBCs
  - pathology examination of tissue biopsies characterized by transmural (full-thickness) inflammation
- Imaging
  - colonoscopy
  - EGD
  - ERCP
  - small bowel endoscopy
  - upper GI series
  - barium enema

Therapeutic Procedures and Services

- Dietary restrictions
- Surgical intervention

Medication List

- Adalimumab (Humira)
- Antibiotics in instances of fulminant disease or abscess
  - ciprofloxacin (in cases of present fistulas) (Cipro)
  - metronidazole
- Antispasmodics
  - hyoscyamine (Anaspaz, Levsin)
- 5-ASA
  - balsalazide (Colazal, Giazo)
  - mesalamine (Asacol, Delzicol)
  - olsalazine (Dipentum)

  - sulfasalazine (Azulfidine, Sulfazine)
- Corticosteroids for acute flare-ups
  - budesonide (Entocort EC)
  - hydrocortisone
  - prednisone
- Infliximab (Remicade)
- Loperamide (Diamide, Imodium A-D)
- Methotrexate (Otrexup)
- Metronidazole (Flagyl)

Clinician Note

Fistulas and abscesses are common complications of Crohn's disease. Carefully review clinical documentation and, if present, assign the appropriate code from category K5Ø as well as the appropriate code indicating the specific type of fistula/abscess.

Clinician Documentation Checklist

Clinician documentation should indicate the following:

- Includes
  - granulomatous enteritis
- Identify
  - manifestations such as pyoderma gangrenosum
  - part of intestinal tract involved
    - small intestine
      - Crohn's disease of duodenum
      - Crohn's disease of ileum
      - Crohn's disease of jejunum
      - regional ileitis
      - terminal ileitis
    - large intestine
      - Crohn's disease of colon
      - Crohn's disease of large bowel
      - Crohn's disease of rectum
      - granulomatous colitis
      - regional colitis
    - both small and large intestine
    - unspecified part
      - Crohn's disease
      - regional enteritis
  - associated
    - without complications

- with complications
  - rectal bleeding
  - intestinal obstruction
  - fistula
  - abscess
  - other complication
  - unspecified complications

Cutaneous Abscess, Furuncle, and Carbuncle

Code Axes

Cutaneous abscess, furuncle and carbuncle of face	**LØ2.Ø-**
Cutaneous abscess, furuncle and carbuncle of neck	**LØ2.1-**
Cutaneous abscess, furuncle and carbuncle of trunk	**LØ2.2-**
Cutaneous abscess, furuncle and carbuncle of buttock	**LØ2.3-**
Cutaneous abscess, furuncle and carbuncle of limb	**LØ2.4-**
Cutaneous abscess, furuncle and carbuncle of hand	**LØ2.5-**
Cutaneous abscess, furuncle and carbuncle of foot	**LØ2.6-**
Cutaneous abscess, furuncle and carbuncle of other sites	**LØ2.8-**
Cutaneous abscess, furuncle and carbuncle, unspecified	**LØ2.9-**

Description of Condition

Cutaneous abscess, furuncle and carbuncle (LØ2)

Clinical Tip
A cutaneous abscess is a collection of pus resulting from an acute or chronic localized skin infection. Pus is the byproduct of tissue damage, fluid, and white blood cells formed by the body's immune response to fight off pathogens (e.g., infection, foreign substances).

A furuncle (boil) is a painful nodule formed by circumscribed inflammation of the skin and subcutaneous tissue that encloses a central core, usually the base of a hair follicle.

Furuncles may be caused by *Staphylococcus* or other bacteria. Accumulation of pus and tissue results in pressure, causing pain that is relieved by drainage.

Carbuncle, furuncle, and abscess are localized, contained pockets of infection. A carbuncle is a collection of pus contained in a cavity or sac, often associated with a hair follicle or groups of hair follicles that form a hardened, circumscribed lump deep in the skin tissues. Carbuncles are commonly associated with *Staphylococcus aureus* infection

A carbuncle is often described as a collection of lesions or boils.

⇨ I-10 ALERT

ICD-10-CM classifies cellulitis (LØ3) and abscess (LØ2) in separate code categories based on whether the infection is encapsulated or contained (i.e., abscess, furuncle, carbuncle) or spread throughout the skin, subcutaneous tissues (cellulitis) and lymph channels (lymphangitis).

Infection of the lymph glands or nodes (LØ4) is classified separately.

CDI ALERT

Abscess and cellulitis are classified separately in ICD-10-CM by severity, anatomic site, and laterality. Ensure documentation is specific regarding extent of infection to avoid misrepresentation of severity.

Documentation of site and laterality should be thorough and specific to avoid reporting unspecified codes.

Code category LØ3 may indicate a severity progression of infection from localized (LØ2) to adjacent tissues that increases the risk for potentially fatal serious systemic infection (sepsis) from circulating pathogens.

Key terms

Key terms found in the documentation may include:

Boil

Folliculitis

Furunculosis

⇨ I-10 ALERT

Category LØ2 Cutaneous abscess, furuncle and carbuncle, includes valid codes that are five or six characters in length. The following axes of classification describe:

Fourth character:
- Anatomic site or region

Fifth character:
- Type of infection: abscess furuncle or carbuncle
- Anatomic site

Sixth character:
- Anatomic site specificity (further specification of site)
- Laterality

Documentation Tip

Specify the nature of the localized infection. Differentiate between abscess, furuncle, and carbuncle. Document the specific anatomic site. For upper limb infections, the axilla is a separately identifiable anatomic site from the upper limb. For paired anatomic sites, specify laterality (right or left).

For example:

Cutaneous abscess of right axilla	(LØ2.411)
Cutaneous abscess of the right upper limb	(LØ2.413)

Clinical Findings

Physical Examination

- Examination of skin for localized infection
- Examination of neck, breasts, face, and buttocks for furuncles
- Examination for carbuncles: may be accompanied by fever and prostration
  - usually described as 1 to 3 cm in size

Diagnostic Procedures and Services

- Laboratory
  - culture for infective agent
  - gram stain

Therapeutic Procedures and Services

- Incision and drainage

Medication List

- Antibiotics
  - clindamycin (Cleocin)
  - doxycycline (Adoxa, Targadox)
  - minocycline (Dynacin, Solodyn)
  - rifampin (Rifadin, Rimactane)
  - trimethoprim (Primsol, Trimpex)
  - vancomycin

Clinician Documentation Checklist

Clinician documentation should indicate the following:

- Identification of
  - infectious organism (e.g., bacterial)

- Furuncle includes
  - boil
  - folliculitis
  - furunculosis
- Document site of cutaneous abscess, furuncle, and carbuncle
  - face
  - neck
  - trunk
    - abdominal wall
    - back (any part except buttock)
    - chest wall
    - groin
    - perineum
    - umbilicus
    - unspecified part
  - buttock
    - gluteal region
  - limb
    - axilla
    - upper limb
    - lower limb
    - unspecified part of limb
  - hand
  - foot
  - other sites
    - head (any part, except face)
    - other site
  - unspecified site
- Identify the laterality of axilla, upper and lower limb, hand, and foot
  - right
  - left

Cystoscopies, Urethroscopies and Cystourethroscopies

Code Axes

Endoscopy—cystoscopy, urethroscopy, cystourethroscopy **52000–52356**

Description of Procedure

These codes represent the endoscopic examination of the urethra, bladder, and ureteric openings into the bladder through an endoscope. Documentation should specify if the procedure is diagnostic or therapeutic, and if therapeutic, what procedures or services were performed.

Clinician documentation should include the following key terms as they apply in order to determine correct code assignment.

Key Term	Code
Biopsy	
Urethra and bladder	52204
Ureter or renal pelvic	52354
Dilation	
Bladder	52260–52265
Intrarenal	52343, 52346
Ureteral	52341, 52344
Urethral	52281, 52285
Ureteropelvic	52342, 52345
Diverticulum	
Bladder	52305
Excision	
Urethra and bladder	
Minor lesions	52224
Small bladder tumor	52234
Medium bladder tumor	52235
Large bladder tumor	52240
Ureteral or renal pelvic tumor	52355
Fulguration	
Bladder neck	52214
Lesions	
Bladder and urethra	52214–52250, 52285
Ureter	52300, 52301

Key Term	Code
Lesions (Continued)	
Periurethral glands	52214
Prostatic fossa	52214
Trigone	52214
Ureteral or renal pelvic lesion	52354
Urethra	52214
Injection	
Chemodenervation, bladder	52287
Radiocontrast, radiologic study, bladder	52281
Into urethral/bladder stricture	52283
Subureteric implant material	52327
Insertion	
Guidewire	52334
Stent	
Urethra	52282
Ureter	52332
Lithotripsy	
Ureter and Pelvis	52353, 52356
Manipulation	
Ureteral calculus	52330, 52352
Pyeloscopy	52351
Radioactive substance	52250
Removal	
Calculus	
Urethra or bladder	52310–52315
Ureter and pelvis	52320–52325, 52352
By litholapaxy	52317–52318
Foreign Body	52310–52315
Stent	
Ureteral	52310–52315, 52356
Sphincterotomy	52277
Tumor	
Bladder	52234–52240
Ureteral or renal pelvic	52355
Ureter Surgery	
Meatotomy	52290
Ureterocele	52300–52301
Urethral syndrome	52285
Ureteroscopy	52351
Urethrotomy	52270–52276

CDI ALERT

Documentation should be reviewed to determine why the procedure was performed (e.g., for removal of foreign body, biopsy, excision of tumor, etc.).

Debridement (Subcutaneous tissue, Muscle and/or Fascia, Bone)

Code Axes

Debridement, subcutaneous tissue	**11Ø42, 11Ø45**
Debridement, muscle and/or fascia	**11Ø43, 11Ø46**
Debridement, bone	**11Ø44, 11Ø47**

Description of Condition

Debridement is the surgical removal of contaminated or devitalized subcutaneous/fascia/muscle/bone tissue or foreign matter that is damaged, necrotic, dead, infected, abscessed, or ischemic, caused by injury, infection, wounds (excluding burn wounds), or chronic ulcers. Using a scalpel or dermatome, the physician excises the affected subcutaneous tissue until viable, bleeding tissue is encountered.

Debridement, subcutaneous tissue (includes epidermis and dermis, if performed); first 2Ø sq cm or less (11Ø42)

Debridement, subcutaneous tissue (includes epidermis and dermis, if performed); each additional 2Ø sq cm, or part thereof (List separately in addition to code for primary procedure) (11Ø45)

CPT Alert

The add-on codes related to the primary codes are to be reported for each additional 20 sq cm debrided. These codes are based on total square centimeters not per wound. For example, if the provider documents 55 sq cm were debrided, a total of three codes should be reported.

Clinical Tip

These procedures include the epidermis and dermis (skin). Subcutaneous tissue contains a sheet or wide band of adipose (fat), areolar connective tissue, and superficial fascia.

Debridement, muscle and/or fascia (includes epidermis, dermis, and subcutaneous tissue, if performed); first 2Ø sq cm or less (11Ø43)

Debridement, muscle and/or fascia (includes epidermis, dermis, and subcutaneous tissue, if performed); each additional 2Ø sq cm, or part thereof (List separately in addition to code for primary procedure) (11Ø46)

Clinical Tip

These procedures include deep fascia and/or muscle, including epidermis, dermis, and subcutaneous tissue, if performed. Deep fascia, also known as muscle fascia, covers, separates, and binds blood vessels, nerves, muscles, bones, and internal organs.

Debridement, bone (includes epidermis, dermis, subcutaneous tissue, muscle and/or fascia, if performed); first 2Ø sq cm or less (11Ø44)

Debridement, bone (includes epidermis, dermis, subcutaneous tissue, muscle and/or fascia, if performed); each additional 2Ø sq cm, or part thereof (List separately in addition to code for primary procedure) (11Ø47)

Clinical Tip

These procedures include bone, including epidermis, dermis, subcutaneous tissue, muscle, and/or fascia, if performed.

Key Terms

Key terms found in the documentation may include:

Bone

Debridement

Dermis

Excision of contaminated or devitalized tissue

Fascia (deep or superficial)

Muscle

Subcutaneous

SubQ

Documentation Tip

Providers should document the size and depth of the debrided area to ensure appropriate reimbursement.

Clinician Documentation Checklist

Clinician documentation should indicate the following:

- The diagnosis for the condition that prompted the procedure
- Depth of the tissue excised by identifying the tissue type (i.e., dermis, subcutaneous, fascia, muscle, bone)
- Total size of the debridement area, preferably in square centimeters

CPT ALERT

These codes report debridement of contaminated or devitalized skin, subcutaneous tissue, fascia, muscle, and bone not associated with open fractures or dislocations.

Depression — Major

Query Note

Excludes 1 note at F31 and F32, F33 indicates that bipolar disorder (depression/hypomania) cannot be reported with major depressive disorder. When both are documented, query for clarification. Additionally, for some types of major depressive disorders such as psychotic, the physician should be queried when documentation does not indicate if the episode is single or recurrent.

Code Axes

Major depressive disorder, single episode, mild	F32.Ø HCC
Major depressive disorder, single episode, moderate	F32.1 HCC
Major depressive disorder, single episode, severe without psychotic features	F32.2 HCC
Major depressive disorder, single episode, severe with psychotic features	F32.3 HCC
Major depressive disorder, single episode, in partial remission	F32.4 HCC
Major depressive disorder, single episode, in full remission	F32.5 HCC
Other depressive episodes	F32.8- HCC
Major depressive disorder, single episode, unspecified	F32.9 HCC
Major depressive disorder, recurrent, mild	F33.Ø HCC
Major depressive disorder, recurrent, moderate	F33.1 HCC
Major depressive disorder, recurrent, severe without psychotic features	F33.2 HCC
Major depressive disorder, recurrent, severe with psychotic symptoms	F33.3 HCC
Major depressive disorder, recurrent, in remission, unspecified	F33.4Ø HCC
Major depressive disorder, recurrent, in partial remission	F33.41 HCC
Major depressive disorder, recurrent, in full remission	F33.42 HCC
Other recurrent depressive disorders	F33.8 HCC
Major depressive disorder, recurrent, unspecified	F33.9 HCC

Description of Condition

Major depressive disorder (F32.-, F33.-)

Major depressive disorder is a disabling condition which impacts social, interpersonal and physical functioning. It is characterized by a combination of traits: pervasive, persistent depressed mood, loss of interest or pleasure in usually enjoyable activities and reduced energy.

Key Terms

Key terms found in the documentation may include:

Depressive disorder, recurrent, severe, without psychotic symptoms

Masked depression (single episode)

MDD

Psychogenic depression, single episode

Reactive depression

Clinical Findings

Physical Examination

History and review of systems may include:

- Interview of patient with no physical findings
- Fatigue
- Sleeping problem
- Loss of appetite or over eating
- Depressed mood that is frequent, persistent, and sad
- Frequent or persistent intense feeling of guilt
- Suicidal thoughts
- Inability to feel pleasure or take interest in things
- Difficulty in concentrating and focusing
- Impaired judgment, planning, or problem-solving
- Low self-esteem
- Pessimism
- Feelings of loneliness
- Unassertiveness
- Difficulty handling conflict
- Social withdrawal

Therapeutic Procedures and Services

- Psychotherapy

Medication List

- Antidepressant medication
  - tricyclic antidepressants (TCA)
  - amitriptyline
  - amoxapine
  - desipramine (Norpramin)
  - doxepin
  - imipramine (Tofranil)
  - nortriptyline (Pamelor)
  - protriptyline (Vivactil)
  - trimipramine (Surmontil)

- Selective serotonin reuptake inhibitors (SSRI)
  - Brintellix
  - Lexapro
  - Luvox
  - Paxil
  - Prozac
  - Zoloft
  - Viibryd

Clinician Note

Documentation should specify whether this is a single episode or recurrent, the current degree of depression, the presence of psychotic features or symptoms, and remission status (i.e., partial, full) when applicable.

Clinician Documentation Checklist

Clinician documentation should indicate the following:

- Type of mood disorder
  - manic episode
  - bipolar disorder
  - major depressive disorder
  - persistent mood (affective) disorder
    - cyclothymic
    - dysthymic
- Frequency of occurrence
  - single episode
  - recurrent episode
  - part of bipolar disorder
- Level of severity
  - hypomanic: for bipolar
  - depressed
  - mild
  - moderate
  - mixed: for bipolar
  - severe
- Psychotic symptoms or features
  - presence of psychotic symptoms or features
    - if present, the level of severity is severe
  - absence of psychotic symptoms or features

Diabetes Mellitus

Code Axes

Note: Subclassifications exist for subcategories EØ8, EØ9, E1Ø, E11, and E13 to represent manifestations including hyperosmolarity, ketoacidosis, kidney complications (e.g., CKD), ophthalmic complications (e.g., retinopathy, cataract), neurological complications (e.g., neuropathy, amyotrophy), circulatory complications (e.g., peripheral angiography, gangrene), skin complications (e.g., dermatitis, foot ulcer), oral complications (e.g., periodontal disease), hypoglycemia, hyperglycemia, other and unspecified complications.

Diabetes mellitus due to underlying condition	**EØ8.-** HCC QPP
Drug or chemical induced diabetes mellitus	**EØ9.-** HCC QPP
Type 1 diabetes mellitus	**E1Ø.-** HCC QPP
Type 2 diabetes mellitus	**E11.-** HCC QPP
Other specified diabetes mellitus	**E13.-** HCC QPP

Description of Condition

Diabetes mellitus due to underlying condition (EØ8.-)

Diabetes or glucose intolerance due to an underlying condition other than genetics or environmental conditions is found in category EØ8.

Clinical Tip

Although rarer than type 1 or type 2 diabetes, it is important to be able to track and classify the type of diabetes due to other underlying conditions. Examples of this type of condition include: chronic pancreatitis; cystic fibrosis; hemochromatosis pancreatic cancers; liver diseases, including hepatitis C; carcinoid tumors of the lungs, intestines or stomach; celiac disease and other autoimmune diseases and malnutrition.

Key Terms

Key terms found in the documentation may include:

Cystic fibrosis-related diabetes (CFRD)

Malnutrition-related diabetes (MRDM) (MMDM)

Clinician Note

Many payers, including Medicare, have quality measures in place to determine that quality and cost effective care is provided to the patient. It is imperative that the diabetes and any associated conditions or complications be documented in the medical record. Documentation should include statements that demonstrate the condition and therapy was monitored, evaluated, assessed/addressed, and/or treated on the current encounter.

I-10 ALERT

Each of the five subcategories for diabetes mellitus follows the same format, with combination codes for the most commonly diagnosed diabetic complications.

CDI ALERT

Ensure that the type of diabetes is clearly documented as it is essential for appropriate classification purposes.

I-10 ALERT

It is uncommon for a provider to document "Borderline Diabetes Mellitus." According to the official ICD-10-CM Official Coding Guidelines when the documentation contains a statement such as "borderline" the diagnosis at the time of discharge is coded as confirmed unless the classification provides a specific entry (e.g., borderline diabetes). The ICD-10-CM index contains the main term "Borderline," subterm "diabetes mellitus," referencing code R73.Ø3. For this reason, documentation in this instance would not support a code from the EØ8 through E11 categories.

Drug or chemical induced diabetes mellitus (EØ9.-)

Diabetes due to drug or chemical ingestion is found in category EØ9. Poisoning would be reported for overdose or substance taken improperly; adverse effect indicates it was properly prescribed and taken but which resulted in an adverse reaction.

Clinical Tip

Some drugs and chemicals, whether considered therapeutic or not, can have unintended consequences and can cause diabetic conditions.

Examples of drugs known to cause diabetes include: hormone supplements, antihypertensive diuretics and beta blockers, antipsychotics and some antidepressants, some anticonvulsants, antiretrovirals, and immunosuppressives.

Key Terms

Key terms found in the documentation may include:

Steroid induced diabetes

Clinician Note

Many payers, including Medicare, have quality measures in place to determine that quality and cost effective care is provided to the patient. It is imperative that the diabetes and any associated conditions or complications be documented in the medical record. Documentation should include statements that demonstrate the condition and therapy was monitored, evaluated, assessed/addressed, and/or treated on the current encounter.

⇨ I-10 ALERT

If the diabetic condition is due to a drug or chemical poisoning, the code for that poisoning should be sequenced first, with the EØ9 code sequenced as a manifestation. If it is due to an adverse reaction to a drug properly administered, the code for the drug with adverse effect (T36–T5Ø) should be assigned as a secondary condition to identify the drug itself; the manifestation (EØ9) will be sequenced first.

⇨ I-10 ALERT

Although a drug or chemical causing a diabetic condition can technically be considered an "underlying condition," there is a separate subcategory for those diabetic conditions caused by drugs or chemicals (EØ9).

CDI ALERT

Diabetes described as "out of control," "inadequately controlled," or "poorly controlled" is reported as the specified type of diabetes with hyperglycemia, fourth character 6. When another diabetic complication is present and the diabetes is stated as poorly controlled, etc., both complications are reported. The exception is diabetes with ketoacidosis: report only the code for diabetes with ketoacidosis as it is inherently uncontrolled.

Type 1 diabetes mellitus (E1Ø.-)

Type 1 diabetes mellitus results from autoimmune destruction of insulin-producing beta cells of the pancreas resulting in little or no insulin production; it is a chronic condition characterized by hyperglycemia; insulin must be taken daily. Triggers can interact with genetic susceptibility at any age to produce type 1 diabetes. Type 1.5 diabetes mellitus has characteristics of both type 1 and type 2 but is autoimmune and manifests in adults, thus it is known as latent autoimmune diabetes of adulthood. Since diabetes type 1.5 is not recognized in ICD-10-CM, query if the diabetes is type 1 or type 2.

Key Terms

Key terms found in the documentation for type 1 diabetes may include:

Diabetes due to autoimmune process

Diabetes due to immune mediated pancreatic islet beta-cell destruction

Idiopathic diabetes

Juvenile onset diabetes

Ketosis-prone diabetes

Latent autoimmune diabetes of adults (Type 1.5)

Slow onset type 1 diabetes

⇨ I-10 ALERT

Codes for typical diabetic type 1 conditions are now presented with more combination code choices, for the most commonly reported diabetic complications. Subcategory codes for hyperosmolarity are not found in this subgroup of codes.

Clinician Note

Many payers, including Medicare, have quality measures in place to determine that quality and cost effective care is provided to the patient. It is imperative that the diabetes and any associated conditions or complications be documented in the medical record. Documentation should include statements that demonstrate the condition and therapy was monitored, evaluated, assessed/addressed, and/or treated on the current encounter.

Type 2 diabetes mellitus (E11.-)

Type 2 diabetes mellitus is a metabolic disorder that involves high blood glucose in the context of insulin resistance and relative insulin deficiency. Unlike type 1 diabetics, those with type 2 diabetes have insulin produced in the pancreas, but it is either in small quantities or their bodies are resistant to it. It is caused by an interaction of lifestyle choices and genetics. This is a chronic condition but can be maintained by anti-diabetic medications, insulin, or diet regimen.

Key Terms

Key terms found in the documentation for type 2 diabetes may include:

Diabetes due to insulin secretory defect

Diabetes NOS

DMII

Insulin resistant diabetes

Clinician Note

Many payers, including Medicare have quality measures in place to determine that quality and cost effective care is provided to the patient. It is imperative that the diabetes and any associated conditions or complication be documented in the medical record. Documentation should include statements that demonstrate the condition and therapy was monitored, evaluated, assessed/addressed, and/or treated on the current encounter.

Other specified diabetes mellitus (E13.-)

There are several other types of diabetes that are caused by various other mechanisms. One type involves the body's tissue receptors not responding to insulin, even when insulin levels are normal, which is what differentiates it from type 2 diabetes. In other cases, genetic mutations (autosomal or mitochondrial) can lead to defects in pancreatic beta cell function. Diseases associated with excessive secretion of insulin-antagonistic hormones can cause diabetes; this condition is typically resolved once the hormone excess is removed.

⇨ I-10 ALERT

Codes for typical diabetic type 2 conditions are now presented with more combination code choices, for the most commonly reported diabetic complications.

CDI ALERT

The age documented in the medical record is not used to select the type of diabetes mellitus unless other documentation is noted. When the documentation does not indicate the type of diabetes, the clinician should be queried. If not, the appropriate code from category E11 Type 2 diabetes mellitus, is reported.

⇨ I-10 ALERT

If the documentation in a medical record does not indicate the type of diabetes but does indicate that the patient uses insulin, a code from category E11 Type 2 diabetes mellitus, should be assigned. A code from category Z79 should also be assigned to identify long-term (current) use of insulin or hypoglycemic drugs. Code Z79.4 should not be assigned if insulin is given temporarily to bring a type 2 patient's blood sugar under control during an encounter.

⇨ I-10 ALERT

Ensure that the medical record documentation does not specify a diabetic disease process that could be classified in one of the other four subcategories of diabetes mellitus codes.

⇨ I-10 ALERT

The ICD-10-CM Official Coding Guidelines state that when documentation indicates postpancreatectomy diabetes mellitus (i.e., lack of insulin due to the surgical removal of all or part of the pancreas), code E89.1 Postprocedural hypoinsulinemia should be reported. Report a code from subcategory Z90.41 Acquired absence of pancreas, and a code from category E13 as additional codes.

Key Terms

Key terms found in the documentation for other specified diabetes may include:

Diabetes mellitus due to genetic defects in insulin action

Diabetes mellitus due to genetic defects of beta-cell function

Postpancreatectomy diabetes mellitus

Postprocedural diabetes mellitus

Secondary diabetes mellitus NEC

Clinical Findings

The table listed below will help differentiate between type1 and type 2 diabetes mellitus.

Finding	Type 1	Type 2
Age of onset	Most commonly 30 years or younger	Most commonly over 30 years
Obesity	Not associated	Associated
Propensity to ketoacidosis	Yes, usually requires insulin	Variable
Associated with HLA-D	Yes	No
Islet pathology	Insulitis	Normal appearing islets
Prone to develop associated complications	Yes	Yes
Hyperglycemia responds to antihyperglycemic drugs	No	Yes

Signs and symptoms include hyperglycemia, urinary frequency, polyuria, and polydipsia. Patients with type 1 diabetes mellitus typically present symptomatic. Patients with type 2 diabetes mellitus are often asymptomatic and the condition is found during routine testing.

Diagnostic Procedures and Services

- Laboratory
  - fasting plasma/serum glucose
  - hemoglobin A1C
  - urine testing for proteinuria and microalbuminuria
  - serum creatinine
  - lipid profile
- Imaging
  - fundoscopy for ophthalmologic disorders
- Other
  - diabetic foot screening
  - Therapeutic Procedures and Services
- Home blood sugar monitoring
- Dietary restrictions (concentrated sugars)

Medication List

- Antihyperglycemics
  - metformin (Glucophage, Fortamet)
  - sitagliptin (Januvia)
- Insulin
- Sulfonylureas
  - chlorpropamide (Diabinese)
  - glimepiride (Amaryl)
  - glipizide (Glucotrol)
  - glyburide (Glycron, DiaBeta)

Clinician Note

Many payers, including Medicare have quality measures in place to determine that quality and cost effective care is provided to the patient. It is imperative that the diabetes and any associated conditions or complications be documented in the medical record. Documentation should include statements that demonstrate the condition and therapy was monitored, evaluated, assessed/addressed, and/or treated on the current encounter.

Clinician Documentation Checklist

Clinician documentation should indicate the following:

- Type 1
  - juvenile onset
  - ketosis-prone
  - idiopathic
  - brittle
  - due to autoimmune process
  - due to immune mediated pancreatic islet beta-cell destruction
- Type 2
  - due to insulin secretory defect
  - insulin resistant
  - insulin use, if any
- Drug or chemical induced
  - the drug
  - insulin use, if any
- Due to underlying condition
  - underlying conditions
    - Cushing syndrome
    - cystic fibrosis
    - malignant neoplasm
    - malnutrition
    - pancreatitis and other diseases of pancreas
  - insulin use, if any

- Other specified causes
  - due to genetic defects of beta-cell function
  - due to genetic defects in insulin action
  - postpancreatectomy
  - postprocedural
  - secondary
- Associated complications
  - ketoacidosis
    - without coma
    - with coma
  - hyperosmolarity
    - without nonketotic hyperglycemic-hyperosmolar coma
    - with coma
- Kidney
  - With diabetic nephropathy
    - intercapillary glomerulosclerosis
    - intracapillary glomerulosclerosis
    - Kimmelstiel-Wilson disease
  - with diabetic chronic kidney disease
    - stage of chronic kidney disease
  - with other diabetic kidney complication
    - renal tubular degeneration
- Ophthalmic
  - with or without macular edema
    - unspecified diabetic retinopathy
    - mild nonproliferative diabetic retinopathy
    - moderate nonproliferative diabetic retinopathy
    - severe nonproliferative diabetic retinopathy
    - proliferative diabetic retinopathy
  - with diabetic cataract
  - with other diabetic ophthalmic complication
- Neurological
  - mononeuropathy
  - polyneuropathy
    - diabetic neuralgia
  - autonomic (poly) neuropathy
  - diabetic gastroparesis
  - amyotrophy

- Circulatory
  - peripheral angiopathy
    - with gangrene
    - without gangrene
- Diabetes mellitus in pregnancy, childbirth, and puerperium
  - type
    - pre-existing diabetes mellitus, type1
    - pre-existing diabetes mellitus, type2
    - gestational diabetes mellitus
    - diet controlled
    - insulin controlled
    - trimester

Drug Dependence

(Opioid F11, Cannabis F12, Sedative F13, Cocaine F14, Other Stimulant F15, Hallucinogen F16, Inhalant F18, Other Psychoactive Substance F19)

Code Axes

Drug/substance dependence, uncomplicated	**F1[1-6, 8-9].20** HCC
Drug/substance dependence, in remission	**F1[1-6, 8-9].21** HCC
Drug/substance dependence with intoxication, uncomplicated	**F1[1-6, 8-9].220** HCC
Drug/substance dependence with intoxication delirium	**F1[1-6, 8-9].221** HCC
Drug/substance dependence with intoxication with perceptual disturbance Note: F16.2 Hallucinogen is not reported in this subcategory.	**F1[1, 3-5, 9].222** HCC
Drug/substance dependence with intoxication, unspecified	**F1[1-6, 8-9].229** HCC
Drug/substance dependence with withdrawal	**F1[1, 4, 5].23** HCC
Drug/substance dependence with withdrawal, uncomplicated	**F1[3, 9].230** HCC
Drug/substance dependence with withdrawal delirium	**F1[3, 9].231** HCC
Drug/substance dependence with withdrawal with perceptual disturbance	**F1[3, 9].232** HCC
Drug/substance dependence with withdrawal, unspecified	**F1[3, 9].239** HCC
Drug/substance dependence with drug-induced mood disorder	**F1[1, 3-6, 8-9].24** HCC
Drug/substance dependence with drug-induced psychotic disorder with delusions	**F1[1- 6, 8-9].250** HCC
Drug/substance dependence with drug-induced psychotic disorder with hallucinations	**F1[1-6, 8-9].251** HCC
Drug/substance dependence with drug-induced psychotic disorder, unspecified	**F1[1, 3-6, 8-9].259** HCC
Drug/substance dependence with drug-induced persisting amnestic disorder	**F1[3, 9].26** HCC
Drug/substance dependence with drug-induced persisting dementia	**F1[3, 8-9].27** HCC
Drug/substance dependence with other drug-induced disorder, anxiety disorder	**F1[2-6, 8-9].280** HCC

Drug/substance dependence with opioid-induced sexual dysfunction **F1[1, 3-5, 9].281** HCC

Drug/substance dependence with drug-induced sleep disorder **F1[1, 3-5, 9].282** HCC

Drug/substance dependence with hallucinogen persisting perception disorder (flashbacks) **F16.283** HCC

Note: this subcategory pertains to Hallucinogen drugs only.

Drug/substance dependence with other drug-induced disorder **F1[1-6, 8-9].288** HCC

Drug/substance dependence with unspecified drug-induced disorder **F1[1-6, 8-9].29** HCC

Description of Condition

Drug dependence (F11.2, F12.2, F13.2, F14.2, F15.2, F16.2, F18.2, F19.2)

Drug/substance dependence is a chronic disorder characterized by use of large amounts of or frequent use of a drug/substance or multiple drugs/substances in which the individual becomes physically and mentally dependent upon to function. Long-term consequences are physical, psychological, and behavioral. Criterion denoting dependence is increased tolerance and continued use despite impairment of health, social life, and job performance. Cessation results in withdrawal symptoms, including early seizures.

CDI ALERT

When a blood test gives evidence of the presence of alcohol/drugs without documentation of substance use, abuse, or dependence and the information is provider-documented and has clinical significance for the encounter and/or meets criteria as an additional diagnosis, report the appropriate code from category R78.[Ø-6].

Key Terms

Key terms found in the documentation may include:

Chronic drug dependence

Drug addiction

Drug dependence

Inhalant dependence

Clinical Findings

Physical Examination

Signs and symptoms reveal intoxication followed by withdrawal from the drug when discontinued. This may be either minor or severe.

Findings of physical withdrawal include:

- Sweating
- Racing heart
- Palpitations
- Muscle tension
- Tightness in the chest
- Difficulty breathing

- Tremor
- Nausea, vomiting, or diarrhea
- Grand mal seizures
- Heart attacks
- Strokes
- Hallucinations
- Delirium tremens (DT)

Emotional withdrawal symptoms include:

- Anxiety
- Restlessness
- Irritability
- Insomnia
- Headaches
- Poor concentration
- Depression
- Social isolation

Diagnostic Procedures and Services

- Laboratory
  - drug screening
  - hepatitis panel
  - laboratory panel
  - CBC
  - HIV screening
  - chemistry panel
- Other
  - EKG

Clinician Note

The provider must state the pattern of harmful usage (dependence, abuse or use) and its current clinical state (uncomplicated, intoxication, remission, etc.) and indicate the relationship to any identified mental, behavioral, or physical disorder or its relevance to the patient's status or encounter including its clinical significance. The specific drug(s) or substance should be identified and documented and in cases of legal medication indicated if it had been prescribed for that individual. Classification should be made according to the most important drug/substance or class of drug/substance used or causing the presenting disorder.

⇨ I-10 ALERT

According to ICD-10-CM Official Coding Guidelines, when documentation indicates the presence of use, abuse, and dependence of the same substance, only one code is reported. The following reporting hierarchy is used when assigning the ICD-10-CM codes:

- If both use and abuse are documented, assign only the code for abuse.
- If both abuse and dependence are documented, the code for dependence only is reported.
- If use, abuse, and dependence are all documented, the code for dependence only is reported
- If both use and dependence are documented, the code for dependence only is reported

Clinician Documentation Checklist

Clinician documentation should indicate the following:

Psychoactive Substance

- Name of substance
  - alcohol
    - blood alcohol level
  - anxiolytics, cannabis, cocaine, hallucinogens, hypnotics, inhalants, nicotine, opioids, sedatives, volatile solvents
  - polysubstance
- Level of substance use
  - use
  - abuse
  - dependence
- Any additional description of use
  - intoxication
  - remission
  - withdrawal
- Associated psychoactive-induced disorders
  - anxiety
  - delirium
  - delusions
  - hallucinations
  - mood disorder
  - perception disturbance
  - persisting amnestic disorder
  - persisting dementia
  - psychotic disorder
  - sexual dysfunction
  - sleep disorder

Nonpsychoactive Substance Abuse

- Name of nonpsychoactive substance
  - antacids
  - herbal/folk remedies
  - laxatives
  - steroids/hormones
  - vitamins
  - other

Drug/Substance Abuse

(Opioid F11, Cannabis F12, Sedative F13, Cocaine F14, Other Stimulant F15, Hallucinogen F16, Inhalant F18, Other Psychoactive Substance F19)

Code Axes

Drug/substance abuse, uncomplicated	**F1[1-6, 8-9].10** HCC
Drug/substance abuse, in remission	**F1[1-6,8-9].11** HCC
Drug/substance abuse with intoxication, uncomplicated	**F1[1-6, 8-9].120** HCC
Drug/substance abuse with intoxication, delirium	**F1[1-6, 8-9].121** HCC
Drug/substance abuse with intoxication with perceptual disturbance	**F1[1-2, 4-6, 9].122** HCC
Drug/substance abuse with intoxication, unspecified	**F1[1-6, 8-9].129** HCC
Drug/substance abuse with drug-induced mood disorder	**F1[1, 3-6, 8-9].14** HCC
Drug/substance abuse with drug-induced psychotic disorder with delusions	**F1[1-6, 8-9].150** HCC
Drug/substance abuse with drug-induced psychotic disorder with hallucinations	**F1[1-6, 8-9].151** HCC
Drug/substance abuse with other drug-induced psychotic disorder, unspecified	**F1[1-6, 8-9].159** HCC
Drug/substance abuse with drug-induced persisting amnestic disorder Note: Psychoactive substance abuse only for this subcategory.	**F19.16** HCC
Drug/substance abuse with drug-induced persisting dementia Note: Only psychoactive substance and inhalant abuse are in this subcategory.	**F1[8-9].17** HCC
Drug/substance abuse with other drug-induced disorder, anxiety disorder	**F1[2-6, 8-9].180** HCC
Drug/substance abuse with other drug-induced disorder, sexual dysfunction	**F1[1, 3-5, 9].181** HCC
Drug/substance abuse with drug-induced sleep disorder	**F1[1, 3, 4-5, 9].182** HCC
Drug/substance abuse with drug-induced persisting perception disorder (flashbacks) Note: Hallucinogen drug abuse only for this subcategory.	**F16.183** HCC
Drug/substance abuse with other drug-induced disorder To use this code, the other drug-related disorder must be specified and not found in any other subcategory.	**F1[1-6, 8-9].188** HCC

Drug/substance abuse with unspecified drug-induced disorder F1[1-6, 8-9].19 HCC

Description of Condition

Drug/substance abuse (F11.1, F12.1, F13.1, F14.1, F15.1, F16.1, F18.1, F19.1)

Drug/substance abuse is characterized by recurring misuse of a drug in excess with identifiable harmful and dysfunctional behaviors and negative consequences for health, psycho-social state, and employment. It lacks the criteria of dependency. Time frame for consideration of abuse would be persisting for at least one month or has occurred repeatedly within a 12 month period.

Key Terms

Key terms found in the documentation may include:

Drug Use Disorder of:

Barbiturate abuse (F13.1-)

Cannabis abuse (F12.1-)

Cocaine abuse (F14.1-)

Crack (cocaine) abuse (F14.1-)

Hallucinogen abuse (F16.1-)

Heroin abuse (F11.1-)

Hypnotic abuse (F13.1-)

Opioid abuse (F11.1-)

Other stimulant abuse (F15.1-)

Sedative abuse (F13.1-)

Clinical Findings

Physical Examination

Signs and symptoms reveal intoxication of the drug, which can differ depending upon the type of substance. Examples may be euphoria, hyperactivity, and sedation. Documentation may indicate flushing or itching of skin. GI complaints including nausea, vomiting, decreased bowel sounds, and constipation may be recorded.

Diagnostic Procedures and Services

- Laboratory
  - drug screen
- Other
  - EKG

⇨ I-10 ALERT

According to ICD-10-CM Official Coding Guidelines, when documentation indicates the presence of use, abuse, and dependence of the same substance, only one code is reported. The following reporting hierarchy is used when assigning the ICD-10-CM codes:

- If both use and abuse are documented, assign only the code for abuse.
- If both abuse and dependence are documented, the code for dependence only is reported.
- If use, abuse, and dependence are all documented, the code for dependence only is reported.
- If both use and dependence are documented, the code for dependence only is reported.

Clinician Note

The provider must state the pattern of harmful usage (dependence, abuse, or use) and its current clinical state (uncomplicated, intoxication, remission, etc.) and indicate the relationship to any identified mental, behavioral, or physical disorder or its relevance to the patient's status or encounter including its clinical significance. The specific drug(s) or substances should be identified and documented and in cases of legal medication indicated if it had been prescribed for that individual. Classification should be made according to the most important drug/substance or class of drug/substance used or causing the presenting disorder.

First Listed Diagnosis Note

Final diagnosis: Drug-seeking with Narcotic Abuse, including past prescription abuse, abdominal pain somatic complaint without organic evidence: The appropriate code from category F11 (F11.1Ø) will be the first listed diagnosis, followed by Z76.5 Person feigning illness (with obvious motivation).

Clinician Documentation Checklist

Clinician documentation should indicate the following:

Psychoactive Substance

- Name of substance
  - alcohol
    - — blood alcohol level
  - anxiolytics, cannabis, cocaine, hallucinogens, hypnotics, inhalants, nicotine, opioids, sedatives, volatile solvents
  - polysubstance
- Level of substance use
  - use
  - abuse
  - dependence
- Any additional description of use
  - intoxication
  - remission
  - withdrawal
- Associated psychoactive-induced disorders
  - anxiety
  - delirium
  - delusions
  - hallucinations
  - mood disorder
  - perception disturbance
  - persisting amnestic disorder
  - persisting dementia
  - psychotic disorder

- sexual dysfunction
- sleep disorder

Nonpsychoactive Substance Abuse

- Name of nonpsychoactive substance
  - antacids
  - herbal/folk remedies
  - laxatives
  - steroids/hormones
  - vitamins
  - other

Drug/Substance Use

(Opioid F11, Cannabis F12, Sedative F13, Cocaine F14, Other Stimulant F15, Hallucinogen F16, Inhalant F18, Other Psychoactive Substance F19)

Code Axes

Drug/substance use, unspecified, uncomplicated	F1[1-6, 8-9].90
Drug/substance use, unspecified with intoxication, uncomplicated	F1[1-6, 8-9].920 HCC
Drug/substance use, unspecified with intoxication, delirium	F1[1-6, 8-9].921 HCC
Drug/substance use, unspecified with intoxication with perceptual disturbance	F1[1-2, 4-5, 9].922 HCC
Drug/substance use, unspecified with intoxication, unspecified	F1[1-6, 8-9].929 HCC
Drug/substance use, unspecified with withdrawal	F1[1, 5].93 HCC
Drug/substance use, unspecified with withdrawal, uncomplicated	F1[3, 9].930 HCC
Drug/substance use, unspecified with withdrawal delirium	F1[3, 9].931 HCC
Drug/substance use, unspecified with withdrawal with perceptual disturbance	F1[3, 9].932 HCC
Drug/substance use, unspecified with withdrawal, unspecified	F1[3, 9].939 HCC
Drug/substance use, unspecified with drug-induced mood disorder	F1[1, 3-6, 8-9].94 HCC
Drug/substance use, unspecified with drug-induced psychotic disorder with delusions	F1[1-6, 8-9].950 HCC
Drug/substance use, unspecified with drug-induced psychotic disorder with hallucinations	F1[1-6, 8-9].951 HCC
Drug/substance use, unspecified with drug-induced psychotic disorder, unspecified	F1[1-6, 8-9].959 HCC
Drug/substance use, unspecified with drug-induced persisting amnestic disorder	F1[3, 9].96 HCC
Drug/substance use, unspecified with other drug-induced persisting dementia	F1[3, 8-9].97 HCC
Drug/substance use, unspecified with other drug-induced disorders, anxiety disorder	F1[2-6, 8-9].980 HCC
Drug/substance use, unspecified with drug-induced sexual dysfunction	F1[1, 3-5, 9].981 HCC

Drug/substance use, unspecified with other drug-induced sleep disorder	**F1[1, 3-5, 9].982** HCC
Drug/substance use, unspecified with other drug-induced disorder	**F1[1-6, 8-9].988** HCC
Drug/substance use, unspecified with unspecified drug-induced disorder	**F1[1-6, 8-9].99** HCC

Description of Condition

Drug/substance use (F11.9, F12.9, F13.9, F14.9, F15.9, F16.9, F18.9, F19.9)

Harmful drug or substance use is characterized by mental, behavioral, and physical disorders due to drug/substance use when dependency or abuse is not documented. Drug/substance use without negative consequences documented, e.g., uncomplicated, is reported with subcategory F1[1-6, 8-9].9Ø. Provider should document the specified drug(s) or substances, when known.

Key Terms

Key terms found in the documentation may include:

Drug intoxication, unknown usage

Drug use with clinical manifestation/state

Clinician Note

The provider must state the pattern of harmful usage (dependence, abuse, or use) and its current clinical state (uncomplicated, intoxication, remission, etc.) and indicate the relationship to any identified mental, behavioral, or physical disorder or its relevance to the patient's status or encounter including its clinical significance. The specific drug(s) or substances should be identified and documented and in cases of legal medication indicated if it had been prescribed for that individual. Classification should be made according to the most important drug/substance or class of drug/substance used or causing the presenting disorder.

Clinician Documentation Checklist

Clinician documentation should indicate the following:

Psychoactive Substance

- Name of substance
  - alcohol
    - blood alcohol level
  - anxiolytics, cannabis, cocaine, hallucinogens, hypnotics, inhalants, nicotine, opioids, sedatives, volatile solvents
  - polysubstance
- Level of substance use
  - use
  - abuse

- dependence
- Any additional description of use
- intoxication
- remission
- withdrawal
- Associated psychoactive-induced disorders
  - anxiety
  - delirium
  - delusions
  - hallucinations
  - mood disorder
  - perception disturbance
  - persisting amnestic disorder
  - persisting dementia
  - psychotic disorder
  - sexual dysfunction
  - sleep disorder

Nonpsychoactive Substance Abuse

- Name of nonpsychoactive substance
  - antacids
  - herbal/folk remedies
  - laxatives
  - steroids/hormones
  - vitamins
  - other

Electrocardiogram

Code Axes

Electrocardiogram **93000–93010**

Description of Procedure

An electrocardiogram is the recording of the electrical activity of the heart on a moving strip of paper that detects and records the electrical potential of the heart during contraction. These may be performed as part of a routine physical examination or due to cardiac symptoms or monitor cardiac conditions.

Electrocardiogram, routine ECG with at least 12 leads; with interpretation and report (93000)

Electrocardiogram, routine ECG with at least 12 leads; tracing only, without interpretation and report (93005)

Electrocardiogram, routine ECG with at least 12 leads; interpretation and report only (93010)

Key Terms

Key terms found in the documentation may include:

ECG

EKG

Clinician Note

Careful documentation is necessary to identify the medical necessity of the procedure, otherwise it is considered routine screening and noncovered by most third-party payers. The following list identifies those conditions which frequently support the medical necessity:

- Acid-base disorders
- Arteriovascular disease including coronary, central, and peripheral disease
- Cardiac hypertrophy
- Cardiac rhythm disturbances
- Chest pain or angina pectoris
- Conduction abnormalities
- Drug cardiotoxicity
- Electrolyte imbalance
- Endocrine abnormalities
- Heart failure

- Hypertension
- Myocardial ischemia or infarction
- Neurological disorders affecting the heart
- Palpitations
- Paroxysmal weakness
- Pericarditis
- Pulmonary disorders
- Sudden lightheadedness
- Structural cardiac conditions
- Syncope
- Temperature disorders

A preoperative EKG may be reasonable and necessary under one of the following conditions:

- In the presence of pre-existing heart disease such as angina, congestive heart failure, coronary artery disease, dysrhythmias, or prior myocardial infarction
- In the presence of known comorbid conditions that may affect the heart, such as chronic pulmonary disease, diabetes, peripheral vascular disease, or renal impairment
- When the pending surgical procedure requires a general or regional anesthetic

CDI ALERT

When reporting the interpretation and report of an EKG, the physician's findings should be clearly documented in the medical record documentation, even when within normal limits. Some payers may require that measurement of all intervals and axis, rhythm and heart rate, as well as an interpretation be recorded and signed by the provider. A notation of "within normal limits" or WNL may not be sufficient.

Clinician Documentation Checklist

Clinician documentation should indicate the following:

- Identify the reason for the test
  - routine screening
  - preoperative EKG
  - monitor cardiac symptoms or cardiac conditions
  - conditions that often support medical necessity
    - acid-base disorders
    - arteriovascular disease including coronary, central, and peripheral disease
    - cardiac hypertrophy
    - cardiac rhythm disturbances
    - chest pain or angina pectoris
    - conduction abnormalities
    - drug cardiotoxicity
    - electrolyte imbalance
    - endocrine abnormalities
    - heart failure
    - hypertension
    - myocardial ischemia or infarction

- — neurological disorders affecting the heart
- — palpitations
- — paroxysmal weakness
- — pericarditis
- — pulmonary disorders
- — sudden lightheadedness
- — structural cardiac conditions
- — syncope
- — temperature disorders
- With interpretation
- Without interpretation

Embolectomy/Thrombectomy

Code Axes

Arterial, with or without catheter	**34001–34203**
Venous, direct or with catheter	**34401–34490**

Description of Procedure

These procedures represent the removal of blood clots or other foreign material from various vessels. The codes are differentiated by arterial and venous procedures as well as the specific vessel. Terms such as anatomical location, embolectomy, or thrombectomy provide guidance.

Clinical Tip

Documentation will indicate that the artery is isolated and dissected from other critical structures and that it may be clamped above and below the clot. If a catheter is required, it is threaded past the clot and a small balloon found at its tip is inflated.

Key Terms

Key terms found in the documentation may include:

Atheroembolism

Atherosclerosis

Occlusion

Steal syndrome

Stenosis

Vessel injury

CPT ALERT

When documentation indicates that an angioscopy was performed during therapeutic intervention, it should be reported in addition to the code for the primary procedure.

Clinician Documentation Checklist

Clinician documentation should indicate the following:

- The medical condition being treated
- Anatomic location
  - artery or vein
    - neck
    - thorax
    - arm
    - abdomen
    - leg
- Type of procedure
  - embolectomy
  - thrombectomy
  - instrumentation (i.e., catheter, balloon)

EMG (Electromyography)

Code Axes

Needle electromyography **95860–95887**

Description of Procedure

Needle electromyography (EMG) records the electrical properties of muscle using an oscilloscope. Recordings, which may be amplified and heard through a loudspeaker, are made during needle insertion, with the muscle at rest, and during contraction. Documentation should clearly indicate the site of the study (e.g., extremity, paraspinal areas, cranial nerve) and if other nerve conduction studies are performed in conjunction with the EMG.

Needle electromyography (95860–95864)

Needle electromyography (95867–95870)

These code ranges represent an EMG when no nerve conduction studies are performed in conjunction with the EMG in the same day. Document the specific nerves being tested and, when appropriate, if the procedure is unilateral or bilateral.

Needle electromyography, each extremity, with related paraspinal areas, when performed with nerve conduction, amplitude and latency/velocity study (95885–95887)

Documentation supporting this series of codes will indicate that other nerve conduction studies were performed during the same encounter.

Clinician Documentation Checklist

Clinician documentation should indicate the following:

- The medical condition or symptoms being treated
  - pain
  - weakness
  - numbness
  - neuropathies
  - dystrophies
  - carpal tunnel syndrome
- Procedure
  - complete procedure (technical and professional)
  - technical component only
  - interpretation (professional) component only
- Nerves being tested

CDI ALERT

Carefully review the medical record documentation to determine if the complete procedure, technical component, or interpretation only was performed as this can affect modifier assignment.

CPT ALERT

When a cervical paraspinal or lumbar paraspinal muscle is tested and there is no corresponding limb study documented on the same day, report code 95887.

- Number of nerves being tested
  - unilateral
  - bilateral
  - paraspinal
- Other nerve conduction studies
- Clinical findings

Emphysema

Code Axes

Unilateral pulmonary emphysema [MacLeod's syndrome]	**J43.Ø** HCC QPP
Panlobular emphysema	**J43.1** HCC QPP
Centrilobular emphysema	**J43.2** HCC QPP
Other emphysema	**J43.8** HCC QPP
Emphysema, unspecified	**J43.9** HCC QPP
Compensatory emphysema	**J98.3** HCC

Clinical Tip
Emphysema is one of several conditions that comprises chronic obstructive pulmonary disease (COPD). Primarily found in tobacco smokers, the lung tissue around the small alveoli are destroyed, thus making them unable to hold their shape on exhalation.

⇨ I-10 ALERT

When emphysema is documented as being present with chronic bronchitis, refer to classification rules at category J44 Other chronic obstructive pulmonary disease. Review documentation carefully to ensure proper classification.

Description of Condition

Unilateral pulmonary emphysema [MacLeod's syndrome] (J43.Ø)

Clinical Tip
MacLeod's syndrome is a rare disorder that is typically diagnosed in childhood, associated with postinfectious bronchiolitis obliterans. The affected lung tissue does not grow normally and consequently is somewhat smaller than the nonaffected lung. The primary radiographic appearance is that of pulmonary hyperlucency. It is an x-linked disorder, meaning that it primarily affects males.

Clinical Tip
Documentation may include terms such as pink puffer (a descriptor for a patient with COPD and severe emphysema, who has a pink complexion and dyspnea) or blue bloater (a descriptor to indicate the appearance of a patient with COPD who has symptoms of chronic bronchitis). Verify with the physician before assigning a code for emphysema.

Key Terms
Key terms found in the documentation for unilateral pulmonary emphysema may include:

Swyer-James-MacLeod syndrome
Unilateral hyperlucent lung syndrome
Unilateral pulmonary artery functional hypoplasia
Unilateral transparency of lung

⇨ I-10 ALERT

As with many pulmonary conditions in ICD-10-CM, a coding instructional note at this category indicates that any exposure to tobacco smoke or smoking behavior should be coded in addition to the code(s) for the conditions themselves.

Panlobular emphysema (J43.1)

Clinical Tip

Panlobular emphysema is the type that involves the entire lung lobule, from the bronchiole to the alveoli, which has expanded. This type of emphysema most commonly involves the lower lobes.

Key Terms

Key terms found in the documentation for panlobular emphysema may include:

Panacinar emphysema

Centrilobular emphysema (J43.2)

Clinical Tip

In this type of emphysema only the proximal and central portions of the bronchiole have expanded. This type of emphysema most commonly involves the upper lobes.

Other and unspecified emphysema (J43.8, J43.9)

Clinical Tip

An emphysematous bleb is caused by damaged alveoli in the lung tissue that can no longer perform oxygen exchange. The air becomes trapped in the adjacent tissue, forming a bleb, and scar tissue accumulates around it.

Key Terms

Key terms found in the documentation may include:

Bullous emphysema
Emphysema NOS
Emphysematous bleb
Vesicular emphysema

Compensatory emphysema (J98.3)

Clinical Tip

Compensatory emphysema is a nonobstructive process in which the unaffected lung tissue adapts and enlarges, due to another portion of the lung being damaged or removed. It does not involve the same destructive lung tissue pattern as the other types of emphysema.

Key Terms

Key terms found in the documentation for other and unspecified emphysema may include:

Bullous emphysema
Emphysema NOS
Emphysematous bleb
Vesicular emphysema

CDI ALERT

Ensure that the appropriate type of emphysema is documented in the medical record.

Clinical Findings

Physical Examination

Patients present with complaints of cough and shortness of breath, which is usually upon exertion. Documentation indicates wheezing and increased expiratory phase of breathing. There are decreased heart and lung sounds. The chest may appear larger in the anteroposterior diameter (barrel chest). Neck vein distention may be present in signs of advanced disease.

Diagnostic Procedures and Services

- Laboratory
  - antitrypsin levels to detect possible deficiency
- Imaging
  - echocardiogram
  - chest x-ray
- Other
  - pulmonary function tests
  - EKG

Clinician Documentation Checklist

Clinician documentation should indicate the following:

- Exposure to environmental tobacco smoke
- History of tobacco use
- Occupational exposure to environmental tobacco smoke
- Tobacco dependence
- Tobacco use
- Type
  - unilateral pulmonary (MacLeod's syndrome)
    - Swyer syndrome
    - unilateral emphysema
    - unilateral hyperlucent lung
    - unilateral pulmonary artery functional hypoplasia
    - unilateral transparency of lung
  - panlobular
    - panacinar
  - centrilobular
  - other
  - unspecified
    - bullous
    - emphysematous bleb
    - vesicular

Encephalopathy

Code Axes

Anoxic encephalopathy	**G93.1** HCC
Metabolic encephalopathy	**G93.41**
Toxic encephalopathy	**G92**
Other encephalopathy	**G93.49**
Encephalopathy, unspecified	**G93.4Ø**

Description of Condition

Encephalopathy is a generalized, or global, alteration in brain function that is typically acute (or subacute) in onset and due to a systemic underlying cause that is usually reversible and resolves when the underlying cause is corrected. Common causes of encephalopathy include fever, infection, dehydration, electrolyte imbalance, acidosis, organ failure, sepsis, hypoxia, drugs, poisons, or toxins.

Anoxic encephalopathy (G93.1)

Anoxic or hypoxic encephalopathy is brain damage due to lack of oxygen.

Clinical Tip

Common causes are cardiopulmonary arrest, prolonged seizures with inadequate breathing, prolonged asthma attacks or exacerbations of COPD.

Key Terms

Key terms found in the documentation may include:

Anoxic brain damage

Anoxic encephalopathy

Metabolic encephalopathy (G93.41)

Potentially reversible encephalopathy due to metabolic causes; most commonly due to infections, fever, dehydration, electrolyte imbalance, acidosis, hypoxia, and organ failure. Metabolic encephalopathy often presents acutely and rapidly and with fluctuating levels of consciousness/alertness.

Clinical Tip

Septic encephalopathy is a clinical term that expresses brain dysfunction as a manifestation of severe sepsis. Metabolic encephalopathy often presents acutely and rapidly and with fluctuating levels of consciousness/alertness.

Key Terms
Key terms in the documentation may include:

Metabolic encephalopathy

Septic encephalopathy

First Listed Diagnosis Note
Admit for encephalopathy due to dehydration: The patient was admitted with mental status changes and diagnostic workup revealed metabolic encephalopathy due to dehydration. Treatment of the metabolic encephalopathy was directed towards reversing the dehydration. However, metabolic encephalopathy may be designated as the first listed diagnosis as it was documented as the condition established after study to be chiefly responsible for the admission of the patient to the hospital for care.

Admit for severe sepsis with septic encephalopathy: Patient was admitted with severe fever, tachycardia, and mental status changes and was documented as having severe *Escherichia coli* sepsis with septic encephalopathy. According to Official Coding Guidelines, the coding of severe sepsis requires a minimum of two codes: first a code for the underlying systemic infection A41.51, followed by a code from subcategory R65.2 Severe sepsis. An additional code is assigned for the associated acute organ dysfunction; in this case septic encephalopathy G93.41.

> **CDI ALERT**
>
> Documentation of the results of blood tests, spinal fluid examination, imaging studies, electroencephalograms, and similar diagnostic studies may be used to differentiate the various causes of encephalopathy and is necessary for reporting specificity.

Toxic encephalopathy (G92)
Toxic encephalopathy is defined as brain tissue degeneration due to a toxic substance and is identified with drugs, poisonings, and chemical substances. Toxic-metabolic can be found in organ failure or intoxication.

Clinical Tip
Toxic and toxic-metabolic encephalopathy generally refer to the effects of drugs, toxins, poisons, and medications, but this term may also be used clinically to refer to encephalopathy caused by fever, sepsis, or other toxic conditions. Review documentation carefully and query if documentation is insufficient to assign the most specific code.

> **CDI ALERT**
>
> The instructional note under G92 states to code first (T51–T65) to identify the toxic agent. Note that T51–T65 identifiy substances that are primarily nonmedicinal, including alcohol, organic solvents, carbon monoxide, smoke, venomous animals, plants, and tobacco.
>
> For encephalopathy due to drugs, the alphabetic index instructs to see also the Table of Drugs and Chemicals.

Key Terms
Key terms found in the documentation may include:

Toxic encephalopathy

Toxic encephalitis

Toxic metabolic encephalopathy

First Listed Diagnosis Note
Admit for toxic encephalopathy due to lead poisoning: Patient was admitted with mental status changes, which after evaluation was determined to be toxic encephalopathy due to accidental toxic lead exposure that occurred while he was removing lead contaminated paint in his home. Toxic encephalopathy should not be sequenced as the first listed diagnosis, as there is an instructional note under code/category G92 instructing to code first the underlying toxic agent. Code T56.ØX1A

Toxic effect of lead and its compounds, accidental (unintentional), initial encounter, would be assigned as the first listed diagnosis, with code G92 assigned as an additional code.

QUERY NOTE

When encephalopathy is documented and the etiology is not identified or clear, query for the underlying cause based on information within the record.

Other encephalopathy (G93.49)

This code is reported when the type of encephalopathy is identified but does not have an alphabetic index entry nor is it an inclusion term in the tabular list for a particular code (e.g., Encephalopathy due to significant burns, multifactorial).

Key Terms

Key terms found in the documentation may include:

Encephalopathy due to (specified; does not fit into any of the index classifications)

CDI ALERT

When a cause cannot be identified, then G93.4Ø Encephalopathy, unspecified, will be reported. When a type of encephalopathy is identified or specified, but does not fit into any of the classifications, G93.49 Other encephalopathy, Encephalopathy NEC, would be reported.

Encephalopathy, unspecified (G93.4Ø)

This code should rarely be reported. Documentation within the record should provide information with which clarification can be queried for specificity.

First Listed Diagnosis Note

Admit for acute mental status changes with a final diagnosis of encephalopathy due to unknown cause: Patient was transferred to another acute care facility for further diagnostic evaluation and treatment. In this case, G93.4Ø Encephalopathy, unspecified, would be reported as the first listed diagnosis.

CDI ALERT

The term encephalopathy is vague, and should generally be preceded by terminology describing the reason, cause, or medical condition of the patient that led to the brain disease or malfunction.

Clinical Findings

Physical Examination

History and review of systems may include:

- Altered mental status
- Dementia
- Seizures
- Tremors
- Muscle twitching
- Poor coordination

Diagnostic Procedures and Services

- Laboratory
  - complete blood count
  - electrolyte level
  - ammonia
  - glucose
  - liver functions
  - drug screening
  - lead level

- blood cultures
- creatinine
- Imaging
  - head CT
  - head MRI
  - Doppler ultrasound
- Other
  - EEG

Clinician Note

For more precise documentation and correct coding, the clinician should make a clinical distinction between encephalopathy and delirium. The diagnostic term encephalopathy is preferred for describing mental status alteration when it is due to toxic or metabolic states. The term delirium is usually classified as a mental disorder or a symptom and is more appropriately documented in psychiatric conditions unrelated to underlying systemic conditions.

Clinician Documentation Checklist

Clinician documentation should indicate the following:

- Other disorders of brain
  - anoxic brain damage
  - toxic encephalopathy
    - includes:
      - toxic encephalitis
      - toxic metabolic encephalopathy
    - identification of the toxic agent
  - benign intracranial hypertension
  - postviral fatigue syndrome
    - benign myalgic encephalomyelitis
  - other and unspecified encephalopathy
    - metabolic encephalopathy
      - septic encephalopathy
    - other encephalopathy
    - unspecified encephalopathy
  - compression of brain
    - Arnold-Chiari type 1 compression of brain
    - compression of brain (stem)
    - herniation of brain (stem)
  - cerebral edema
  - Reye's syndrome
    - also identification of, if salicylates-induced

- other specified disorders of brain
  - temporal sclerosis
    - hippocampal sclerosis
    - mesial temporal sclerosis
  - brain death
  - other disorders of brain
    - postradiation encephalopathy
- unspecified disorder of brain

- Other disorders of brain in diseases
  - the underlying disease

Endoscopy — Lower GI

Code Axes

Colonoscopy	**45378–45398** QPP
Flexible sigmoidoscopy	**45330–45350**

Description of Procedure

These codes represent the examination of the colon by flexible fiberoptic endoscope. Since code selection is based upon the portion of the intestine being examined as well as any other services and procedures performed during the surgical encounter, it is critical that the documentation be clear and complete. As with any other endoscopic procedures, this procedure can be performed for either diagnostic or therapeutic purposes.

A flexible sigmoidoscopy is reported when the documentation indicates that the provider examined only the lower one third of the intestine and documentation does not include notation that the splenic flexure was examined. Report a colonoscopy when the entire colon, including the cecum is examined according to the documentation. When the documentation does not indicate that the cecum is examined, report the appropriate colonoscopy code with modifier 52 Reduced services.

Clinical Tip

Control of bleeding that is the result of a biopsy or polypectomy is considered part of the main service and is not reported separately; however, it should be clearly documented.

Key Terms

Key terms found in the documentation may include:

Colo
Colo with bx
Colo w/polypectomy
Flex sig
Flex sig w/bx
Flex sig w/polypectomy

Clinician Documentation Checklist

Clinician documentation should indicate the following:

- Type of sedation provided
- Quality of bowel preparation
- Clearly indicate the anatomical structures examined
  - colonoscopy
    - examination of cecum or terminal ileum (or small bowel proximal to an anastomosis)

  - sigmoidoscopy
    - examination of sigmoid colon (may include a portion of descending colon)
- The medical condition being treated
- Flexible sigmoidoscopy
  - biopsy
  - removal of foreign body
  - removal of tumor
  - control of bleeding
  - submucosal injection
  - decompression
  - snare technique used
  - ablation
  - balloon dilation
  - ultrasound examination
  - fine needle aspiration
  - placement of stent
  - band ligation
- Colonoscopy
  - removal of foreign body
  - biopsy
  - mucosal injection
  - control of bleeding
  - ablation
  - removal of tumor-hot biopsy forceps
  - removal of tumor-snare technique
  - balloon dilation
  - stent placement
  - ultrasound
  - fine needle aspiration
  - decompression
  - band ligation
- Summary of findings and recommendations

Endoscopy — Upper GI

Code Axes

Esophagoscopy	**43180–43232**
Esophagogastroduodenoscopy	**43233–43259, 43266, 43270**

Description of Procedure

These codes represent the examination of the esophagus and stomach by endoscope. Code selection is dependent upon the anatomical structures examined.

An esophagoscopy is the examination of the stomach with either a rigid or flexible endoscope. Documentation should indicate that the esophagus from the cricopharyngeus muscle to gastroesophageal junction was visualized. When the documentation indicates that the esophagus, stomach, duodenum, and/or jejunum are visualized, an esophagogastroduodenoscopy is supported.

Like other endoscopic procedures, these can be performed for either diagnostic or therapeutic reasons. The table below helps identify key terms in the documentation and cross-walks to the code that is supported by those terms.

Physician documentation should include the following key terms as they apply in order to determine correct code assignment.

Key Term	Esophagus Only	EGD
Brushing and washings	43191, 43197, 43200	43235
Submucosal injections	43192, 43201	43236
Biopsy	43193, 43198, 43202	43239
Diverticulectomy	43180	
Injection varices	43204	43243
Band varices	43205	43244
Foreign body removal	43194, 43215	43247
Lesion removal or destruction		
hot biopsy or bipolar	43216	43250
snare	43217	43251
ablation	43229	43270
Insertion		
tube or stent	43212	43266
intraluminal tube or catheter		43241
Percutaneous gastrostomy tube		43246

Key Term	Esophagus Only	EGD
Dilation		
balloon less than 30 mm	43195, 43220	43249
balloon greater than 30 mm	43214	43233
balloon or dilator, retrograde		43213
over guidewire	43196, 43226	43248
gastric/duodenal stricture		43245
Control of bleeding	43227	43255
Ultrasound examination		
intramural or transmural fine needle aspiration/biopsy	43232	43238, 43242
transmural injection of diagnostic or therapeutic substance		43253
esophagus only	43231	
esophagus, stomach or duodenum, and adjacent structures		43237
esophagus, stomach and either duodenum or jejunum distal to anastomosis of surgical altered stomach		43259
Drainage of pseudocyst		43240
Mucosal resection	43211	43254
Optical endomicroscopy	43206	43252
Thermal energy for gastroesophageal reflux		43257
Esophagogastric fundoplasty		43210

Key Terms

Key terms found in the documentation may include:

EGD

Esophagoscopy

Clinician Documentation Checklist

Clinician documentation should indicate the following:

- The medical condition being treated
- The type of sedation including medications
- The anatomical structures examined including esophagus (cricopharyngeus muscle [upper esophageal sphincter]), the stomach, and the duodenum. If duodenum is not deliberately examined, the clinical reason should be described.
  - washings
  - biopsy
  - ultrasound examination and aspiration, etc. performed
  - removal of foreign body
  - destruction of lesion including instrumentation used
  - control of bleeding
  - injection varices

- insertion of tube, stent or intraluminal tube or catheter
- placement of percutaneous gastrostomy tube
- dilation including type of instrumentation
- drainage of pseudocyst
- mucosal resection
- optical endomicroscopy
- thermal energy
- esophagogastric fundoplasty

- Summary of findings and recommendations

Epilepsy and Recurrent Seizures

Code Axes

Localization-related (focal) (partial) idiopathic epilepsy and epileptic syndromes with seizures of localized onset	**G40.0-** HCC
Localization-related (focal) (partial) symptomatic epilepsy and epileptic syndromes with simple partial seizures	**G40.1-** HCC QPP
Localization-related (focal) (partial) symptomatic epilepsy and epileptic syndromes with complex partial seizures	**G40.2-** HCC QPP
Generalized idiopathic epilepsy and epileptic syndromes	**G40.3-** HCC QPP
Absence epileptic syndrome	**G40.A-** HCC QPP
Juvenile myoclonic epilepsy (impulsive petit mal)	**G40.B-** HCC
Other generalized epilepsy and epileptic syndromes	**G40.4-** HCC
Epileptic seizures related to external causes	**G40.5-** HCC
Other epilepsy and recurrent seizures	**G40.8-** HCC QPP
Epilepsy, unspecified	**G40.9-** HCC **G40.909** HCC QPP **G40.911** HCC **G40.919** HCC

⇨ I-10 Alert

There is an additional classification axis for the presence of status epilepticus. Sixth characters are found throughout the subcategory representing this condition.

Clinical Tip

The following definitions should be used for all subclassifications related to epilepsy and epileptic syndromes:

Status epilepticus: Typically defined as one continuous, unremitting seizure lasting longer than 30 minutes, or recurrent seizures without regaining consciousness between seizures for greater than 30 minutes. The condition is always considered a medical emergency.

Intractable epilepsy: There is not a universal definition for this complication, but it appears that most agree that a definition of drug-resistant epilepsy is a failure of adequate trials of two tolerated and appropriately chosen and used antiepileptic drug (AED) schedules.

CDI Alert

Ensure that not only is the type of epilepsy or recurrent seizure documented, but that the details related to status epilepticus and intractable epilepsy are also present in the medical record.

Key Terms

Key terms found in the documentation for intractable epilepsy may include:

- Focal epilepsy
- Pharmacoresistant (pharmacologically) resistant epilepsy
- Poorly controlled epilepsy
- Refractory (medically) epilepsy
- Treatment resistant epilepsy

Description of Condition

Localization-related (focal) (partial) idiopathic epilepsy and epileptic syndromes with seizures of localized onset (G4Ø.Ø-)

Clinical Tip

Localization-related epilepsy also referred to as a focal or partial syndrome, is either symptomatic (i.e., the cause is known) or cryptogenic, which means there is a presumed focal structural cause that cannot be identified historically or be seen with current imaging techniques. Localization-related epilepsy arises from an epileptic focus, a small portion of the brain that serves as the irritant driving the epileptic response.

Key Terms

Key terms found in the documentation for localization-related epilepsy may include:

Benign childhood epilepsy with centrotemporal EEG spikes

Childhood epilepsy with occipital EEG paroxysms

Localization-related idiopathic epilepsy and epileptic syndromes with seizures of localized onset

Clinician Note

Many types of procedures are used to treat specific forms of epilepsy. For example, vagus nerve stimulation and stereotaxic depth electrode implantation are used to treat focal epilepsy. However, medical necessity must be clearly indicated by the type of epilepsy the patient has. Careful attention to the documentation indicating the specific type of epilepsy is, therefore, crucial in supporting the medical necessity of these procedures.

Localization-related (focal) (partial) symptomatic epilepsy and epileptic syndromes with simple partial seizures (G4Ø.1-)

Clinical Tip

Simple partial seizures (SPS) are those that are not associated with any impairment of consciousness. The seizures may also include experiences of unusual feelings or sensations.

Key Terms

Key terms found in the documentation for localization-related epilepsy with simple partial seizures may include:

Attacks without alteration of consciousness

Epilepsia partialis continua [Kozhevnikov]

Simple partial seizures developing into secondarily generalized seizures

Clinician Note

Many types of procedures are used to treat specific forms of epilepsy. For example, vagus nerve stimulation and stereotaxic depth electrode implantation are used to treat focal epilepsy. However, medical necessity must be clearly indicated by the type of epilepsy the patient has. Careful attention to the documentation indicating the specific type of epilepsy is, therefore, crucial in supporting the medical necessity of these procedures.

Localization-related (focal) (partial) symptomatic epilepsy and epileptic syndromes with complex partial seizures (G40.2-)

Clinical Tip

Complex partial seizures (CPS) usually start in a small area of the temporal lobe or frontal lobe of the brain, but quickly involve other areas of the brain that affect alertness and awareness. Some CPS seizures (typically starting in the temporal lobe) begin with a simple partial seizure. Also called an aura, this warning seizure often includes an odd feeling in the stomach. Then the person loses awareness and stares blankly. Complex partial seizures starting in the frontal lobe tend to be shorter and are also more likely to include automatisms like bicycling movements of the legs or pelvic thrusting.

Key Terms

Key terms found in the documentation for localization-related epilepsy with complex partial seizures may include:

Attacks with alteration of consciousness, often with automatisms

Complex partial seizures developing into secondarily generalized seizures

Clinician Note

Many types of procedures are used to treat specific forms of epilepsy. For example, vagus nerve stimulation and stereotaxic depth electrode implantation are used to treat focal epilepsy. However, medical necessity must be clearly indicated by the type of epilepsy the patient has. Careful attention to the documentation indicating the specific type of epilepsy is, therefore, crucial in supporting the medical necessity of these procedures.

CDI ALERT

MERRF (Myoclonic epilepsy with ragged-red fibers) syndrome (E88.42) is related to this (G40.3) classification subcategory. If present in the medical record, it should clearly be documented as a part of the epilepsy classification.

Generalized idiopathic epilepsy and epileptic syndromes (G40.3-)

Clinical Tip

Generalized epilepsies arise from many independent foci (multifocal epilepsies) or from epileptic circuits that involve the whole brain. One third of all epilepsies are classified as idiopathic generalized epilepsy (IGE), which are genetically determined and affect otherwise normal people of both sexes and all races. They involve typical absences, myoclonic jerks, and generalized tonic-clonic seizures, alone or in varying combinations and severity. The condition is usually life-long, although some are age-related. A major advance in recent epileptology is the recognition of different epileptic syndromes that allows an accurate diagnosis and management of seizure disorders. This is important because the short- and long-term treatment strategies are entirely different for each disorder.

Clinician Note
Many types of procedures are used to treat specific forms of epilepsy. For example, vagus nerve stimulation and stereotaxic depth electrode implantation are used to treat focal epilepsy. However, medical necessity must be clearly indicated by the type of epilepsy the patient has. Careful attention to the documentation indicating the specific type of epilepsy is, therefore, crucial in supporting the medical necessity of these procedures.

Absence epileptic syndrome (G4Ø.A-)

Clinical Tip
This condition is idiopathic generalized epilepsy that affects children between the ages of 10 and 17 years of age, typically beginning at or near puberty. It involves recurrent absence seizures, which are brief episodes of unresponsive staring, sometimes with minor motor features such as eye blinking or subtle chewing. Some patients go on to develop generalized tonic-clonic seizures, but for some, the prognosis is favorable with no decline in cognition or any other neurological defects, and the seizures spontaneously cease with age.

Key Terms
Key terms found in the documentation for absence epileptic syndrome may include:

Absence epileptic syndrome

Childhood absence epilepsy (pyknolepsy)

Juvenile absence epilepsy

Clinician Note
Many types of procedures are used to treat specific forms of epilepsy. For example, vagus nerve stimulation and stereotaxic depth electrode implantation are used to treat focal epilepsy. However, medical necessity must be clearly indicated by the type of epilepsy the patient has. Careful attention to the documentation indicating the specific type of epilepsy is, therefore, crucial in supporting the medical necessity of these procedures.

Juvenile myoclonic epilepsy (impulsive petit mal) (G4Ø.B-)

Clinical Tip
This condition involves idiopathic generalized epilepsy that develops in patients aged 8 to 20 years and continues for the rest of their lives. Patients have normal cognition and are otherwise neurologically intact. Myoclonic jerks (quick little jerks of the arms, shoulder, or occasionally the legs) are the most common type of seizure, although generalized tonic-clonic seizures and absence seizures may occur as well. Sleep deprivation is a common triggering mechanism for this type of seizure.

Key Terms

Key terms found in the documentation for juvenile myoclonic epilepsy may include:

Janz syndrome

Clinician Note

Many types of procedures are used to treat specific forms of epilepsy. For example, vagus nerve stimulation and stereotaxic depth electrode implantation are used to treat focal epilepsy. However, medical necessity must be clearly indicated by the type of epilepsy the patient has. Careful attention to the documentation indicating the specific type of epilepsy is, therefore, crucial in supporting the medical necessity of these procedures.

Other generalized epilepsy and epileptic syndromes (G4Ø.4-)

Clinical Tip

Generalized epilepsies arise from many independent foci (multifocal epilepsies) or from epileptic circuits that involve the whole brain.

Key Terms

Key terms found in the documentation for other generalized epilepsy and epileptic syndromes may include:

Epilepsy with grand mal seizures on awakening
Epilepsy with myoclonic absences
Epilepsy with myoclonic-astatic seizures
Doose syndrome epilepsy
Drop attacks
Grand mal seizure NOS
MAE
Nonspecific atonic epileptic seizures
Nonspecific clonic epileptic seizures
Nonspecific myoclonic epileptic seizures
Nonspecific tonic epileptic seizures
Nonspecific tonic-clonic epileptic seizures
Symptomatic early myoclonic encephalopathy

Clinician Note

Many types of procedures are used to treat specific forms of epilepsy. For example, vagus nerve stimulation and stereotaxic depth electrode implantation are used to treat focal epilepsy. However, medical necessity must be clearly indicated by the type of epilepsy the patient has. Careful attention to the documentation indicating the specific type of epilepsy is, therefore, crucial in supporting the medical necessity of these procedures.

Epileptic seizures related to external causes (G40.5-)

Clinical Tip

Seizures may be caused by an exposure to several external causes, such as lead or carbon monoxide, or from alcohol or drugs taken internally, such as antidepressants. The seizure disorder may also be triggered by environmental factors, such as stress, lack of sleep, or hormonal changes related to the menstrual cycle. In some patients, lights flashing at a certain speed can trigger seizures.

Key Terms

Key terms found in the documentation for epileptic seizures related to external causes may include:

Epileptic seizures related to alcohol

Epileptic seizures related to drugs

Epileptic seizures related to hormonal changes

Epileptic seizures related to sleep deprivation

Epileptic seizures related to stress

> **⇨ I-10 ALERT**
>
> Combination codes are available in ICD-10-CM that indicate seizure activity due to a number of external causes. These codes are differentiated by the presence of intractability and status epilepticus as are the other codes in the epilepsy subcategories. Additional codes should be assigned for drug adverse effects, and to clearly classify the type of epilepsy, if documented.

Other epilepsy and recurrent seizures (G40.8-)

Clinical Tip

Lennox-Gastaut syndrome is a generalized epilepsy that is characterized by a developmental delay or childhood dementia, mixed generalized seizures, and EEG demonstrating a pattern of approximately 2 Hz "slow" spike-wave. Onset typically occurs between the ages of 2 and 18, and different types of seizures may be associated with the condition, such as astatic seizures (drop attacks), tonic seizures, tonic-clonic seizures, atypical absence seizures, and sometimes, complex partial seizures.

West's syndrome is a rare epileptic disorder that affects infants, with a triad of infantile spasms, a characteristic EEG pattern called hypsarrhythmia, and developmental regression. Patients are generally between the third and the twelfth month of age, most often around five months of age. The syndrome is typically caused by an organic brain dysfunction whose origins may be prenatal, perinatal (caused during birth), or postnatal.

Landau–Kleffner syndrome (LKS) is a neurological syndrome that involves the sudden or gradual development of aphasia (the inability to understand or express language) and an abnormal electroencephalogram (EEG). Patients are typically between the ages of 3 and 7 years old and because this syndrome appears during such a critical period of language acquisition in a child's life, speech production may be affected just as severely as language comprehension.

Key Terms

Key terms found in the documentation for Lennox-Gastaut syndrome may include:

Lennox syndrome

> **⇨ I-10 ALERT**
>
> This is a residual subcategory that includes all types of epileptic seizures that are not included in the previous subcategories in G40.-. Also included here are epilepsies and epileptic syndromes that are undetermined as to whether they are focal or generalized.

Key terms found in the documentation for West's syndrome may include:

Epileptic spasms

Generalized flexion epilepsy

Infantile epileptic encephalopathy

Infantile myoclonic encephalopathy

Infantile spasms

Jackknife convulsions

Massive myoclonia

Salaam spasms or attacks

Key terms found in the documentation for Landau–Kleffner syndrome may include:

Acquired epileptic aphasia

Aphasia with convulsive disorder

Infantile acquired aphasia

Clinical Findings

Physical Examination

The history and review of systems may include:

- Seizures
  - Bitten tongue
  - Incontinence
  - Lost consciousness
- Generalized seizures
  - followed by postictal state

Clinical indicators on physical examination that may indicate the cause of a seizure include:

- Fever and stiff neck
- Papilledema
- Asymmetry of muscle strength
- Hyperreflexia
- Skin lesions

Diagnostic Procedures and Services

- Laboratory
  - glucose
  - BUN
  - electrolytes
  - creatinine
  - liver function
- Imaging
  - head CT

  - head MRI
- Other
  - EEG

Clinician Note
Many types of procedures are used to treat specific forms of epilepsy. For example, vagus nerve stimulation and stereotaxic depth electrode implantation are used to treat focal epilepsy. However, medical necessity must be clearly indicated by the type of epilepsy the patient has. Careful attention to the documentation indicating the specific type of epilepsy is, therefore, crucial in supporting the medical necessity of these procedures.

Medication List
If the cause of the seizure cannot be identified or altered, anticonvulsants may be required. In many cases medication may be withheld until a second seizure occurs, particularly in children. However, for acute seizures and status epilepticus with most seizures lasting > 5 minutes, medication is required to stop the seizures.

- Anticonvulsant
  - benzodiazepines (Clonazepam, Diazepam, Klonopin)
  - carbamazepine (Carbatrol, Tegretol)
  - divalproex (Depakote)
  - ezogabine (Potiga)
  - fosphenytoin (Cerebyx)
  - gabapentin (Neurontin)
  - lamotrigine (Lamictal)
  - levetiracetam (Keppra)
  - phenytoin (Dilantin)
  - pregabalin (Lyrica)
  - vigabatrin (Sabril)

Clinician Documentation Checklist

Clinician documentation should indicate the following:

- Type
  - localization-related (focal) (partial) idiopathic epilepsy and epileptic syndromes with seizures of localized onset
    - includes
      - ♦ benign childhood epilepsy with centrotemporal EEG spikes
      - ♦ childhood epilepsy with occipital EEG paroxysms
  - localization-related (focal) (partial) symptomatic epilepsy and epileptic syndromes with simple partial seizures
    - includes
      - ♦ attacks without alteration of consciousness
      - ♦ epilepsia partialis continua (Kozhevnikov)

- simple partial seizures developing into secondarily generalized seizures
- Bravais Jacksonian epilepsy

- localization-related (focal) (partial) symptomatic epilepsy and epileptic syndromes with complex partial seizures
  - includes
    - attacks with alteration of consciousness, often with automatisms
    - complex partial seizures developing into secondarily generalized seizures
- generalized idiopathic epilepsy and epileptic syndromes
  - MERRF (myoclonic epilepsy with ragged red fibers) syndrome, if applicable
- absence epileptic syndrome
  - includes
    - childhood absence epilepsy (pyknolepsy)
    - juvenile absence epilepsy
- Juvenile myoclonic epilepsy (impulsive petit mal)
- other generalized epilepsy and epileptic syndromes
  - includes
    - epilepsy with grand mal seizures on awakening
    - epilepsy with myoclonic absences
    - epilepsy with myoclonic-astatic seizures
    - grand mal seizure
    - nonspecific atonic epileptic seizures
    - nonspecific clonic epileptic seizures
    - nonspecific myoclonic epileptic seizures
    - nonspecific tonic epileptic seizures
    - nonspecific tonic-clonic epileptic seizures
    - symptomatic early myoclonic encephalopathy
- epileptic seizures related to external causes
  - associated epilepsy and recurrent seizures
  - includes
    - epileptic seizures related to alcohol
    - epileptic seizures related to drug
      - identify the drug
    - epileptic seizures related to hormonal changes
    - epileptic seizures related to sleep deprivation
    - epileptic seizures related to stress
- other specified epilepsy and recurrent seizures
  - includes
    - epilepsies and epileptic syndromes undetermined as to whether they are focal or generalized

        - Landau-Kleffner syndrome
        - infant benign myoclonic epilepsy
    - subtype
        - Lennox-Gastaut syndrome
        - epileptic spasms
            - infantile spasms
            - salaam attacks
            - West's syndrome
        - other epilepsy
        - other seizures
  - unspecified epilepsy
- Identification of the above type of epilepsy and seizures as:
  - not intractable
  - intractable
    - includes
      - pharmacoresistant (pharmacologically resistant)
      - treatment resistant
      - refractory (medically)
      - poorly controlled
  - with status epilepticus
  - without status epilepticus

Esophagitis

Code Axes

Esophagitis **K2Ø.-, K21.Ø HCC**

Description of Condition

Esophagitis is an inflammation, irritation or swelling of the esophagus. Causes include esophageal reflux, autoimmune disorder, radiation or chemotherapy, medications, and/or ingestion of caustic agents.

Eosinophilic esophagitis (K2Ø.Ø)

Eosinophilic esophagitis is an increasingly recognized disease with typical onset any time between infancy and young adulthood. It is a chronic autoimmune disease that results in eosinophil-predominant inflammation of the esophagus that may cause reflux-like symptoms, food impaction, and the inability to swallow.

Clinical Tip

Eosinophilic esophagitis is often considered when gastro-esophageal reflux symptoms do not respond to acid-suppression therapy.

Other and unspecified esophagitis (K2Ø.8, K2Ø.9)

Clinical Tip

Other esophagitis includes inflammation and swelling of the esophagus due to an infection that has resulted in an abscess formation

Esophagitis, unspecified

Esophagitis NOS includes chemical, necrotic, chronic, and postoperative esophagitis. Although relatively rare, it also includes esophagitis caused by infection.

Gastro-esophageal reflux disease with esophagitis (K21.Ø)

The development of esophagitis in patients with gastroesophageal reflux disease (GERD) may be attributed to some of the following factors; the lack of ability to clear the refluxate from the esophagus, the volume of gastric contents, the corrosive nature of the refluxate, and local mucosal protective functions.

Clinical Tip

Esophagitis may cause severe pain when swallowing and even esophageal bleeding, which is typically occult but can be massive.

Key Terms

Key terms found in the documentation may include:

Abscess of esophagus

Esophagitis NOS

Reflux esophagitis

Clinical Findings

Physical Examination

History and review of systems may include:

- Cough
- Dysphagia
- Heartburn
  - while lying down
  - when bending over
- Hematemesis
- Hoarseness
- Midsternal or substernal pain or pressure
- Painful swallowing
- Wheezing

Diagnostic Procedures and Services

- Imaging
  - Bernstein test
  - esophageal manometry
  - esophagoscopy with or without biopsy
  - upper GI series

Therapeutic Procedures and Services

- Surgical
  - fundoplication procedure
- Other
  - elevate head of the bed
  - eliminate certain food and beverages that exacerbate reflux
  - smoking cessation

Medication List

- Antacids to neutralize stomach acids
  - calcium carbonate (Maalox, Tums)
  - calcium carbonate and magnesium hydroxide (Mylanta, Rolaids)
  - magnesium hydroxide (milk of magnesia)
  - sodium bicarbonate (Alka-Seltzer)
- Histamine -2 blockers to decrease gastric acid production
  - anitidine (Zantac)

  - cimetidine (Tagamet)
  - famotidine (Pepcid)
  - nizatidine (Axid)
- Proton pump inhibitors to prevent gastric acid secretion
  - omeprazole (Prilosec)
  - lansoprazole (Prevacid)
  - rabeprazole sodium (AcipHex)
  - pantoprazole (Protonix)
  - esomeprazole magnesium (Nexium)

Antibiotics, antifungals, and antivirals may also be used when the esophagitis is caused by bacteria, yeast, or other infection.

Clinician Documentation Checklist

Clinician documentation should indicate the following:

- Identify risk factors
  - alcohol abuse
  - alcohol dependence
  - cigarette use
  - medication without drinking appropriate amount of water
    - doxycycline
    - tetracycline
    - potassium
    - vitamin C
  - surgery or radiation to the chest
  - vomiting
- Type
  - eosinophilic esophagitis
  - other esophagitis
    - abscess of esophagus
  - reflux esophagitis

Facet Joint Injections

Code Axes

Injection(s), diagnostic or therapeutic agent, paravertebral facet (zygapophyseal) joint (or nerves innervating that joint) with image guidance (fluoroscopy or CT), cervical or thoracic	**64490–64492**
Injection(s), diagnostic or therapeutic agent, paravertebral facet (zygapophyseal) joint (or nerves innervating that joint) with image guidance (fluoroscopy or CT), lumbar or sacral	**64493–64495**

CDI ALERT

The documentation should be carefully reviewed to determine what exact procedures were performed. There are times when the procedure performed listed at the beginning of the operative report will not be the actual procedure described in the body of the report.

Description of Procedure

Facet joint injections should be reported using the appropriate codes from range 64490–64495. Correct code selection is dependent upon:

- Level of the spine injected
- Number of levels reported
- Whether the service was performed unilaterally or bilaterally

Single level: A single level injection occurs when the physician administers one or more substances to a level using one or more needles. A physician may insert a needle and attach a small tube through which the first substance is administered via a syringe. The physician may then change out the syringe and administer a second substance. However, only one needle puncture is performed.

In another method, the physician inserts the needle, administers a substance, and then removes the needle and makes a second puncture with a new needle and syringe to administer an additional substance. Despite the fact that there are two puncture sites, only a single level is being treated.

Multiple levels: When the physician documentation clearly indicates that multiple levels of the spine were injected, add-on codes 64491–64492 and 64494–64495, respectively, are reported.

Bilateral injections: Modifier 50 should be appended when the documentation states that injections were made on the same level but on different sides. Add-on codes 64491–64492 or 64494–64495 are not appropriate when the documentation indicates that the injections were performed bilaterally.

Anesthetic/steroids: Examine the documentation for the name and dosage of the anesthetic agent and/or steroid agent administered. List the appropriate HCPCS Level II code separately.

Clinician Note

Documentation must indicate if the procedure was performed unilaterally or bilaterally. This supports the use of modifier 50 when documentation indicates that the injection was performed bilaterally.

CDI ALERT

Medical record documentation should contain information regarding the preoperative evaluation leading to suspicion of the presence of facet joint pathology, as well as the provider's postoperative conclusions. In addition, the anatomical area of the spine and the exact location of the injection site should be clearly notated, as well as the specific name and dosage of the anesthetic agent and/or steroid administered.

Clinical Tip

Medicare considers facet joint blocks to be reasonable and necessary for chronic pain (persistent pain for three (3) months or greater) suspected to originate from the facet joint. Facet joint block is one of the methods used to document/confirm suspicions of posterior element biomechanical pain of the spine. Hallmarks of posterior element biomechanical pain are as follows:

- The pain does not have a strong radicular component.
- There is no associated neurological deficit and the pain is aggravated by hyperextension, rotation, or lateral bending of the spine, depending on the orientation of the facet joint at that level.
- A paravertebral facet joint represents the articulation of the posterior elements of one vertebra with its neighboring vertebrae; it is further noted that there are two (2) facet joints at each level, left and right.

During a paravertebral facet joint block procedure, a needle is placed in the facet joint or along the medial branches that innervate the joints under fluoroscopic guidance and a local anesthetic and/or steroid is injected. After the injection(s) has been performed, the patient is asked to indulge in the activities that usually aggravate his/her pain and to record his/her impressions of the effect of the procedure. Temporary or prolonged abolition of the pain suggests that the facet joints are the source of the symptoms and appropriate treatment may be prescribed in the future. Some patients have long-lasting relief with local anesthetic and steroid; others require a denervation procedure for more permanent relief. Before proceeding to a denervation treatment, the patient should experience at least a 50 percent reduction in symptoms for the duration of the local anesthetic effect.

Diagnostic or therapeutic injections/nerve blocks may be required for the management of chronic pain. It may take multiple nerve blocks targeting different anatomic structures to establish the etiology of the chronic pain in a given patient. It is standard medical practice to use the modality most likely to establish the diagnosis or treat the presumptive diagnosis. If the first set of procedures fails to produce the desired effect or to rule out the diagnosis, the provider should proceed to the next logical test or treatment indicated. For the purpose of this paravertebral facet joint block, an anatomic region is defined per CPT as cervical/thoracic (64490, 64491, 64492) or lumbar/sacral (64493, 64494, 64495).

Clinician Documentation Checklist

Clinician documentation should indicate the following:

- Medical condition being treated
- Anatomic region
  - cervical/thoracic
  - lumbar/sacral
- Exact location of the injection
- Name and dosage of medication
  - anesthetic agent
  - steroid administered

- Level of spine injected
  - single level
  - second level
  - third or additional levels
- Number of levels injected
  - single
  - multiple
- Laterality
  - unilateral
  - bilateral
- Imaging guidance
  - fluoroscopy
  - CT

Foodborne Intoxication and Infection

Code Axes

ICD-10-CM codes for bacterial foodborne intoxication (i.e., bacterial food poisoning) are located in category AØ5 with the exceptions of *Clostridium difficile* (AØ4.7), *E. coli* (AØ4.Ø-4), *Salmonella* with gastroenteritis (AØ2.Ø), listeriosis (A32.89) and *Norovirus* enteritis (AØ8.11).

Salmonella with gastroenteritis	**AØ2.Ø**
E. coli intestinal infection	**AØ4.[Ø-4]**
Campylobacter enteritis	**AØ4.5**
Clostridium difficile enterocolitis	**AØ4.7[1,2]**
Bacterial foodborne intoxication	**AØ5.[Ø-5, 8]**
Unspecified bacterial foodborne intoxication	**AØ5.9**
Other form of Listeriosis	**A32.89**
Norovirus enteritis	**AØ8.11**

⇨ I-10 ALERT

ICD-10-CM includes a new concept in category AØ5: bacterial foodborne intoxications. A foodborne intoxication involves a toxin caused by a microorganism in the food causing the illness. There are eight codes for foodborne intoxications in ICD-10-CM, differentiated by toxin.

Description of Condition

Food poisoning is foodborne infection, intoxication or toxin-mediated infection due to ingested bacterium that produces toxins or virus or parasite which causes intestinal illness (dysentery). The food or water is either contaminated externally (e.g., Salmonella) or the bacterium is present in the food and produces an exotoxin as a byproduct (e.g., Botulism).

(AØ5) Other bacterial foodborne intoxications, not elsewhere classified, including that due to staphylococcal intoxication (AØ5.Ø), botulism food poisoning (AØ5.1), foodborne Clostridium perfringens intoxication (AØ5.2), Vibrio parahaemolyticus intoxication (AØ5.3), Bacillus cereus intoxication (AØ5.4), Vibrio vulnificus intoxication (AØ5.5), and other and unspecified foodborne intoxications (AØ5.8, AØ5.9)

Toxins are produced by harmful microorganisms, the result of a chemical contamination, or are naturally part of a plant or seafood. When these toxins are ingested and invade the gastrointestinal tract, they are considered bacterial foodborne intoxications. Viruses and parasites do not cause foodborne intoxications.

Key Terms

Key terms found in the documentation may include:

Botulism (AØ5.1)

Classical foodborne intoxication due to *Clostridium botulinum* (AØ5.1)

Enteritis necroticans (AØ5.2)

Pig-bel (AØ5.2)

(AØ2.Ø) Salmonella enteritis, (AØ4.[Ø-4]) E. coli intestinal infection, (AØ4.5) Campylobacter enteritis, (AØ4.7[1,2]) Clostridium difficile enterocolitis, (A32.89) Other forms of Listeriosis, and (AØ8.11) Norovirus enteritis represents foodborne intoxications

Key Terms

Key terms found in the documentation may include:

C difficile enterocolitis

E. coli (EHEC)

E. coli (EIEC) (EPEC) (ETEC) (EAEC/EAgEC)

(STEC) other Shiga toxin producing *E. coli*

Clinical Findings

The following clinical information may primarily be found in *E. coli* and *Salmonella.*

Physical Examination

History and review of systems may include:

- Copious, watery diarrhea
- Fever
- Ingestion of potentially tainted food
- Contact with an ill person
- GI bleeding with little stool

Diagnostic Procedures and Services

- Laboratory
  - stool culture
  - blood culture
  - serum electrolytes
  - BUN
  - creatinine

Therapeutic Procedures and Services

- Oral or IV hydration

Medication List

- Antidiarrheal medication, if appropriate
- Antiemetics
- Antibiotics, if appropriate
  - azithromycin
  - ceftriaxone (Rocephin)
  - ciprofloxacin (Cipro)

Clinician Documentation Checklist

Clinician documentation should indicate the following:

- Listeriosis
  - cutaneous
  - meningitis
  - meningoencephalitis
  - sepsis
  - oculoglandular
  - endocarditis

Fracture Care

Code Axes

Fracture care codes are contained in the musculoskeletal subsection of the CPT® manual and are classified according to the anatomical location.

Description of Procedure

There are numerous types of fracture care. Clear and concise documentation is required for the procedures to be reported appropriately. Codes are categorized by the type of reduction and the method of stabilization (fixation or immobilization) and may be either open or closed.

Documentation for fractures should include the type and location of the fracture performed to correct it, including percutaneous skeletal fixation when applicable.

It should be noted that careful documentation is required as it is sometimes difficult to differentiate between the type of fracture and the type of treatment. For example, a closed fracture may require closed or open treatment while an open fracture requires open treatment. When documenting fracture care include:

- The site of the fracture
- If the treatment was open or closed
- If manipulation was performed (reduction)
- Type of fixation if any

Key Terms

Manipulation

Open treatment

Percutaneous fixation

Reduction

Skeletal traction

Clinician Note

Terms such as open, closed, pins, or wires provide the guidance needed to ensure correct code assignment.

CDI ALERT

Internal fixation involves wires, pins, screws, and plates placed through the skin or within the fractured area to stabilize and immobilize the injury. It is often described as open reduction with internal fixation (ORIF).

Fracture of Femur

Code Axes

Fracture of unspecified part of neck of femur **S72.ØØ-** HCC

Unspecified intracapsular fracture of femur **S72.Ø1-** HCC

Fracture of epiphysis (separation) (upper) of femur **S72.Ø2-** HCC
(Displaced and non-displaced)

Midcervical fracture of femur **S72.Ø3-** HCC
(Displaced and non-displaced)

Fracture of base of neck of femur **S72.Ø4-** HCC
(Displaced and non-displaced)

Unspecified fracture of head of femur **S72.Ø5-** HCC

Articular fracture of head of femur **S72.Ø6-** HCC
(Displaced and non-displaced)

Other fracture of head and neck of femur **S72.Ø9-** HCC

Unspecified trochanteric fracture of femur **S72.1Ø-** HCC

Fracture of greater trochanter of femur **S72.11-** HCC
(Displaced and non-displaced)

Fracture of lesser trochanter of femur **S72.12-** HCC
(Displaced and non-displaced)

Apophyseal fracture of femur **S72.13-** HCC
(Displaced and non-displaced)

Intertrochanteric fracture of femur **S72.14-** HCC
(Displaced and non-displaced)

Subtrochanteric fracture of femur **S72.2-** HCC
(Displaced and non-displaced)

⇨ I-10 ALERT

Part of the expansion of fracture codes is due to laterality issues (i.e., right, left, unspecified), but many of the codes are also differentiated by whether or not the fracture was displaced. Codes are also available to classify hip articular and apophyseal fractures as well.

Classification Note

Many diverse types of care can be provided to patients with fracture injuries; ICD-10-CM allows the easy classification of each type of visit in a seventh-character format. Many fracture classifications include seventh-character definitions similar to the one below, which is related to hip fractures (category S72).

Character	Description
A	initial encounter for closed fracture
B	initial encounter for open fracture type I or II
C	initial encounter for open fracture type IIIA, IIIB, or IIIC
D	subsequent encounter for closed fracture with routine healing
E	subsequent encounter for open fracture type I or II with routine healing

Character	Description
F	subsequent encounter for open fracture type IIIA, IIIB, or IIIC with routine healing
G	subsequent encounter for closed fracture with delayed healing
H	subsequent encounter for open fracture type I or II with delayed healing
J	subsequent encounter for open fracture type IIIA, IIIB, or IIIC with delayed healing
K	subsequent encounter for closed fracture with nonunion
M	subsequent encounter for open fracture type I or II with nonunion
N	subsequent encounter for open fracture type IIIA, IIIB, or IIIC with nonunion
P	subsequent encounter for closed fracture with malunion
Q	subsequent encounter for open fracture type I or II with malunion
R	subsequent encounter for open fracture type IIIA, IIIB, or IIIC with malunion
S	sequela

It is essential that the type of encounter be clearly documented, along with timeframes, history of initial injury and prior treatment, and current encounter treatment plan. Initial encounter is defined as the period of time in which the patient is receiving active treatment for the fracture (surgical treatment, emergency department encounter, and evaluation and treatment by a new physician). When the patient is receiving subsequent care for encounters after the patient has completed active treatment of the fracture and it is routine care for the fracture during the healing or recovery phase, a seventh character for subsequent encounter should be reported. Examples of fracture aftercare are: cast change or removal, removal of external or internal fixation device, medication adjustment, and follow-up visits following fracture treatment. If a code is not specified as open or closed, it should be classified as closed; if not specified as displaced or nondisplaced, it should be classified as displaced.

CDI ALERT

Ensure that each fracture site is described in its entirety, including the specific site (including laterality) and whether or not it is displaced. The circumstances of the encounter should be clearly documented, such as initial encounter for closed fracture, etc.

Other official guidelines related to fractures that affect documentation include:

- Fractures in patients with known osteoporosis whose injury would not usually break a normal, healthy bone should not be classified with a traumatic injury code, but with a combination code from category M8Ø Osteoporosis with current pathological fracture.
- When malunion or nonunion complications of fractures are present, the injury is classified with an injury code, but with the appropriate seventh character. All other complications should be classified separately with the appropriate complication codes.
- The reason and provision of fracture aftercare should be clearly documented and should not be classified to a separate aftercare (Z code) code. The appropriate injury seventh character is to be used instead.

Clinician Note

Careful review of medical record documentation is necessary because the type of fracture (severity) may or may not support the medical necessity of the service provided. Additionally, coordination of benefits is often required for payment from third-party payers for fracture codes so the documentation should indicate how the fracture occurred (auto accident, fall from ladder at work, fall when riding a bike).

Clinician Documentation Checklist

Clinician documentation should indicate the following:

The 7th character in fractures is based on the Gustilo classification. The following information is important to assign the appropriate 7th character:

- Episode of care: initial, subsequent, sequela
  - initial encounter: patient is receiving active treatment for the fracture
    - examples: surgical treatment, emergency department encounter, evaluation by new physician
  - subsequent encounter: patient has completed active treatment for the condition
    - examples: cast change/removal, medication adjustment, follow-up visits
  - sequela: complication or condition that arises as a direct result of a condition
    - example: scar from a burn. (The scar would be coded separately, but the burn would be assigned the S seventh character as the injury responsible for the scar.)
- Open or closed fracture
  - if open, type I or type II (Gustilo classification)
  - if open, type IIIA, IIIB, or IIIC
- Healing
  - routine healing
  - delayed healing
  - malunion
  - nonunion

Fracture — Nontraumatic of Spine/Vertebra

Code Axes

Fatigue fracture of vertebra, site unspecified	**M48.40 QPP**
Fatigue fracture of vertebra, cervical regions	**M48.41, M48.42, M48.43 QPP**
Fatigue fracture of vertebra, thoracic regions	**M48.44, M48.45 QPP**
Fatigue fracture of vertebra, lumbosacral regions	**M48.46, M48.47, M48.48 QPP**
Collapsed vertebra, NEC, site unspecified	**M48.50 HCC**
Collapsed vertebra, NEC, cervical regions	**M48.51, M48.52, M48.53 HCC**
Collapsed vertebra, NEC, thoracic regions	**M48.54, M48.55 HCC**
Collapsed vertebra, NEC, lumbosacral regions	**M48.56, M48.57, M48.58 HCC**
Age-related osteoporosis with current pathological fracture, vertebra(e)	**M80.08 HCC**
Other osteoporosis with current pathological fracture, vertebra(e)	**M80.88 HCC**
Pathological fracture in neoplastic disease, vertebrae	**M84.58 HCC**
Pathological fracture in other disease, other site	**M84.68 HCC**
Personal history of (healed) osteoporosis fracture	**Z87.310**

I-10 Alert

Codes for nontraumatic fractures have been vastly expanded in ICD-10-CM, with specific codes related to cause and type of fracture (e.g., collapsed vertebra, etc.). These codes require the addition of seventh characters that specify the episode of care, such as that for initial or subsequent encounter, or that for sequela (late effect) of the fracture.

CDI Alert

Any nontraumatic fracture must be documented specifically, including the type, cause, and age of fracture (new versus old). Specificity of site is also necessary in order to classify these cases appropriately.

Description of Condition

Fatigue fracture of vertebra (M48.4-)

Clinical Tip

A fatigue fracture is one that results from excessive activity rather than from a specific injury. This type of fracture is most commonly found in people who have engaged in unaccustomed, repetitive, vigorous activity. It is important to note that this type of fracture is not a result of a disease process and is typically found in younger patients than that involving a disease. These fractures may also be referred to as stress fractures, but the mechanism causing the fracture should be indicated.

Key Terms

Stress fracture

I-10 Alert

The category for collapsed vertebra(e) should only be used when the underlying cause of the fracture has not been documented.

CDI Alert

Ensure that the underlying cause of any stress or fatigue fracture is clearly documented for appropriate classification.

Clinician Note
When documentation indicates that an admission or encounter is for a procedure aimed at treating an underlying condition, the code for the underlying condition (such as a vertebral fracture) should be the first listed diagnosis. It is not necessary to indicate any signs or symptoms such as pain or neuropathy that may also be documented.

Collapsed vertebra, NEC (M48.5-)

CDI ALERT

Review documentation carefully for mention of collapsed vertebra(e) underlying cause. For patients under the age of 50, the condition is most often due to trauma; for patients over age 60, a common cause for females is postmenopausal (age-related) osteoporosis. In elderly patients, other common causes include malignancy and/or infection, and may be the presenting clinical symptom in multiple myeloma patients.

Key Terms
Key terms found in the documentation for collapsed vertebra may include:

- Collapsed vertebra NOS
- Compression fracture
- Wedging of vertebra NOS

Clinician Note
Review the medical record for terms such as osteoporosis, fatigue fracture, pathological fracture, stress fracture, or traumatic fracture. If present, query the physician to determine if a more specific type of vertebral fracture code is appropriate.

Age-related osteoporosis with current pathological fracture, vertebra(e) (M8Ø.Ø8-)

I-10 ALERT

Codes in the subcategory for age-related osteoporosis are differentiated by the presence of a current pathological fracture and then by site, including laterality. Seventh characters are required that represent the episode of care, whether initial or subsequent, or whether healing has been routine or delayed, whether any nonunion or malunion has occurred, or whether any sequela (late effect) conditions are present.

Clinical Tip
Osteoporosis, or a weakened state of bone density, may be caused by a number of conditions. Primary osteoporosis, which includes that designated as "age-related," may relate to a lower level of estrogen in postmenopausal women; men with decreased testosterone levels are also at risk for increased bone loss.

Key Terms
Key terms found in the documentation for age-related osteoporosis with current pathological fracture may include:

- Involutional osteoporosis with current pathological fracture
- Osteoporosis NOS with current pathological fracture
- Osteoporosis with current fragility fracture
- Osteoporotic fracture
- Postmenopausal osteoporosis with current pathological fracture
- Senile osteoporosis with current pathological fracture

Clinician Note
Documentation should be reviewed to determine if any major osseous defect is present as this should be reported separately. Look for terms such as bone loss or bone fragility. However, before assigning a code from M89.7- verify that this is indeed a major osseous defect.

Other osteoporosis with current pathological fracture, vertebra(e) (M8Ø.88-)

Clinical Tip

Osteoporosis that is not age-related may be related to several other conditions, such as rheumatoid arthritis, hyperparathyroidism, Cushing's disease, chronic kidney disease, multiple myeloma or other malignancy, or drugs such as anti-epileptics, glucocorticoids, or lithium.

Key Terms

Key terms found in the documentation for other osteoporosis with current pathological fracture may include:

Drug-induced osteoporosis with current pathological fracture

Idiopathic osteoporosis with current pathological fracture

Osteoporosis of disuse with current pathological fracture

Post-oophorectomy osteoporosis with current pathological fracture

Postsurgical malabsorption osteoporosis with current pathological fracture

Post-traumatic osteoporosis with current pathological fracture

Clinician Note

Documentation should be reviewed to determine if any major osseous defect is present as this should be reported separately. Look for terms such as bone loss or bone fragility. However, before assigning a code from M89.7- verify that this is indeed a major osseous defect.

> **I-10 ALERT**
>
> Codes in the subcategory for other osteoporosis are differentiated by the presence of a current pathological fracture and then by site, including laterality. Seventh characters are required that represent the episode of care, whether initial or subsequent, or whether healing has been routine or delayed, whether any nonunion or malunion has occurred, or whether any sequela (late effect) conditions are present.

> **CDI ALERT**
>
> Ensure that the underlying cause of the pathological fracture is documented. If it is not due to age-related osteoporosis but an osteoporotic condition is present, it should be classified to subcategory M8Ø.8-. Any condition that is drug-induced should also be classified with an additional code from the T36–T5Ø code range.

Pathological fracture in neoplastic disease, vertebrae (M84.58-)

Clinical Tip

The majority of bony metastases involves the axial skeleton (skull, vertebral column, ribs, and sternum), the proximal femur and the proximal humerus. Patients with bony lesions are at increased risk for pathological fracture and treatment typically consists of providing pain relief and stability of the area involved.

> **I-10 ALERT**
>
> Codes for pathological fracture in the setting of neoplastic disease are differentiated by site, including laterality. Seventh characters are required that represent the episode of care, whether initial or subsequent, or whether healing has been routine or delayed, whether any nonunion or malunion has occurred, or whether any sequela (late effect) conditions are present. To appropriately capture the full diagnosis, additional codes should be assigned for the neoplastic disease process.

Clinical Findings

The following are specific to fatigue or stress fractures but may apply to other listed diagnosis within this topic.

Physical Examination

History and review of systems may include:

- History of back pain associated with a specific activity
- Pain with palpation of the affected site
- Localized swelling of the area
- Leg alignment
- Motor function
- Flexibility

Diagnostic Procedures and Services

- Imaging
  - x-ray
  - ultrasound
  - MRI
  - CT scan
  - scintigraphy

Therapeutic Procedures and Services

- Physical therapy
- Restricted activity and rest

Medication List

- Analgesics: narcotic analgesics combinations contain a narcotic analgesic, such as codeine or hydrocodone, with one or more other analgesic, such as acetaminophen, aspirin, or ibuprofen
- NSAIDs

CDI ALERT

If a pathological fracture is documented for a case involving a neoplastic disease process, query the physician to determine whether the fracture is due to bony metastasis. These cases are classified to subcategory M84.5-, with an additional code for the neoplastic process.

Clinician Note

The pathological fracture due to neoplastic disease should not be reported when documentation indicates bone loss but not a fracture of the bone.

The affected bone may be upper or lower end, but if the portion of the bone is at the joint, the clinician should designate the site as the bone, not the joint.

Clinician Documentation Checklist

Clinician documentation should indicate the following:

- Osteoporosis with pathologic fracture
  - excludes: acute traumatic fractures
  - history of healed pathologic fracture
- Osteoporosis without pathologic fracture
  - history of healed pathologic fracture
- Age-related osteoporosis
  - postmenopausal
  - senile
  - involutional
- Other osteoporosis
  - idiopathic
  - drug-induced
  - postsurgical malabsorption
  - post-traumatic
  - disuse

Gastroenteritis (Viral, Bacterial, Protozoal)

Code Axes

The majority of the ICD-10-CM viral, bacterial, protozoal, and gastroenteritis codes are in categories AØ2 through AØ9:

Salmonella enteritis	**AØ2.Ø**
Shigellosis	**AØ3.Ø** **AØ3.[1-3, 8-9]**
Other bacterial intestinal infections	**AØ4-**
Other protozoal intestinal diseases	**AØ7-**
Viral and other specified intestinal infections	**AØ8-** **AØ8.Ø** **AØ8.1[1, 9]** **AØ8.2** **AØ8.3[1-2, 9]** **AØ8.[4, 8]**
Infectious gastroenteritis and colitis, unspecified	**AØ9**

⇨ I-10 Alert

Viral infections are the most common cause of gastroenteritis but bacteria, parasites, and food-borne illnesses are also common causes. CDC statistics indicate that deaths from gastroenteritis have increased dramatically. In 2007, the most recent statistics available from the CDC, 17,000 people died from gastroenteritis; overwhelmingly, these people were older and the most common infections were *Clostridium difficile* and norovirus.

Description of Condition

(AØ4) Other bacterial intestinal infections, including specific codes for various types of Escherichia coli (E. coli) infections (AØ4.Ø–AØ4.4), enteritis due to Campylobacter (AØ4.5), Yersinia enterocolitica (AØ4.6), Clostridium difficile (AØ4.71, AØ4.72), and other and unspecified bacterial intestinal infections (AØ4.8, AØ4.9)

E. coli is one of the most commonly reported causes of human infections, particularly of the urinary and digestive tracts. The infections are classified to the following groups:

Enteropathogenic (AØ4.Ø): These bacteria are typically ingested through contaminated drinking water or through meat. The *E. coli* bacteria interfere with signal transduction of cells in the colon.

Enterotoxigenic (AØ4.1): This type of bacteria is ingested through contaminated water or food and invades the intestinal mucosa.

Enteroinvasive (AØ4.2): This strain of *E. coli* causes dysentery-like diarrhea by invading and multiplying on epithelial cells in the colon and then destroying those cells. It is transmitted solely by infected humans.

Enterohemorrhagic (AØ4.3): This is one of the most serious strains of the bacteria, causes bloody diarrhea, and, if left untreated, can cause hemolytic uremic syndrome, which can be fatal. It releases toxins into the lumen of the GI tract. The sources are mostly from water or food, such as raw meat, unpasteurized milk, fruits, and vegetables.

CDI ALERT

Ensure that the organism responsible for the gastroenteritis (if known) is documented. If the organism is presumed, suspected, etc., documentation should indicate the signs, symptoms, manifestations, clinical scenario, work-up, and treatment that support the probable diagnosis.

Documentation Tip

It is important to translate the terms the physician documents to the correct main term in the index. For example, if the physician documents the term gastroenteropathy the ICD-10-CM index includes entries related to this section and has a "see also" instructional note indicating that the main term gastroenteritis should also be referenced.

Clinical Tip

Another serious form of bacterial intestinal infection is that caused by *Clostridium difficile*, which is typically found as a result of extended antibiotic use: antibiotic associated diarrhea (AAD). It causes severe diarrhea when competing bacteria in the gut have been destroyed by antibiotics. The bacterium releases toxins that cause the diarrhea, bloating, and abdominal pain. The antibiotics most commonly associated with AAD include the following:

- Clindamycin (e.g., Cleocin)
- Fluoroquinolones (e.g., levofloxacin [Levaquin])
- Ciprofloxacin (Cipro, Cipro XR, Proquin XR)
- Penicillins
- Cephalosporins

Key Terms

Key terms found in the documentation may include:

Bacterial dysentery

Bacterial enteritis

Diffusely adherent *E. coli* (enteropathogenic)

E. coli O157:H7 (enterohemorrhagic)

Enterotoxigenic *E. Coli* (ETEC)

Pseudomembranous colitis (*C. difficile*)

Travelers' diarrhea

(AØ8) Viral and other specified intestinal infections, including rotaviral enteritis (AØ8.Ø), acute gastroenteropathy due to Norwalk agent and other small round viruses (AØ8.1-), adenoviral enteritis (AØ8.2), calicivirus (AØ8.31), astrovirus (AØ8.32), and other and unspecified viral intestinal infections (AØ8.39, AØ8.4)

CDI ALERT

The term enteritis relates to an inflammation of the small bowel and can be caused by a number of factors including but not limited to bacterial infection, viral infection, and immune responses. Medical documentation should be reviewed to determine if bacterial or viral infection is the cause of the inflammation before a code from this chapter of the ICD-10-CM system is assigned.

Key Terms

Key terms found in the documentation may include:

Coxsackie virus enteritis

Echovirus enteritis

Enterovirus enteritis

Norovirus

Norwalk-like agent

Small round virus (SRV) gastroenteropathy

Torovirus enteritis

Clinical Findings

Physical Examination

History and review of systems may include:

- Copious, watery diarrhea
- Ingestion of potentially tainted food
- Contact with an ill person
- GI bleeding with little stool
- Fever
- Nausea
- Vomiting
- Abdominal pain

Diagnostic Procedures and Services

- Laboratory
  - stool culture
  - blood culture
  - serum electrolytes
  - BUN
  - creatinine

Therapeutic Procedures and Services

- Oral or IV hydration

Medication List

- Antidiarrheal medication, if appropriate
- Antiemetics
- Antibiotics, if appropriate
  - azithromycin
  - ceftriaxone (Rocephin)
  - ciprofloxacin (Cipro)

Clinician Documentation Checklist

Clinician documentation should indicate the following:

- Suspected cause
  - viral
  - bacterial
    - *Salmonella*
    - *Staphylococcus*
    - *Escherichia coli*
    - *Clostridium*
    - *Shigella*
    - *Campylobacter jejuni*
    - *Yersinia*

- parasitic
- food poisoning
- drug reactions
- food allergies
- colitis
- short bowel syndrome
- obstructing tumors
- ingestion of toxins

- In the absence of a specific organism, indicate signs, symptoms, manifestations, etc.
  - duration of illness
  - location of pain
  - stools
    - frequency
    - blood/mucous
  - primary symptoms
    - diarrhea
    - nausea
    - vomiting
    - abdominal cramps
    - fever
    - malaise
- Associated pathology
  - dehydration
  - hypokalemia
  - acidosis
  - metabolic alkalosis
  - hyponatremia
- Therapies
  - hydration
  - medications
  - antibiotics
  - antiemetics
  - antimotility agents
  - antispasmodics

Gastrointestinal Hemorrhage

Code Axes

Other diseases of the digestive system **K92.-**

Description of Condition

Gastrointestinal (GI) Bleeding

GI bleeding can originate anywhere along the GI tract from the mouth to the anus and may be overt or occult. Overt bleeding is seen without aid and is referred to as "gross." Occult bleeding is visible only by microscopic exam or laboratory test. Upper GI origin is demonstrated by hematemesis, occult positive stool, or melena from small bowel. Lower GI origin is demonstrated by melena, occult positive stool, and hematochezia.

Hematemesis (K92.Ø)

Vomiting of red blood indicates acute upper GI bleeding, usually from gastric or duodenal ulcer, gastric or duodenal erosions, erosive esophagitis, varices, and Mallory-Weiss tear. Vomitus described as coffee-ground emesis results from upper GI bleeding that has slowed or stopped.

Melena (K92.1)

Black, tarry stool due to dark colored blood which may persist for several days after bleeding has stopped. Hematochezia is overt bright-colored blood passed from the anus, usually in or with stool and usually indicates lower GI bleeding.

Clinical Tip
Certain foods and medications may cause black stools, these should be ruled out to determine if the cause of the melena is blood.

Key Terms
Key terms found in the documentation may include:

- Black stool
- Hematochezia
- Occult positive stool
- Tarry stool

Gastrointestinal hemorrhage, unspecified (K92.2)

Key Terms
Key terms found in the documentation may include:

- Colon hemorrhage
- Duodenal hemorrhage

⇨ I-10 ALERT

Code assignment should not be based on ancillary test results or clinical criteria alone. A diagnosis and its clinical significance must be supported and documented by the clinician. When it is unclear or there is conflicting information, query the physician for clarification.

Gastric hemorrhage
Gastrointestinal bleeding
Intestinal hemorrhage
Stomach hemorrhage

Clinical Findings

Physical Examination

History and review of systems may include:

- Abdominal discomfort
- Anemia
- Diaphoresis
- Dizziness
- Easily bruising
- Fatigue
- Frequency of blood passage
- Hematemesis
- Hematochezia
- Hypotension
- Melena
- Pallor
- Quantity of blood passage
- Syncope
- Tachycardia
- Weakness
- Weight loss

Diagnostic Procedures and Services

- Laboratory
  - CBC
  - coagulation profile
  - fecal occult blood test
  - hematocrit
  - hypovolemia
- Imaging
  - angiography
  - barium enema
  - barium swallow
  - capsule endoscopy
  - colonoscopy/endoscopy
  - nasogastric aspiration
  - upper GI series

- Other
  - digital rectal exam (DRE)

Therapeutic Procedures and Services

- Coagulation
- Embolization
- Endotracheal intubation to prevent aspiration
- IV hydration
- Nasogastric lavage
- Oxygen for respiratory distress
- Polypectomy
- Sclerotherapy
- Surgical resection
- Transfusions

Medication List

- H2 antagonist/blocker
- Iron therapy

Clinician Documentation Checklist

Clinician documentation should indicate the following:

- Type:
  - hematemesis
  - melena
  - unspecified gastrointestinal hemorrhage
    - unspecified gastric hemorrhage
    - unspecified intestinal hemorrhage

Glaucoma

Code Axes

Glaucoma suspect	H4Ø.Ø-
Open-angle glaucoma	H4Ø.1- QPP
Primary angle-closure glaucoma	H4Ø.2Ø-
Acute angle-closure glaucoma	H4Ø.21-
Glaucoma secondary to eye trauma	H4Ø.3-
Glaucoma secondary to eye inflammation	H4Ø.4-
Glaucoma secondary to other eye disorders	H4Ø.5-
Glaucoma secondary to drugs	H4Ø.6-
Other glaucoma	H4Ø.8-
Unspecified glaucoma	H4Ø.9
Glaucoma in diseases classified elsewhere	H42

I-10 ALERT

ICD-10-CM classifications for glaucoma include combination codes with the stage of disease specified in the seventh character for certain categories requiring reporting of disease stage.

Multiple codes should be reported, as appropriate to report the type of glaucoma, the affected eye and stage (when required).

Note: Conditions classified to chapter 7 include laterality (right, left, bilateral) within the code structure. All ophthalmic conditions should specify the affected eye(s).

Description of Condition

CDI ALERT

Ensure that the type of glaucoma is documented and the laterality of the affected eye or eyes (i.e., right, left, bilateral).

Ensure documentation of type, severity and status of disease is complete and specific.

Glaucoma (H4Ø.----)

Clinical Tip

Glaucoma is an eye disease that gradually causes peripheral vision degradation caused by an increase in intraocular pressure (IOP) from abnormal aqueous humor outflow from the anterior chamber or decreased aqueous humor production by the ciliary body. If untreated, increased pressure leads to optic nerve damage and blindness. Prognosis and treatment depends on the type of disease, the underlying cause and whether the disease is a primary or secondary condition.

Borderline glaucoma is a condition indicative of the clinical signs and symptoms associated with glaucoma, such as borderline high IOP with associated visual field deficits.

Open angle glaucoma is an increase in IOP due to free access of the aqueous humor to the trabecular network in the angle of the anterior chamber causing progressive "tunnel vision," photophobia, and poor night vision Heredity, trauma, and chronic intraocular disease are contributing factors.

Acute closed angle glaucoma entails a sudden onset of severe eye pain and visual disturbances. The severe rise in IOP due to aqueous obstruction necessitates immediate intervention to preserve sight.

Therapies vary according to the type and severity of glaucoma, and include topical, systemic and numerous surgical procedures to reduce intraocular pressure.

Key Terms

Key terms found in the documentation for glaucoma vary depending on the type of disease, and may include:

- Acute angle-closure glaucoma:
  - Acute angle closure attack (crisis)
- Anatomic narrow angle:
  - Angle closure suspect
  - Primary angle closure suspect
- Glaucoma suspect:
  - Borderline glaucoma
  - Ocular hypertension
  - Pre-glaucoma
- Primary open angle glaucoma:
  - Chronic simple glaucoma
- Aqueous misdirection:
  - Malignant glaucoma

Documentation Tip

Borderline open angle glaucoma: level of risk (low or high) should be specifically documented to report appropriate severity level.

Ensure complete documentation that specifies the underlying causal condition as required by ICD-10-CM coding conventions for the following types of glaucoma:

H40.3 Glaucoma secondary to eye trauma

Documentation must specify nature of trauma.

H40.4 Glaucoma secondary to eye inflammation

Documentation must specify type and nature of inflammatory disorder.

H40.5 Glaucoma secondary to other eye disorders

Documentation must specify underlying eye disorder.

H40.6 Glaucoma secondary to drugs

Documentation must specify the causal drug or agent and intent (e.g., poisoning, overdose, adverse effect of drug in therapeutic use, underdosing, assault).

H42 Glaucoma in disease classified elsewhere

(This code cannot be reported alone or sequenced first.)

Documentation must specify the underlying causal disease.

Indeterminate stage of disease (seventh character 4) is not interchangeable with unspecified disease stage (seventh character Ø). An indeterminate stage of disease should only be reported if the stage of disease cannot be clinically determined.

⇨ I-10 ALERT

Subcategory H40 includes valid codes that are five or six characters in length. Code H42 is a valid three-digit manifestation code that requires the associated underlying disease to be sequenced first.

The following axes of classification in category H40 describe:

- Fifth character:
  - Type of glaucoma (suspect, angle closure, primary, secondary, other)
- Sixth character:
  - Laterality (right, left, bilateral, unspecified)
- Seventh character (where required):
  - Disease stage

Clinical Findings

Physical Examination

History and review of systems may include:

- Visual examination
  - optic nerve changes on ophthalmoscopy
  - typical visual field defects
  - elevated intraocular pressure (IOP)
- Family history of glaucoma

Therapeutic Procedures and Services

- Decrease IOP
  - laser
  - medication
  - surgery

Medication List

- Oral medications
  - acetazolamide (Diamox)
  - methazolamide (Neptazane)
- Topical including drops
  - beta-blocker to reduce IOP
    - betaxolol (Kerlone)
    - carteolol (Ocupress)
    - levobunolol (AKBeta, Betagan)
    - metipranolol (OptiPranolol)
  - reduce IOP
    - bimatoprost (Lumigan)
    - latanoprost (Xalatan)
    - tafluprost (Zioptan)
    - travoprost (Travatan)
    - unoprostone (Rescula)

CDI ALERT

Specify laterality of affected eye for all ophthalmic conditions.

Clinician Documentation Checklist

Clinician documentation should indicate the following:

- Specifiy laterality of affected eye
  - right
  - left
  - bilateral
- Document the stage of disease as
  - mild
  - moderate
  - severe

  - indeterminate
- Document the specific type of glaucoma, underlying cause and significant findings, such as:
  - glaucoma suspect
    - open angle (specify high or low risk)
    - anatomic narrow angle (primary angle closure suspect)
    - steroid responder
    - ocular hypertension
    - primary angle closure glaucoma without glaucoma damage
  - open angle glaucoma
    - low tension
    - pigmentary
    - capsular (with pseudoexfoliation of lens)
    - residual stage
- Primary angle-closure glaucoma; specify stage as
  - acute (attack) (crisis)
  - chronic
  - intermittent
  - residual
- Glaucoma secondary to eye trauma
  - specify underlying (causal) trauma and residual complications
- Glaucoma secondary to eye inflammation
  - specify underlying chronic inflammatory condition
- Glaucoma secondary to other eye disorder
  - specify underlying eye disorder
- Glaucoma secondary to drugs
  - specify drug, medication or substance, and intent (poisoning, adverse effect in therapeutic use, assault, underdosing)
- Other glaucoma
  - glaucoma with increased episcleral venous pressure
  - hypersecretion glaucoma
  - aqueous misdirection (malignant glaucoma)

When glaucoma is associated with an ocular disorder, adverse effects of drugs or medications, or sequel of previous trauma, relate the glaucoma to the causal or underlying condition or factor.

Document any associated or underlying chronic or systemic disease processes. If conditions are inter-related, document the cause-and-effect relationship.

Hearing Loss

Code Axes

Noise effects on inner ear	**H83.3-**
Conductive and sensorineural hearing loss	**H9Ø.-**
Other and unspecified hearing loss	**H91.-**
Transient ischemic deafness	**H93.Ø1-**

> ⇨ **I-10 ALERT**
>
> ICD-10-CM classifies hearing loss in separate code categories based on the type or underlying cause of hearing loss; whether the hearing loss is caused by mechanical, sensory, vascular, neurological, or other causes such as noise-induced trauma.
>
> Noise-induced (acoustic) hearing loss is classified to subcategory H83 Other diseases of inner ear. Category H9Ø Conductive and sensorineural hearing loss, includes auditory disorders of the external, middle, or inner ear of specific or mixed type. Category H91 Other and unspecified hearing loss, includes expanded subcategories, which include specific classifications for ototoxic hearing loss, sudden idiopathic hearing loss, and presbycusis. Subcategory H93.Ø Degenerative and vascular disorders of ear, includes classifications for transient ischemic deafness.
>
> **Note:** Conditions classified to chapter 8 include laterality (right, left, bilateral) within the code structure. All conditions should specify the affected ear(s).

Description of Condition

Hearing loss

Clinical Tip

Acquired hearing loss (deafness) can be clinically categorized according to the type or underlying cause. The central nervous system, organs of the ear, and related structures are vulnerable to damage, disease, tumor and deterioration from multiple possible causes, and pathologies including genetic predisposition, drugs, trauma, infection, disease, and other inter-related or overlapping factors. Types of hearing loss include:

Conductive: mechanical external and middle ear malfunction

Sensory: cochlear or inner ear disorders

Neural: auditory nerve trauma, disease or other disorder

Sensorineural: damage to cochlea or inner ear pathways to the central nervous system

Combination (mixed): overlapping causal factors (e.g., conductive and sensorineural)

Otosclerosis: genetic-related bony overgrowth (hardening) of the stapes

Transient ischemic: circulatory compromise of the small cerebrovascular vessels that supply the cochlea in the inner ear

Presbycusis: normal, degenerative age-related hearing loss of high-frequency stimuli

Sudden idiopathic: abrupt onset of unilateral hearing loss without apparent cause with spontaneous recovery of hearing within two weeks.

Key Terms

Key terms found in the documentation may include:

Acoustic trauma of inner ear (noise-induced)

Central hearing loss

Congenital deafness

Deafness

High frequency/low frequency hearing loss

Neural hearing loss

Perceptive deafness

Presbyacusia

Clinical Findings

Physical Examination

History and review of systems may include:

- Gradual or acute hearing loss
- Ear pain
- Ear discharge
- Tinnitus
- Vertigo
- Exposure to an acute event (e.g., head trauma)
- Exposure to chronic loud noise
- External ear exam
  - obstruction
  - infection
- TM perforation or drainage
- Otitis media
- Neurologic examination
- Cholesteatoma

Diagnostic Procedures and Services

- Imaging
  - MRI or CT
- Other
  - audiologic tests

Therapeutic Procedures and Services

- Drainage of fluid from middle ear effusion
- Surgery for damaged TM or ossicles
- Hearing aid

Documentation Tip

Documentation must include the underlying cause or type of hearing loss to avoid reporting nonspecific diagnoses. The provider should qualify the loss as:

- Noise-induced
- Conductive
- Sensorineural (or mixed type; with conductive)
- Conductive (or mixed type; with sensorineural)
- Vascular (ischemic)

⇨ I-10 ALERT

ICD-10-CM classifies hearing loss to separate categories, based on the underlying cause or pathology, for example:

H83	Other diseases of inner ear
H9Ø	Conductive and sensorineural hearing loss
H91	Other and unspecified hearing loss
H93.Ø	Degenerative and vascular disorders of ear includes classifications for transient ischemic deafness

Note: Conditions classified to chapter 8 include laterality (i.e., right, left, bilateral) within the code structure. All conditions should specify the affected ear(s).

Subcategory H83.3 Noise effects on inner ear, and H91.8 Other specified hearing loss, contain placeholders X to allow for future code expansion, without disturbing the code structure.

- Ototoxic
- Presbycusis (age related; degenerative)
- Idiopathic (sudden)
- Other (specify)

Documentation of laterality and status of hearing on contralateral side should be thorough and specific to avoid reporting unspecified codes.

Ototoxic hearing loss requires documentation of the causal drug or agent and intent (e.g., poisoning, overdose, adverse effect of drug in therapeutic use, underdosing, assault) to support complete, accurate reporting.

Ensure that all related conditions are coded appropriately, particularly if hearing loss is related to other underlying diseases or disorders (e.g., vascular disease, metabolic disturbances, congenital anomalies, infection).

Clinician Note

Specify the type of hearing loss. Differentiate between noise-induced, conductive, sensory, neural, ischemic, idiopathic and other. Document whether a combination of types or pathologies exist (e.g., sensorineural, mixed conductive and sensorineural).

Document the specific anatomic site affected. For example, for transient ischemic deafness, document whether the ischemia is related to inner ear or other cerebrovascular disease. Specify the site of ischemia and underlying pathology, if known.

Document the laterality of the affected site (left, right, bilateral), and the status of hearing on the contralateral side.

For example:

H9Ø.3 Sensorineural hearing loss, bilateral

H9Ø.42 Sensorineural hearing loss, unilateral, left ear, with unrestricted hearing on the contralateral side

Clinician Documentation Checklist

Clinician documentation should indicate the following:

Noise effects on inner ear

- Type
  - labyrinthitis
  - labyrinthine fistula
  - labyrinthine dysfunction
    - includes
      - labyrinthine hypersensitivity
      - labyrinthine hypofunction
      - labyrinthine loss of function
  - noise effects of inner ear
    - includes

        - ♦ acoustic trauma of inner ear
        - ♦ noise-induced hearing loss of inner ear
    - other specified diseases of inner ear
    - unspecified disease of inner ear
- Identification of laterality of ear
    - right
    - left
    - bilateral

Conductive and sensorineural hearing loss

- Conductive hearing loss, bilateral
- Conductive hearing loss, unilateral with unrestricted hearing on contralateral side
    - identification of laterality of ear
        - — right
        - — left
- Unspecified conductive hearing loss
    - conductive deafness
- Sensorineural hearing loss, bilateral
- Sensorineural hearing loss, unilateral with unrestricted hearing on contralateral side
    - identification of laterality of ear
        - — right
        - — left
- Unspecified sensorineural hearing loss
    - includes
        - — central hearing loss
        - — congenital deafness
        - — neural hearing loss
        - — perceptive hearing loss
        - — sensorineural deafness
        - — sensory hearing loss
- Mixed conductive and sensorineural hearing loss, bilateral
- Mixed conductive and sensorineural hearing loss, unilateral with unrestricted hearing on contralateral side
    - identification of laterality of ear
        - — right
        - — left
- Unspecified mixed conductive and sensorineural hearing loss

Other and unspecified hearing loss

- Type
    - ototoxic hearing loss
        - — identification of the drug

 — presbycusis
 — presbyacusia
- sudden idiopathic hearing loss
 — sudden hearing loss
- deaf nonspeaking
- other specified hearing loss
- unspecified hearing loss
 — high frequency
 — low frequency
 — deafness
 — complete deafness
 — partial deafness

- Identification of laterality of ear
  - right
  - left
  - bilateral

Heart Failure

Code Axes

Left ventricular failure, unspecified	**I5Ø.1** HCC
Systolic (congestive) heart failure	**I5Ø.2-** HCC
Diastolic (congestive) heart failure	**I5Ø.3-** HCC
Combined systolic (congestive) and diastolic (congestive) heart failure	**I5Ø.4-** HCC
Other heart failure	**I5Ø.8**
Heart failure, unspecified	**I5Ø.9** HCC
Postprocedural heart failure	**I97.13-**
Heart failure due to hypertension	**I11.Ø** HCC
Heart failure due to hypertension with chronic kidney disease (CKD)	**I13.Ø, I13.2** HCC
Rheumatic heart failure	**IØ9.81** HCC

Key Terms
Key terms found in the documentation may include:

Biventricular (heart) failure
Cardiac asthma
Cardiac, heart or myocardial failure
CHF
Congestive heart disease
Congestive heart failure
Edema of lung with heart disease
Edema of lung with heart failure
Left heart failure
Pulmonary edema with heart disease
Pulmonary edema with heart failure
Right ventricular failure (secondary to left heart failure)

⇨ I-10 ALERT

When documentation indicates that the patient has congestive heart failure (CHF), review for any hypertensive heart or hypertensive heart and kidney disease. Combination classifications (e.g., I11.Ø) may be required to fully describe the condition. This classification assumes a cause-and-effect relationship because the two conditions are linked by the term "with" in the index. Per 2017 guidelines, code these conditions as related even if provider documentation does not specifically link them, unless the provider clearly states the conditions are not related. ICD-10-CM codes contain the word "congestive" in their code titles; therefore, it is not necessary to assign a separate code for CHF.

Description of Condition

Systolic (congestive) heart failure (I5Ø.2-)

Systolic heart failure is characterized by impairment of myocardial contraction, resulting in inadequate emptying of the ventricle and associated ventricular dilation. Documentation that describes an "exacerbation" of congestive heart failure indicates an acute flare-up of the condition. If the patient also carries a chronic CHF diagnosis, classify the case to one of the "acute on chronic" CHF codes.

⇨ I-10 ALERT

Results of an echocardiogram will assist in differentiating between systolic and diastolic heart failure. Systolic heart failure (I5Ø.2-) shows a decreased ejection fraction while diastolic heart failure (I5Ø.3-) has a normal or nearly normal ejection fraction.

Diastolic (congestive) heart failure (I5Ø.3-)

Diastolic heart failure occurs in patients with CHF symptoms, yet with preserved left ventricular ejection fraction (> 0.50) in the absence of major valvular disease. Filling defect occurs as a result of impaired myocardial relaxation, resulting in increased diastolic pressure. Diastolic dysfunction accounts for 40 percent to 60 percent of patients with CHF.

Other forms of heart failure

When heart failure is documented as due to hypertension (I11.Ø), hypertension and CKD (I13.Ø, I13.2), rheumatic heart disease (IØ9.81), or is due to an obstetric (O75.4) or other procedure (I97.13-), the documentation should clearly indicate whether CHF is the precipitating factor. In these cases, a separate code should be assigned to appropriately classify the heart failure.

Clinical Findings

Physical Examination

History and review of systems may include:

- Myocardial infarction
- Hypertension
- Heart murmur
- Dyspnea
- Fatigue
- Reflecting low cardiac output
- Ankle swelling
- LV Failure
  - tachycardia
  - tachypnea
  - cyanosis
  - hypotension
  - LV systolic dysfunction
- RV failure
  - pitting edema of feet and ankles
  - enlarged liver
  - abdominal swelling
  - ascites
  - elevated jugular venous pressure

Diagnostic Procedures and Services

- Laboratory
  - CBC

  - creatinine
  - BUN
  - electrolytes
  - albumin
  - liver function
- Imaging
  - chest x-ray
  - echocardiogram
  - radionuclide imaging
  - cardiac MRI
- Other
  - ECG
  - coronary angiography
  - cardiac catheterization

Therapeutic Procedures and Services

- Treatment for the cause of heart failure
- Diet and lifestyle changes
- Device therapy, if applicable (i.e., pacemakers, ICD)
- Percutaneous intervention or surgery

Medication List

Choice of medications depends on the type of heart failure and individual patient characteristics.

Medications for symptom relief include:

- Digitalis preparation (Digoxin)
- Diuretics
- Nitrates

Medications for long-term management include:

- ACE inhibitors
- Aldosterone antagonists
- Angiotensin II receptor blockers (ARB)
- Beta blockers
- Vasodilators (nitroglycerin)

The lists of medications used to treat heart failure are numerous, for more detail go to:
http://www.merckmanuals.com/professional/cardiovascular-disorders/heart-failure/drugs-for-heart-failure.

Clinician Note

Code assignment for congestive heart failure is dependent upon both the type of failure (e.g., left systolic, diastolic, combined) as well as severity (e.g., acute chronic, acute on chronic). Documentation should be carefully reviewed for this type of information and, if not present, the physician should be queried. Code I5Ø.9 should only be reported if the type of heart failure can be further specified.

Clinician Documentation Checklist

Clinician documentation should indicate the following:

- Types
  - left ventricular
  - systolic
  - diastolic
  - combined systolic and diastolic
  - unspecified
- Severity
  - acute
  - chronic
  - acute on chronic
- Also document
  - associated hypertension
  - associated renal disease
  - congestive
  - neonatal

Postprocedural Heart Failure

- Postcardiotomy syndrome
- Postmastectomy lymphedema syndrome
- Postprocedural hypertension
- Type of surgery
  - following heart catheterization
  - following cardiac bypass
  - following cardiac surgery
  - following other circulatory surgery
  - following other surgery
- Timing
  - intraoperative
  - postoperative
- Other functional disturbances
  - cardiac insufficiency
  - cardiac arrest
  - heart failure
  - other functional disturbances
- Hemorrhage and/or hematoma
- Accidental puncture and laceration
- Cerebrovascular infarction

Hematuria in Glomerular Disease

Code Axes

Recurrent and persistent hematuria with minor glomerular abnormality	**NØ2.Ø**
Recurrent and persistent hematuria with focal and segmental glomerular lesions	**NØ2.1**
Recurrent and persistent hematuria with diffuse membranous glomerulonephritis	**NØ2.2**
Recurrent and persistent hematuria with diffuse mesangial proliferative glomerulonephritis	**NØ2.3**
Recurrent and persistent hematuria with diffuse endocapillary proliferative glomerulonephritis	**NØ2.4**
Recurrent and persistent hematuria with diffuse mesangiocapillary glomerulonephritis	**NØ2.5**
Recurrent and persistent hematuria with dense deposit disease	**NØ2.6**
Recurrent and persistent hematuria with diffuse crescentic glomerulonephritis	**NØ2.7**
Recurrent and persistent hematuria with other morphologic changes	**NØ2.8**
Recurrent and persistent hematuria with unspecified morphologic changes	**NØ2.9**

Clinical Tip
Glomerular disease affects the glomerulus, which is responsible for filtering toxins out of the blood and excreting them in the urine, while keeping red blood cells and proteins in the bloodstream. Hematuria (blood in the urine) may be a precursor to more serious renal disorders.

Note: The following definitions are related to the glomerular diseases discussed in this section:

Global: Affecting the whole of the glomerulus uniformly.

Segmental: Affecting one glomerular segment, leaving other segments unaffected.

Diffuse: Affecting all glomeruli in both kidneys.

Focal: Affecting a proportion of glomeruli, with others unaffected

⇨ I-10 ALERT

Hematuria has been found to be a far more important symptom in the diagnosis and treatment of renal diseases than previously thought. When it is recurrent and persistent and diagnosed with several various glomerular diseases, combination codes are available in ICD-10-CM in category NØ2 to report the condition.

Description of Condition

Recurrent and persistent hematuria with minor glomerular abnormality (NØ2.Ø)

Clinical Tip

As the name implies, this form of glomerular disease is minor, but requires treatment to avoid further disease progression to nephrotic syndrome. The most common symptom is massive fluid accumulation, edema, and proteinuria. It affects the pediatric population at higher rates than that for adults and typically responds after three months of steroid treatment.

Key Terms

Key terms found in the documentation for recurrent and persistent hematuria with minor glomerular abnormality may include:

Minimal change disease

Minimal change lesion

Nil disease (lipoid nephrosis)

Nil lesions

Clinician Note

Documentation such as laboratory results should support the presence of blood in the urine.

Recurrent and persistent hematuria with focal and segmental glomerular lesions (NØ2.1)

Clinical Tip

This condition usually presents as nephrotic syndrome, especially in children, and is a cause of acute kidney failure in adults. Focal and segmental refer to the presentation of the kidney tissue on biopsy: focal—only some of the glomeruli are involved (as opposed to diffuse), and segmental refers to the fact that only part of each glomerulus is involved (as opposed to global).

Key Terms

Key terms found in the documentation for recurrent and persistent hematuria with focal and segmental glomerular lesions may include:

Focal glomerular sclerosis

Focal nodular glomerulosclerosis

Focal segmental glomerulosclerosis (FSGS)

Recurrent and persistent hematuria with focal and segmental hyalinosis

Recurrent and persistent hematuria with focal and segmental sclerosis

Recurrent and persistent hematuria with focal glomerulonephritis

Clinician Note

Documentation such as laboratory results should support the presence of blood in the urine.

Recurrent and persistent hematuria with diffuse membranous glomerulonephritis (NØ2.2)

Clinical Tip
This is a slowly progressive disease of the kidney affecting mostly patients between the ages of 30 and 50 years, characterized by inflammation of the basement membrane but not the mesangium (a structure in the glomerulus of the kidney, between the capillaries). It is the second most common cause of nephrotic syndrome in adults, with focal segmental glomerulosclerosis (FSGS) being the most common.

Key Terms
Key terms found in the documentation for recurrent and persistent hematuria with diffuse membranous glomerulonephritis may include:

Membranous glomerulopathy

Membranous nephritis

Membranous nephropathy

Clinician Note
Terms such as nephritic and nephrosis are often used when documenting glomerular diseases and require careful attention to the medical record documentation.

Recurrent and persistent hematuria with diffuse mesangial proliferative glomerulonephritis (NØ2.3)

Clinical Tip
This disease process is a form of glomerulonephritis associated primarily with the mesangium, a supportive structure in the glomerulus of the kidney, between the capillaries that assists with filtration. The condition also causes antibody deposits in the mesangium layer, which increases in size and number, giving the glomeruli a lumpy appearance. It usually causes nephrotic syndrome and may progress to chronic kidney failure.

Key Terms
Key terms found in the documentation for recurrent and persistent hematuria with diffuse mesangial proliferative glomerulonephritis may include:

Glomerulonephritis — mesangial proliferative

Mesangial proliferative GN

Clinician Note
Documentation such as laboratory results should support the presence of blood in the urine.

Recurrent and persistent hematuria with diffuse endocapillary proliferative glomerulonephritis (NØ2.4)

Clinical Tip

This condition is characterized by endocapillary hypercellularity, which is defined by the presence and proliferation of cells within the capillary lumina, affecting kidney function. Proliferating cells are mesangials, endothelials, and circulating inflammatory cells that have migrated to the capillary tuft. There is occlusion of capillary lumens due to cellular proliferation and endothelial cells edema. The lesion is usually diffuse, but, in some cases, it is segmental and focal.

Key Terms

Key terms found in the documentation for recurrent and persistent hematuria with diffuse endocapillary proliferative glomerulonephritis may include:

Diffuse proliferative endocapillary glomerulonephritis (EPGN)

Clinician Note

Documentation such as laboratory results should support the presence of blood in the urine.

Recurrent and persistent hematuria with diffuse mesangiocapillary glomerulonephritis (NØ2.5)

Clinical Tip

This condition is a chronic form of glomerulonephritis characterized by mesangial cell proliferation, irregular thickening of glomerular capillary walls, and thickening of the mesangial matrix and glomerular basement membrane.

Key Terms

Key terms found in the documentation for recurrent and persistent hematuria with diffuse mesangiocapillary glomerulonephritis may include:

Membranoproliferative glomerulonephritis

Clinician Note

Documentation such as laboratory results should support the presence of blood in the urine.

Recurrent and persistent hematuria with dense deposit disease (NØ2.6)

Clinical Tip

This is a type of glomerulonephritis caused by deposits in the kidney glomerular mesangium and basement membrane (GBM) thickening, which damages the glomeruli. The distinctive factor involves deposits at the intraglomerular mesangium.

Key Terms

Key terms found in the documentation for recurrent and persistent hematuria with dense deposit disease may include:

Membranoproliferative glomerulonephritis type II (MPGNII)

Clinician Note

Documentation such as laboratory results should support the presence of blood in the urine.

Recurrent and persistent hematuria with diffuse crescentic glomerulonephritis (NØ2.7)

Clinical Tip

This is an uncommon form of acute glomerulonephritis characterized by heavy proteinuria, microaneurysms, and hypertension. The primary distinguishing characteristic is crescent formation in the glomeruli; prognosis is related to the proportion of affected glomeruli. In true crescentic glomerulonephritis, crescents are present in 50 percent or more of the glomeruli. Crescents in 80 percent to 100 percent of the glomeruli have been described as rapidly progressive glomerulonephritis. This lesion usually progresses to renal insufficiency and/or failure in less than six months.

Key Terms

Key terms found in the documentation for recurrent and persistent hematuria with diffuse crescentic glomerulonephritis may include:

Extracapillary glomerulonephritis

Clinical Findings

Physical Examination

History and review of systems may include:

- Dark-colored urine
- Recent strep throat
- Fatigue
- Weight gain
- Vomiting
- Hypertension
- Edema
- Oliguria
- Fever
- Periorbital edema
- Respiratory crackles
- Elevated jugular venous pressure
- Abdominal pain
- Palpable kidneys
- Diagnostic Procedures and Services

- Laboratory
  - urinalysis
  - BUN
  - serum creatinine
  - CBC
  - serologic testing
  - urine culture
- Imaging
  - ultrasonography
  - CT scan
  - voiding cystourethrograms
  - radionuclide study

Clinician Note

Documentation such as laboratory results should support the presence of blood in the urine.

Medication List

Treatment is directed at the cause of the hematuria and may include:

- Antibiotics
- Antihypertensive
- Diuretics

Clinician Documentation Checklist

Clinician documentation should indicate the following:

- Type of glomerular disease
  - global
  - segmental
  - diffuse
  - focal
  - mesangial/mesangium
  - endocapillary hypercellularity

Hemorrhoids and Perianal Venous Thrombosis

Code Axes

First degree hemorrhoids	**K64.Ø**
Second degree hemorrhoids	**K64.1**
Third degree hemorrhoids	**K64.2**
Fourth degree hemorrhoids	**K64.3**
Residual hemorrhoidal skin tags	**K64.4**
Perianal venous thrombosis	**K64.5**
Other and unspecified hemorrhoids	**K64.8, K64.9**

Clinical Tip
The definitions for the degrees of hemorrhoids are as follows:

First degree: No prolapse outside of the anal canal

Second degree: Prolapse with straining, but retract spontaneously

Third degree: Prolapse with straining and require manual replacement back inside the anal canal

Fourth degree: Prolapsed tissue that cannot be manually replaced

Key Terms
Key terms found in the documentation may include:

External hemorrhoids

External hemorrhoid with thrombosis

First degree internal hemorrhoid

Fourth degree internal hemorrhoid

Internal hemorrhoids

Perianal hematoma

Piles

Second degree internal hemorrhoid

Third degree internal hemorrhoid

Thrombosed hemorrhoids

Clinician Documentation Checklist
Clinician documentation should indicate the following:

- Piles
- Combined
- Hemorrhoid skin tag

I-10 ALERT

The classification axis for hemorrhoids is completely revised in ICD-10-CM. It has been moved from the circulatory chapter to the digestive system chapter. Instead of internal/external and bleeding/other complication axes, ICD-10-CM classifies these conditions according to degree, first through fourth.

CDI ALERT

Alert the medical staff to the need for documentation of the degree or stage of hemorrhoids and provide ICD-10-CM definitions, if necessary. Additionally, documentation often will indicate the location of the hemorrhoid using clock positioning.

CDI ALERT

Carefully examine the medical record documentation for indications of thrombosis. Thrombosis is a condition arising from the presence or formation of blood clots within a blood vessel that may cause vascular obstruction and insufficient oxygenation.

- Type
  - first-degree hemorrhoids
    - grade/stage I hemorrhoids
    - hemorrhoids (bleeding) without prolapse outside of anal canal
  - second-degree hemorrhoids
    - grade/stage II hemorrhoids
    - hemorrhoids (bleeding) that prolapse with straining, but retract spontaneously
  - third-degree hemorrhoids
    - grade/stage III hemorrhoids
    - hemorrhoids (bleeding) that prolapse with straining and require manual replacement into anal canal
  - fourth-degree hemorrhoids
    - grade/stage IV hemorrhoids
    - hemorrhoids (bleeding) with prolapsed tissue that cannot be manually replaced
  - residual hemorrhoids skin tags
    - external hemorrhoids
    - skin tags of anus
  - perianal venous thrombosis
    - external hemorrhoids with thrombosis
    - perianal hematoma
    - thrombosed hemorrhoids
  - other hemorrhoids:
    - internal hemorrhoids, without mention of degree
    - prolapsed hemorrhoids, degree not specified
  - unspecified hemorrhoids
    - hemorrhoids (bleeding)
    - hemorrhoids (bleeding) without mention of degree

Human Immunodeficiency Virus (HIV) Disease

Code Axes

Human immunodeficiency virus (HIV) disease **B2Ø** HCC

Clinical Tip

Some conditions are considered opportunistic infections and are routinely associated with HIV disease; it is vitally important that these conditions be coded when documented.

Condition	ICD-10-CM Code
Tuberculosis, all types	A15–A19.-
Strep and other sepsis	A4Ø.9, A41.-
Herpesviral infections	A6Ø.Ø[Ø-4,9], A6Ø.1, A6Ø.9, BØØ.-
Candidal infections	B37.-
Cryptococcal infections	B45.-
Pneumocystosis	B59
Kaposi's sarcoma	C46.-
Non-follicular lymphoma	C83.-
Mature T/NK-cell lymphoma	C84.-
Other specified and unspecified non-Hodgkin lymphoma	C85.-
Unspecified dementia	FØ3.9-
Other and unspecified encephalopathy and disorder of brain	G93.4-, G93.9
Acute and subacute endocarditis	I33.-
Flu due to identified influenza A virus with pneumonia	JØ9.X1
Other and unspecified viral pneumonia	J12.8-, J12.9
Bacterial pneumonia, NEC	J15.-
Lobar and other pneumonia	J18.[1,8,9]

Note: The codes in the table above are not all-inclusive.

Clinical Tip

According to the Centers for Disease Control and Prevention (CDC), in order to be diagnosed with AIDS, a person with HIV must have an AIDS-defining condition or have a baseline CD4 count less than 200 cells/mm.

Ensure that the patient's HIV status is clearly documented. If a patient has inconclusive serologic evidence of an HIV infection, code R75 should be assigned. A patient that has tested positive for HIV, but as of yet has had no symptoms or AIDS-defining conditions, should be classified to code Z21. The documentation differentiating these three HIV status positions should be clear in the medical record.

I-10 ALERT

The guidelines for ICD-10-CM indicate that the code for HIV disease should only be assigned for confirmed cases, which may consist of a physician's diagnostic statement. Positive serology or culture is not specifically required in order to assign the HIV code. If the reason for the encounter is for treatment of an HIV-related disease, the HIV code (B2Ø) should be assigned as the first-listed/principal diagnosis. Because of this guideline, it is essential that those staff members participating in the coding and/or documentation improvement efforts become knowledgeable about the disorders that are considered AIDS-defining conditions.

CDI ALERT

Carefully examine the medical record documentation. Terms such as "HIV positive," "known HIV," or "HIV test positive" refer to the patients' asymptomatic human immunodeficiency virus (HIV) status and do not refer to an HIV-related illness.

Key Terms

Key terms found in the documentation may include:

Acquired immune deficiency syndrome (AIDS)

AIDS related complex (ARC)

HIV infection, symptomatic

Primary HIV infection

Clinical Findings

Diagnostic Procedures and Services

- Laboratory
  - HIV antibody test
  - nucleic acid amplification assays
  - ELISA
  - Western blot
- Associated pathology
  - malignancies such as Kaposi's sarcoma, lymphoma and squamous cell carcinoma
  - fungal diseases such as candidiasis, cryptococcosis and penicilliosis
  - bacterial diseases such as tuberculosis, *Mycobacterium avium* complex, bacterial pneumonia, and septicemia
  - protozoal diseases such as *Pneumocystis carinii* pneumonia (PCP), toxoplasmosis, microsporidiosis, cryptosporidiosis, isosporiasis, and leishmaniasis
  - viral diseases such as those caused by cytomegalovirus, herpes simplex, and herpes zoster virus

Therapeutic Procedures and Services

- Therapy for opportunistic infections and malignancies: antibiotics for opportunistic infections and chemotherapy for malignancies
- Antiretroviral treatment: drugs that suppress the HIV infection. A combination of drugs is standard and using a single drug is discouraged.
- Hematopoietic stimulating factors: treatment of anemia
- Prophylaxis for opportunistic infections: prevention of certain infections before they develop. This should be offered to patients with CD4 counts below 200 cells/µl, weight loss, or oral candidiasis.
- Surgical procedures
  - placement of a vascular access device

Medication List

- Antiretroviral treatment: nucleoside reverse transcriptase inhibitors (NRTI)
  - Combivir
  - Emtriva
  - Videx, Videx EC
  - Retrovir (AZT)
  - Epzicom

- Nonnucleoside reverse transcriptase inhibitors (NNRTI)
  - Viramune
  - Rescriptor
  - Sustiva
- Prophylaxis treatment
  - Trimethoprim-sulfamethoxazole
  - Dapsone
  - aerolized pentamidine
  - Clarithromycin
  - Rifabutin
- Hematopoietic stimulating factors
  - erythropoietin
- Treatment of opportunistic infections
  - Trimetrexate
  - Primaquine
  - Clindamycin

Hypertension Complicating Childbirth, Pregnancy, and the Puerperium

CDI ALERT

Documentation must indicate if the hypertension is pre-existing or gestational as well as the following:

- Trimester
- Hypertensive heart disease when present
- Chronic kidney disease when present
- Pre-eclampsia if present

Code Axes

Pre-existing hypertension complicating pregnancy, childbirth and the puerperium	**O10.0- O10.42 O10.43**
Pre-existing hypertension with pre-eclampsia	**O11.-**
Gestational (pregnancy-induced) hypertension without significant proteinuria	**O13.-**
Unspecified maternal hypertension	**O16.-**

CDI ALERT

In addition to identifying any conditions associated with the hypertension as shown in the Key Terms section, the documentation should also indicate whether the hypertension is essential, secondary, or unspecified. If unspecified, query the physician as to the type.

Description of Condition

The Pregnancy, Childbirth and the Puerperium chapter of the ICD-10-CM system contains codes which describe pregnancy complicated by hypertension.

I-10 ALERT

Category O10 Pre-existing hypertension complicating pregnancy, childbirth and the puerperium, includes codes for hypertensive heart and hypertensive chronic kidney disease. When assigning one of the O10 codes that includes hypertensive heart disease or hypertensive chronic kidney disease, it is necessary to add a secondary code from the appropriate hypertension category to specify the type of heart failure or chronic kidney disease.

Pre-existing hypertension complication pregnancy, childbirth and the puerperium (O10.01–O10.93)

Documentation should indicate pre-existing hypertension affecting the management of the pregnancy.

Key Terms

Key terms found in the documentation may include:

Eclampsia complicated by pre-existing hypertension
Pre-eclampsia complicated by pre-existing hypertension
Pregnancy complicated by hypertension due to ______________
Pregnancy complicated by hypertensive arteriosclerosis of kidney
Pregnancy complicated by hypertensive cardiovascular disease
Pregnancy complicated by hypertensive chronic kidney disease
Pregnancy complicated by hypertensive chronic nephritis
Pregnancy complicated by hypertensive chronic renal disease
Pregnancy complicated by hypertensive heart disease
Pregnancy complicated by hypertensive heart failure
Pregnancy complicated by hypertensive interstitial nephritis
Pregnancy complicated by hypertensive nephropathy
Pregnancy complicated by hypertensive nephrosclerosis
Pregnancy complicated by hypertensive renal disease
Pregnancy complicated by secondary hypertension

Pre-existing hypertension with pre-eclampsia (O11.1–O11.9)

Pre-eclampsia is a complication of pregnancy manifesting in the development of borderline hypertension, protein in the urine, and unresponsive swelling between the 20th week of pregnancy and the end of the first week following birth in mild to moderate cases. Severe pre-eclampsia presents with hypertension (blood pressure greater than 150/100) associated with marked swelling, proteinuria, abdominal pain, and/or visual changes. Documentation must support that the patient had pre-existing hypertension or this code is not supported. ***Synonym(s):*** mild toxemia.

> **I-10 ALERT**
>
> When reporting a code from O11, an additional code from category O10 must be assigned to indicate the type of hypertension.

Key Terms

Key terms found in the documentation may include:

Essential hypertension (pre-eclampsia)

Hypertension with pre-eclampsia

Maternal hypertension superimposed with pre-eclampsia

Pre-existing hypertension (pre-eclampsia)

> **CDI ALERT**
>
> Documentation should indicate the type of hypertension present (i.e., essential, secondary) as well as any organ involvement (i.e., hypertensive heart disease, chronic kidney disease)

Gestational (pregnancy-induced) hypertension without significant proteinuria (O13.1–O13.9)

Gestational hypertension is a form of hypertension that forms during pregnancy. Gestational hypertension is diagnosed when blood pressure readings are higher than 140/90 mm Hg after 20 weeks of pregnancy with normal blood pressure.

Key Terms

Key terms found in the documentation may include:

Gestation hypertension

Gestational hypertension without proteinuria

Hypertension during pregnancy

Hypertension with pregnancy

> **CDI ALERT**
>
> When the physician documentation indicates that the patient has significant amounts of protein in the urine (i.e., proteinuria), query the physician to see if the patient may be pre-eclamptic.

Unspecified maternal hypertension (O16.1–O16.9)

Hypertension during pregnancy; documentation does not indicate if the hypertension is pre-existing or gestational.

> **CDI ALERT**
>
> Query the physician to determine if a more specific diagnosis is available.

Clinical Findings

Physical Examination

History and review of systems may include:

- Rapid weight gain
- Swelling of hands, face and feet that persists
- Decreased/no urine output
- Severe headaches
- Bloody urine
- Dizziness

- Excessive nausea and vomiting
- Visual disturbance
- Hypertension severity
- Reflex changes
- Abdominal pain

Diagnostic Procedures and Services

- Laboratory
  - urinalysis
  - urine dip
  - CBC
  - glucose levels
  - liver enzymes
  - creatinine clearance
  - serum creatinine
  - BUN
  - albumin
  - uric acid
  - TSH
- Other
  - fetal ultrasound transducer

Therapeutic Procedures and Services

- Home BP monitoring
- Patient education
- Bed rest
- Fetal monitoring
- Antihypertension medication if applicable

Clinician Documentation Checklist

Clinician documentation should indicate the following:

- At time of visit
  - antepartum (trimester #)
  - childbirth
  - puerperium
- Type
  - pre-existing
    - essential
    - secondary
      - etiology when known
    - hypertensive heart disease
      - type of heart disease
      - hypertensive chronic kidney disease

- stage of kidney disease
  - hypertensive heart and chronic kidney disease
    - type of heart disease
    - stage of kidney disease
  - unspecified
  - with pre-eclampsia
    - type of heart disease
- gestational
  - without significant proteinuria
- unspecified maternal hypertension

Pre-existing Hypertension with Pre-eclampsia

- Trimester
- Gestational edema only
- Pre-eclampsia
  - Severity
    - mild
    - moderate
    - severe
  - HELLP syndrome, if present
  - with hypertension
    - gestational
    - pre-existing

Hypertensive Diseases

Code Axes

Essential (primary) hypertension	**I1Ø**
Hypertensive heart disease	**I11.-** HCC
Hypertensive chronic kidney disease	**I12.-** HCC
Hypertensive heart and chronic kidney disease	**I13.-** HCC
Secondary hypertension	**I15.-**
Postoperative hypertension	**I97.3**

Description of Condition

Essential (primary) hypertension (I1Ø)

Elevated arterial blood pressure that occurs without an apparent organic cause. In the benign form, the blood pressure is mildly elevated. In the malignant form, the elevation is severe and may result in necrosis of the kidneys or retinas. Hemorrhage and death may occur, most often due to uremia or rupture of cerebral vessels.

⇨ I-10 ALERT

Hypertension no longer uses type as an axes of classification. Therefore, terms such as "malignant," "benign," or "unspecified" no longer require a different code assignment and are included in the essential (primary) hypertension category (I1Ø).

Key Terms

Key terms found in the documentation may include:

- Arterial hypertension
- Benign hypertension
- Controlled hypertension
- Essential hypertension
- HBP
- High blood pressure
- HTN
- Hypertension
- Malignant hypertension
- Primary hypertension
- Uncotrolled hypertension

Hypertensive heart disease (I11.Ø–I11.9)

A causal relationship is stated (due to hypertension) or implied (hypertensive).

The same heart conditions (I5Ø.-, I51.4–I51.9) with hypertension are also assigned a code from this category.

CDI ALERT

Documentation containing an elevated BP without mention of hypertension does not support a diagnosis of hypertension.

Key terms
Key terms found in the documentation may include:

Hypertensive cardiovascular disease
Hypertensive heart disease
Hypertensive heart failure

Hypertensive chronic kidney disease (I12.Ø–I12.9)

Documentation indicates that both hypertension and a condition classifiable to category N18 Chronic kidney disease (CKD), are present. Since a cause-and-effect relationship is presumed, when documentation indicates both chronic kidney disease with hypertension this category is supported.

> **I-10 ALERT**
> When documentation states the hypertension is due to kidney disease, the hypertension is considered secondary.

Key Terms
Key terms found in the documentation may include:

Hypertension and arteriosclerosis of kidney
Hypertension and chronic kidney disease
Hypertension and chronic nephritis
Hypertension and chronic renal disease
Hypertension and interstitial nephritis
Hypertension and nephrosclerosis
Hypertensive chronic kidney disease
Hypertensive nephropathy
Hypertensive renal disease

> **CDI ALERT**
> Documentation should also identify the stage of chronic kidney disease. This is reported separately.

Hypertensive heart and chronic kidney disease (I13.1–I13.9)

When both hypertensive kidney disease and hypertensive heart disease are stated in the diagnosis, the appropriate code from category I13 is supported. The ICD-10-CM system assumes a relationship between the hypertension and the chronic kidney disease, whether or not the condition is documented as related.

Key Terms
Key terms found in the documentation may include:

Hypertensive chronic heart and kidney disease
Hypertensive heart and renal disease
Hypertensive heart disease and arteriosclerosis of kidney
Hypertensive heart disease and chronic kidney disease
Hypertensive heart disease and chronic nephritis
Hypertensive heart disease and chronic renal disease
Hypertensive heart disease and interstitial nephritis
Hypertensive heart disease and nephrosclerosis
Hypertensive nephropathy and hypertensive heart disease

> **CDI ALERT**
> When documentation indicates that heart failure is present, an additional code from category I5Ø to identify the type of heart failure is assigned.

Secondary Hypertension (I15.Ø-I15.9)

Secondary hypertension is hypertension that is due to an underlying condition.

> ➩ **I-10 ALERT**
>
> Two codes are required: one to identify the underlying etiology and one from category I15 to identify the hypertension. Sequencing is determined by the reason for admission/encounter.

Key Terms

Key terms found in the documentation may include:

Hypertension due to ___________

Renovascular hypertension

Secondary hypertension [condition causing the hypertension]

Postoperative hypertension (I97.3)

Documentation indicates that hypertension as the complication of a procedure is present.

Key Terms

Key terms found in the documentation may include:

Postprocedure hypertension

Clinical Findings

Physical Examination

Hypertension is typically asymptomatic until complications arise in other organ systems. History and review of symptoms may include:

- Dizziness
- Headache
- Epistaxis
- Flushed face
- Fatigue

Severe hypertension may cause major cardiovascular and renal symptoms including:

- Shortness of breath with minimal exertion
- Swollen ankles, legs, and feet
- Swelling in abdomen
- Pitting edema
- Jugular vein distention
- Confusion
- Blurry or double vision
- Bloody urine
- Decrease in urine output
- Exam
  - funduscopic exam
  - auscultation for bruits (neck and abdomen)
  - peripheral pulses
  - complete cardiac, neurologic and respiratory exam

Diagnostic Procedures and Services

- Laboratory
  - urinalysis
  - albumin
  - creatinine
  - fasting plasma glucose
  - Na
  - TSH
  - lipid profile
- Imaging
  - chest x-ray
  - Doppler ultrasound
  - angiography
  - cardiac MRI
  - cardiac cath
  - echocardiogram
- Other
  - EKG
  - Holter monitor
  - stress test

Therapeutic Procedures and Services

- Low-salt diet
- Lifestyle changes
- Smoking cessation
- Implantable cardioverter defibrillator (ICD)
- Left ventricular assist device

Medication List

- diuretic
- beta blocker
- ACE inhibitor
- Ca channel blockers
- angiotensin II receptor blockers (ARB)
- digoxin
- aldosterone antagonists
- direct vasodilators

Clinician Documentation Checklist

Clinician documentation should indicate the following:

- Hypertension
- Heart disease
- Heart failure
  - diastolic
    - acute
    - chronic
  - systolic
    - acute
    - chronic
- Chronic kidney disease (CKD)
  - CKD stage

Hysterectomy

Code Axes

Hysterectomy procedures	**58150–58294**
Laparoscopic hysterectomy	**58541–58554**

Description of Procedure

A hysterectomy is the removal of the uterus. The tubes and/or ovaries may or may not be removed at the time of a hysterectomy procedure. There are three surgical approaches that can be used to perform a hysterectomy (abdominal incision or open, vaginal approach, or laparoscopic approach) and other services may be performed during the surgical encounter such as urethrocystopexy for urinary incontinence or lymph node sampling. It is also important to note that the size of the uterus may also affect code assignment.

Open Approach

Total abdominal hysterectomy (corpus and cervix), with or without removal of tube(s), with or without removal of ovary(s) (58150)

Total abdominal hysterectomy (corpus and cervix), with or without removal of tube(s), with or without removal of ovary(s); with colpourethrocystopexy (e.g., Marshall-Marchetti-Krantz, Burch) (58152)

Documentation will indicate a horizontal incision just within the pubic hairline. The physician removes the uterus including the cervix and may elect to remove one or both of the ovaries and one or both of the fallopian tubes (salpingo-oophorectomy). The supporting pedicles containing the tubes, ligaments, and arteries are clamped and cut free. The uterus and cervix are removed along with a narrow rim or cuff of vaginal lining. The vaginal defect may be left open for drainage.

At the time of a total hysterectomy, it may also be necessary to perform a colpourethrocystopexy for urinary incontinence. Documentation will indicate that the bladder neck is suspended by placing sutures through the tissue surrounding the urethra and into the back of the symphysis pubis, which is the midline junction of the pubic bones in the front (Marshall-Marchetti-Krantz or MMK), or sutures may be placed in the fascia on either side of the bladder and then through the Cooper's ligaments above. The sutures are then tied which elevates the vesical neck (the junction of the bladder and urethra) in the direction of the Cooper's ligament (Burch procedure). The sutures are pulled tight so that the tissues are tacked to the symphysis pubis and the urethra is moved forward.

Supracervical abdominal hysterectomy (subtotal hysterectomy), with or without removal of tube(s), with or without removal of ovaries (58180)

CDI ALERT

When the documentation states that the uterus weighs more than 250 grams, see codes 58543–58544.

Documentation for a supracervical abdominal hysterectomy will indicate the removal of the uterus above the cervix and may elect to remove one or both of the ovaries and one or both of the fallopian tubes (salpingo-oophorectomy) via a horizontal incision just within the pubic hairline. It is important to note that the uteri cervix is not removed during this service.

LAPAROSCOPIC APPROACH

Laparoscopy, surgical, supracervical hysterectomy, for uterus greater than 250 g (58543)

Laparoscopy, surgical, supracervical hysterectomy, for uterus greater than 250 g; with removal of tube(s) and ovary(s) (58544)

Key terms in the documentation for these procedures will indicate that the patient is placed in the dorsal lithotomy position, that a speculum is placed in the vagina so that the clinician may grasp the cervix with an instrument to manipulate the uterus during the surgery, and that trocars are inserted periumbilically in the right and left lower quadrants of the abdomen. Documentation will also indicate that the uterus is morcellized and removed using endoscopic tools. In 58544, one or both ovaries and/or one or both fallopian tubes are removed in similar fashion. Once the excisions are complete, the abdominal cavity is deflated and instruments and trocars removed. The fascia and skin are closed with sutures.

Vaginal hysterectomy, with total or partial vaginectomy (58275)

Vaginal hysterectomy, with total or partial vaginectomy; with repair of enterocele (58280)

Vaginal hysterectomy, radical (Schauta type operation) (58285)

Schauta procedure

The Schauta procedure is the surgical removal through a vaginal approach of the uterus, cervix, upper vagina, and parametrium. This procedure does not permit pelvic lymph node dissection but is useful in certain patients, such as in obese patients. Other parts such as the lymph nodes, ovaries, and fallopian tubes are also usually removed if clinically indicated. It is usually performed for early malignancy of the cervix but can also be performed on patients who have severe uterine prolapse or prolapse accompanied by stress incontinence and for patients with pelvic relaxation, history of myomata, and irregular uterine bleeding.

Vaginal hysterectomy for uterus greater than 250 g (58290–58294)

Vaginal Hysterectomy

A vaginal hysterectomy is the removal of the uterus through the vagina. During a vaginal hysterectomy, the surgeon detaches the uterus from the ovaries, fallopian tubes, and upper vagina, as well as from the blood vessels and connective tissue that support it. The uterus is then removed through the vagina. This service can be done either open (by incision) or laparoscopically.

When reviewing the clinical documentation for vaginal hysterectomies it is important to determine:

- Size of the uterus
- If the procedure was open or laparoscopic
- If the ovaries and/or tubes were removed
- Any additional services performed at the time of the procedure (such as urethrocystopexy or vaginectomy)

Below are some key items to look for in documentation for specific procedures.

- Codes 58260–58264 are used to report an open vaginal hysterectomy of a uterus 250 grams or less. Correct code assignment is determined based on whether the ovaries and/or fallopian tubes were removed or not and what additional services were performed during the same operative session.
- Codes 58275 and 58280 are used to report a vaginal hysterectomy with a total or partial vaginectomy. Report 58280 when documentation indicates that an enterocele was also performed.
- When the uterine weight is over 250 grams, codes 58290–58294 are reported. As with codes 58260–58270, appropriate code selection is dependent upon what, if any, other procedures are performed during the surgical encounter.

Clinician Documentation Checklist

Clinician documentation should indicate the following:

- Medical condition being treated
- Surgical approach
  - abdominal or open
  - vaginal
  - laparoscopic
- Weight of uterus (g)
- Vaginectomy performed
  - total
  - partial
  - radical

- Other procedures performed
  - removal of tubes
  - removal of ovary(s)
  - removal of bladder
  - urethral transplantations
  - resection of rectum
  - resection of colon
  - colostomy
  - repair of enterocele
  - lymph node sampling (biopsy)

Influenza

Code Axes

Influenza due to identified novel influenza A virus with pneumonia **J09.X1**

Influenza due to identified novel influenza A virus with other respiratory manifestations **J09.X2**

Influenza due to identified novel influenza A virus with gastrointestinal manifestations **J09.X3**

Influenza due to identified novel influenza A virus with other manifestations **J09.X9**

Influenza due to other identified influenza virus with unspecified type of pneumonia **J10.00**

Influenza due to other identified influenza virus with the same other identified influenza virus pneumonia **J10.01**

Influenza due to other identified influenza virus with other specified pneumonia **J10.08**

Influenza due to other identified influenza virus with other respiratory manifestations **J10.1**

Influenza due to other identified influenza virus with gastrointestinal manifestations **J10.2**

Influenza due to other identified influenza virus with other manifestations **J10.8-**

Subcategories represent conditions with encephalopathy, myocarditis, otitis media, and other manifestations.

Influenza due to unidentified influenza virus with pneumonia **J11.0-**

Subcategories identify whether the pneumonia is unspecified or specified.

Influenza due to unidentified influenza virus with other respiratory manifestations **J11.1**

Influenza due to unidentified influenza virus with gastrointestinal manifestations **J11.2**

Influenza due to unidentified influenza virus with other manifestations **J11.8-**

Subcategories represent conditions with encephalopathy, myocarditis, otitis media, and other manifestations.

⇨ I-10 ALERT

Codes in these categories representing specific forms of influenza should only be assigned if the specific disease process (e.g., novel influenza A virus) is documented as confirmed. The specific codes in these categories should not be assigned if the corresponding documentation contains terminology such as "possible," "suspected," or "probable." In those instances, assign the appropriate code(s) for the presenting symptoms.

> **CDI Alert**
>
> Ensure that the medical record indicates the causal agent or virus, if possible. If the condition is due to influenza A virus, treatment typically involves oseltamivir or zanamivir.

Description of Condition

Influenza (all types) with pneumonia (JØ9.X1, J1Ø.Ø[Ø,1,8], J11.Ø[Ø,8])

Clinical Tip

Influenza due to novel virus A is most commonly isolated from birds, whether domestic poultry or wild birds, which act as asymptomatic carriers of influenza A virus. The category also includes influenza designated as that due to swine or other animals. The course of the disease largely depends on the manifestations, which can range from pneumonia or other respiratory conditions, to encephalopathy or myocarditis.

Key Terms

Key terms found in the documentation for novel influenza A virus may include:

- Avian flu
- Avian influenza
- Bird flu
- Bird influenza
- H5N1
- Influenza A/H5N1
- Influenza of other animal origin, not bird or swine
- Swine influenza (viruses that normally cause infections in pigs)

Clinician Note

Documentation must indicate the presence of pneumonia to support code assignment. When documentation does not specifically indicate pneumonia, see Influenza (all types) with other respiratory manifestations.

Influenza (all types) with other respiratory manifestations (JØ9.X2, J1Ø.1, J11.1)

Clinical Tip

Patients with influenza may demonstrate respiratory conditions other than pneumonia, which may include laryngitis, pharyngitis, or other upper respiratory symptoms. Ensure that any associated pleural effusion and/or sinusitis is documented and coded separately.

Key Terms

Key terms found in the documentation for influenza-related respiratory manifestations may include:

- Influenzal laryngitis
- Influenzal pharyngitis
- Influenzal upper respiratory symptoms

Clinical Tip

Chest pain, cough, fever, hiccups, rapid breathing, or shortness of breath are symptoms of pleural effusion; however, unless specifically indicated by the physician the code for pleural effusion should not be reported.

Influenza (all types) with other manifestations (JØ9.X9, J1Ø.8-, J11.8-)

CDI ALERT

Conditions such as encephalopathy, myocarditis, and other serious clinical conditions are very rare when associated with the influenzal virus. Ensure that documentation clearly links the conditions before assigning the condition to this classification.

Key Terms

Key terms found in the documentation for influenza-related manifestations may include:

Influenzal encephalopathy

Influenzal myocarditis

Influenzal otitis media

Clinical Findings

Physical Examination

History and review of symptoms include fever, cough, sudden onset of chills, headache sometimes with photophobia, and general aches and pains. In mild cases symptoms may resemble a common cold. Respiratory symptoms may start as a scratchy sore throat and nonproductive cough and progress to a persistent, productive cough.

Diagnostic Procedures and Services

- Reverse transcriptase assays
- Rapid diagnostic testing
- Pulse oximetry
- Imaging
  - chest x-ray

Therapeutic Procedures and Services

- Treat symptoms
- Rest
- Hydration

Medication List

- Antiviral drugs
  - adamantanes
    - amantadine (Symmetrel)
    - rimantadine (Flumadine)
  - neuraminidase inhibitors
    - oseltamivir (Tamiflu)
    - zanamivir (Relenza)
- Vaccination against seasonal influenza

Clinician Documentation Checklist

Clinician documentation should indicate the following:

- Influenza due to
  - novel influenza a virus (certain identified virus)
    - avian influenza
    - bird influenza
    - influenza a/h5n1
    - influenza of other animal origin, not bird or swine
    - swine influenza virus
  - other identified influenza virus
    - identification of the virus
  - unidentified influenza virus
- Influenza with
  - pneumonia
    - identify for
      - associated lung abscess
      - type of pneumonia
        - same as other identified influenza virus
        - other specified
        - unspecified
  - other respiratory manifestations
    - laryngitis
    - pharyngitis
    - upper respiratory symptoms
    - identify for associated
      - pleural effusion
      - sinusitis
  - gastrointestinal manifestations
    - gastroenteritis
  - other manifestations
    - encephalopathy
    - myocarditis
    - otitis media
      - identify for associated perforated tympanic membrane
    - other
      - identify the manifestations

Injections and Infusions (Non-chemotherapy)

Code Axes

Hydration, therapeutic, prophylactic, and diagnostic injections and infusions (nonchemotherapy) **96360–96379**

Key Terms

Key terms found in the documentation may include:

IM Inj

Inf

Inj

Intradermal Inj

IV Inf

SQ Inj

> **CDI ALERT**
>
> Documentation should state why the patient required these services to support the medical necessity.

Clinician Documentation Checklist

Clinician documentation should indicate the following:

- The site of the injection or infusion
- The route of administration
  - subcutaneous
  - intramuscular
  - intravenous
  - intradermal
- The substance administered
  - fluids
  - medication
  - sequential
  - combined
  - the number of units

> **CDI ALERT**
>
> The volume of hydration therapy and the doses of nonchemotherapy drugs administered should be clearly documented.

In the instance of infusions the documentation should also include:

- If the IV therapy was the main service
- The amount of time
- Technique (i.e., push or drip)
- If for hydration

> **CDI ALERT**
>
> The stop and start time of infusion therapy should be documented in order to support code assignment.

Intracranial Injury

Code Axes

Concussion	**SØ6.ØX-** HCC
Traumatic cerebral edema	**SØ6.1X-** HCC
Diffuse traumatic brain injury	**SØ6.2X-** HCC
Focal traumatic brain injury, unspecified	**SØ6.3Ø-** HCC
Contusion and laceration of cerebrum (right, left, unspecified)	**SØ6.3[1,2,3]-** HCC
Traumatic hemorrhage of cerebrum (right, left, unspecified)	**SØ6.3[4,5,6]-** HCC
Contusion, laceration, and hemorrhage of cerebellum	**SØ6.37-** HCC
Contusion, laceration, and hemorrhage of brainstem	**SØ6.38-** HCC
Epidural hemorrhage	**SØ6.4X-** HCC
Traumatic subdural hemorrhage	**SØ6.5X-** HCC
Traumatic subarachnoid hemorrhage	**SØ6.6X-** HCC
Injury of [right, left] internal carotid artery, intracranial portion, NEC	**SØ6.8[1,2]-** HCC
Other specified and unspecified intracranial injury	**SØ6.89-** HCC, **SØ6.9X-** HCC

Classification Note

All of the code subcategories listed above are also differentiated along two additional code axes: one related to duration of loss of consciousness and one related to type of encounter. The additional character choices are as follows:

Sixth character: Loss of consciousness:

Ø without loss of consciousness

1 with loss of consciousness of 30 minutes or less

2 with loss of consciousness of 31 minutes to 59 minutes

3 with loss of consciousness of 1 hour to 5 hours 59 minutes

4 with loss of consciousness of 6 hours to 24 hours

5 with loss of consciousness greater than 24 hours with return to pre-existing conscious level

6 with loss of consciousness greater than 24 hours without return to pre-existing conscious level with patient surviving

7 with loss of consciousness of any duration with death due to brain injury prior to regaining consciousness

8 with loss of consciousness of any duration with death due to other cause prior to regaining consciousness

9 with loss of consciousness of unspecified duration

Seventh character: Type of encounter:

A initial encounter

D subsequent encounter

S sequela

Concussion (SØ6.ØX-)

Clinical Tip

A concussion is the most common and mildest form of traumatic brain injury (TBI) with a variety of symptoms, including somatic (e.g., headache), cognitive (e.g., feeling dazed), and emotional (e.g., increased irritability). In addition, some patients experience physical signs, such as loss of consciousness or amnesia, cognitive impairment, such as slowed reaction times, or sleep disturbances. Patients with a personal history of concussion are at higher risk for another, particularly if the new injury occurs before symptoms from the initial injury have resolved. Symptoms typically resolve within seven to 10 days, with no serious long-term effects. Varying definitions exist, but it is thought that a concussion is a functional state, meaning that symptoms are caused primarily by temporary biochemical changes in neurons, taking place at their cell membranes and synapses.

CDI ALERT

If a concussion is documented along with a more specific intracranial injury, the case should be classified to that specific intracranial injury.

Key Terms

Key terms found in the documentation for concussion may include:

Commotio cerebri

Mild brain injury

Mild head injury (MHI)

Minor head trauma

Mild traumatic brain injury (MTBI)

Traumatic cerebral edema (SØ6.1X-)

Clinical Tip

Cerebral edema following a traumatic event can lead to an expansion of brain volume and has a crucial impact on morbidity and mortality as it increases intracranial pressure, impairs cerebral perfusion and oxygenation, and contributes to additional ischemic injuries. It has been determined that the formation of cerebral edema is one of the major factors leading to the high mortality and morbidity in a traumatic brain injury (TBI) patient. Recently, significant progress has been made toward identifying factors that contribute to edema formation after TBI, most notably both vasogenic and cytotoxic cerebral edema that causes the blood brain barrier (BBB) to remain open. Managing BBB permeability has increasingly become a promising approach to managing brain edema and associated swelling.

CDI ALERT

Ensure that any connection between cerebral swelling or edema and the patient's personal history of trauma are documented clearly in the medical record.

Key Terms
Key terms found in the documentation for traumatic cerebral edema may include:

Diffuse traumatic cerebral edema

Focal traumatic cerebral edema

Diffuse traumatic brain injury (SØ6.2X-)

Clinical Tip
Diffuse traumatic brain injury occurs over a widespread area of the brain as opposed to focal brain injury, which is confined to one specific area. It is common for both focal and diffuse damage to occur as the result of the same event; many traumatic brain injuries have aspects of both focal and diffuse injury. Diffuse injuries are most often found in acceleration/deceleration injuries in which the head does not necessarily hit anything, but brain tissue is damaged because tissue types with varying densities accelerate at different rates. This also includes brain injury due to hypoxia, meningitis, or damage to blood vessels. Diffuse injuries may be difficult to detect and define because often, much of the damage is microscopic.

Key Terms
Key terms found in the documentation for diffuse traumatic brain injury may include:

Acceleration/deceleration brain injury

Diffuse axonal brain injury

Unspecified focal traumatic brain injury (SØ6.3Ø-)

Clinical Tip
Focal brain injury occurs in a specific location and it is common for both focal and diffuse damage to occur as the result of the same event; many traumatic brain injuries have aspects of both focal and diffuse injury. Focal injuries are most commonly associated with an injury in which the head strikes or is struck by an object and is usually associated with brain tissue damage visible to the naked eye. The manifestations associated with this type of injury generally relate to the area that has been damaged.

Key Terms
Key terms found in the documentation for focal traumatic brain injury may include:

Focal neurological deficit brain injury

Contusion and laceration of cerebrum (right, left, unspecified) (SØ6.3[1,2,3]-)

Clinical Tip

A cerebral laceration is a type of traumatic brain injury that involves the tissue of the brain being mechanically cut or torn, while a cerebral contusion does not involve the tears. Lacerations are very common in penetrating and perforating head trauma injuries and in many cases accompany skull fractures. They are particularly common in the inferior frontal lobes and the poles of the temporal lobes. Both conditions are considered more serious than concussions and can cause bleeding or swelling in the brain. Intracranial pressure is monitored and surgical treatment may be required.

CDI ALERT

Ensure that any signs of either contusion and/or laceration are documented clearly in the medical record, with differentiation of each.

Traumatic hemorrhage of cerebrum (right, left, unspecified) (SØ6.3[4,5,6]-)

Clinical Tip

Three criteria that are typically used to classify cerebral hemorrhages are: location (i.e., subarachnoid, extradural, subdural), kind of vessel involved (i.e., arterial, venous, capillary), and origin (i.e., traumatic, degenerative). Each kind of cerebral hemorrhage has distinctive clinical characteristics. The hemorrhage may lead to displacement or destruction of brain tissue and in some cases an extensive hemorrhage can be fatal.

Key Terms

Key terms found in the documentation for traumatic hemorrhage of cerebrum may include:

Traumatic cerebral hematoma

Traumatic intracerebral hemorrhage

Contusion, laceration, and hemorrhage of cerebellum (SØ6.37-)

Clinical Tip

The cerebellum is located at the base of the skull and controls coordination, balance, and equilibrium. Hemorrhaging into this area causes dizziness, loss of coordination, and/or vomiting. In most cases, a patient who is awake and has a Glasgow coma scale score of 14 or greater with a small hemorrhage, without hydrocephalus, may be a candidate for conservative supportive care with close monitoring. Ventriculostomy may be indicated in patients with hemorrhage and hydrocephalus, but is controversial.

CDI ALERT

Ensure that any signs of either contusion and/or laceration are documented clearly in the medical record, with differentiation of each.

Contusion, laceration, and hemorrhage of brainstem (SØ6.38-)

Clinical Tip

Traumatic brainstem hemorrhage after blunt head injury is an uncommon event, although the most frequent site of hemorrhage is the midline rostral brainstem. The prognosis of these patients is poor because of its critical location. Traumatic brainstem hemorrhage typically results in coma, decerebrate posturing, and autonomic nervous system dysfunction.

Epidural hemorrhage (SØ6.4X-)

Clinical Tip

An epidural or extradural hematoma is a type of traumatic brain injury (TBI) in which a buildup of blood occurs between the dura mater, the tough outer membrane of the central nervous system) and the skull. The condition can be life threatening because the buildup of blood may increase pressure in the intracranial space, compress delicate brain tissue, and cause brain shift. There may be a lucid period of time after the injury and a time lag before symptoms appear, which may rapidly progress to coma. This typically occurs at six to eight hours post injury.

Traumatic subdural hemorrhage (SØ6.5X-)

> **CDI ALERT**
>
> Ensure that documentation of the timing between injury and symptoms is clearly defined in the medical record, particularly if the patient has a history of both acute and chronic subdural hematoma.

Clinical Tip

A subdural hematoma is a collection of blood in the space between the outer layer (dura) and middle layers of the covering of the brain (the meninges). The time between the injury and the appearance of symptoms can vary from less than 48 hours to several weeks or more. Symptoms appearing in less than 48 hours are due to an acute subdural hematoma. This type of bleeding is often fatal and results from tearing of the venous sinus. If more than two weeks have passed before symptoms appear, the condition is called a chronic subdural hematoma resulting from tearing of the smaller vein.

Key Terms

Key terms found in the documentation for traumatic subdural hemorrhage may include:

Extradural hemorrhage

Clinician Note

Coordination of benefits is often required for payment from third-party payers; therefore, the documentation should indicate how the injury occurred (e.g., auto accident, fall from ladder at work, fall when riding a bike).

Traumatic subarachnoid hemorrhage (SØ6.6X-)

Clinical Tip

Traumatic subarachnoid hemorrhage refers to bleeding into the subarachnoid space that is found between the middle (arachnoid) and the innermost (pia mater) membranes that cover the brain. The condition occurs as the result of severe blunt head trauma. In this condition the brain may be subject to severe twisting and torsion that can shear blood vessels between the arachnoid and pia mater resulting in subarachnoid hemorrhage. Swelling of brain tissue with an increase in pressure in the brain may result. A blood clot and increased intracranial pressure can obstruct the flow of cerebrospinal fluid resulting in hydrocephalus.

Clinician Note

Coordination of benefits is often required for payment from third-party payers; therefore, the documentation should indicate how the injury occurred (e.g., auto accident, fall from ladder at work, fall when riding a bike).

Injury of [right, left] internal carotid artery, intracranial portion, NEC (SØ6.8[1,2]-)

Clinical Tip

Carotid artery injury is relatively rare and is reported to occur in approximately 1 percent of individuals who experience severe blunt head trauma. Arterial dissections in the head and neck usually are associated with deceleration and shear injuries and treatment of carotid and vertebral arterial dissections remains somewhat controversial. The most conservative approach includes medical management, with ongoing debate as to whether anticoagulation with heparin and/or antiplatelet therapy is more effective. Stents have been used to treat patients who have contraindications to anticoagulation or antiplatelet therapy.

CDI ALERT

Ensure that documentation clearly indicates the site of the injury, particularly the portion of the carotid artery involved.

Clinician Note

Coordination of benefits is often required for payment from third-party payers; therefore, the documentation should indicate how the injury occurred (e.g., auto accident, fall from ladder at work, fall when riding a bike).

Clinical Findings

Physical Examination

History and review of symptoms may include:

- Rapid trauma assessment
- Glasgow coma scale (GCS)
- Neurological examination
- Common symptoms
  - fatigue
  - headache
  - memory loss
  - sleep disturbance
  - irritability
  - vision problems (blurred, loss of, sensitivity to light, diplopia)
  - depression
  - poor concentration
  - seizures
  - confusion
  - nausea
  - loss of smell
  - lack of concentration

- slurred speech
- difficulty conversing
- tinnitus
- sensitivity to sound
- impaired hearing
- papilledema

Diagnostic Procedures and Services

- Laboratory
  - blood test
  - toxicology
- Imaging
  - CT
  - MRI
  - PET scan
- Other
  - EEG
  - sensor to monitor intracranial pressure (ICP)

Therapeutic Procedures and Services

- Monitor pupillary reaction, BP, pulse frequently
- Discharge home if TBI is mild
- Patients with moderate TBI are observed in the hospital
- Patients with severe TBI are admitted to a critical care unit
- Surgery
- Mechanical ventilation
- Oxygen therapy

Medication List

- Antiseizure medication
  - phenytoin (Dilantin)
  - thiopental (Pentothal)
- Barbiturates to lower intracranial pressure
  - hypertonic saline solution
- Corticosteroids
- Sedation in critical cases
  - etomidate (Amidate)
  - lorazepam (Ativan)
  - propofol (Diprivan)

Intraoperative and Postprocedural Complications and Disorders of Ear and Mastoid Process

Code Axes

Recurrent cholesteatoma of postmastoidectomy cavity	**H95.Ø-**
Chronic inflammation of postmastoidectomy cavity	**H95.11-**
Granulation of postmastoidectomy cavity	**H95.12-**
Mucosal cyst of postmastoidectomy cavity	**H95.13-**
Intraoperative hemorrhage and hematoma of ear and mastoid process complicating a procedure	**H95.2-**
Accidental puncture and laceration of ear and mastoid process during a procedure	**H95.3-**
Postprocedural hemorrhage of ear and mastoid process following a procedure	**H95.4-**
Postprocedural hematoma of ear and mastoid process following a procedure	**H95.5-**
Postprocedural stenosis of external ear canal	**H95.81-**

Description of Condition

Intraoperative and postprocedural complications and disorders of the ear and mastoid process

Clinical Tip

Surgical intervention on the external, middle, or inner ear entails certain operative and postoperative risks. Similar to other surgery, these risks include intraoperative or postoperative (delayed) hemorrhage, intraoperative puncture or laceration and infection. However, certain procedures (e.g., mastoidectomy) carry risk for certain delayed complications which may require further care and treatment. Such specific complications include:

Cholesteatoma (recurrent): Abnormal growth of keratinous squamous epithelial cells forming a mass within the middle ear extending to the external meatus.

Granulation: Accumulation of fibrous, collagen-rich connective tissue that provides a barrier against infectious microorganisms to facilitate healing.

Mucosal cyst: Mucous-lined cyst cavity following removal of mastoid bone.

I-10 ALERT

ICD-10-CM classifies postoperative complications to (typically) the end of the body system classification chapter, where possible. Chapter 8 contains multiple specific intraoperative and postoperative complication codes.

Note: Conditions classified to chapter 8 include laterality (i.e., right, left, bilateral) within the code structure. All conditions should specify the affected ear(s).

CDI ALERT

Documentation must include the specific nature of the complication to avoid reporting nonspecific diagnoses. The documentation should qualify the disorder as:

- Intraoperative (i.e., complication during surgery requiring care, correction)
- Postoperative (i.e., complication developing after surgery for which the patient seeks care)

Documentation should state whether the procedure that resulted in a complication was:

- Performed on the ear or mastoid process
- Other (non-ear/mastoid process) procedure

Documentation should specify the nature of the complication as:

- Recurrent cholesteatoma
- Chronic inflammation
- Granulation of postmastoidectomy cavity
- Mucosal cyst of postmastoidectomy cavity
- Hemorrhage or hematoma
- Accidental puncture or laceration
- Stenosis
- Other (provider must document specifics)
- A separate or additional code may be reported, if necessary, to specify the nature of the complication.

Documentation of laterality (i.e., right, left, bilateral) should be present to avoid reporting unspecified codes.

Stenosis of ear canal: Narrowing of ear canal due to trauma, scar tissue, surgery, osteoma (bony overgrowth).

Key Terms

Key terms found in the documentation may include:

Cholesteatoma (middle ear postmastoidectomy cavity):

- Cholesterosis
- Keratosis

Granulation:

- Granuloma
- Proud flesh

Clinical Findings

Physical Examination

History and review of systems may include:

- Hearing loss
- Vertigo
- Balance issues
- Facial nerve paralysis
- Tinnitus
- Altered taste
- Chronic drainage
- Fistula
- Dural injury

Diagnostic Procedures and Services

- Long-term monitoring
- MRI

Therapeutic Procedures and Services

- Second surgery

Clinician Note

Specify the nature of the complication. Document a link or otherwise clearly associate the complicating condition/manifestation to the causal procedure. Specify the causal/precipitating procedure.

Document whether complications exist in combination with other systemic disease or auditory disorder. Specify any contributory history of trauma, infection or other related condition or status (e.g., deafness).

Document the laterality of the affected site (left, right, bilateral).

Clinician Documentation Checklist

Clinician documentation should indicate the following:

- Type
  - recurrent cholesteatoma of postmastoidectomy cavity
  - other disorders of ear and mastoid process following mastoidectomy
    - subtype
      - chronic inflammation of postmastoidectomy cavity
      - granulation of postmastoidectomy cavity
      - mucosal cyst of postmastoidectomy cavity
      - other disorders following mastoidectomy
  - intraoperative hemorrhage and hematoma of ear and mastoid process complicating a procedure
    - identify the procedure as
      - procedure on ear and mastoid process
      - other procedure
  - accidental puncture and laceration of ear and mastoid process during a procedure
    - identify the procedure as
      - procedure on ear and mastoid process
      - other procedure
  - postprocedural hemorrhage and hematoma of ear and mastoid process following a procedure
    - identify the procedure as
      - procedure on ear and mastoid process
      - other procedure
  - other intraoperative and postprocedural complications and disorders of ear and mastoid process
    - postprocedural stenosis of external ear canal
    - other intraoperative complications and disorders of ear and mastoid process
      - specify the disorder
    - other postprocedural complications and disorders of ear and mastoid process
      - specify the disorder
- Identification of laterality of ear
  - right
  - left
  - bilateral

Intraoperative and Postprocedural Complications and Disorders of Genitourinary System

Code Axes

Postprocedural (acute) (chronic) kidney failure	**N99.Ø**
Postprocedural urethral stricture	**N99.1-**
Postprocedural adhesions of vagina	**N99.2**
Prolapse of vaginal vault after hysterectomy	**N99.3**
Postprocedural pelvic peritoneal adhesions	**N99.4**
Complications of stoma of urinary tract	**N99.5-** HCC

Note: Official coding guideline I.B.16 indicates: Code assignment is based on the provider's documentation of the relationship between the condition and the care or procedure, unless otherwise instructed by the classification. The guideline extends to any complications of care, regardless of the chapter in which the code is located. It is important to note that not all conditions that occur during or following medical care or surgery are classified as complications. There must be a cause-and-effect relationship between the care provided and the condition, and an indication in the documentation that it is a complication. Query the provider for clarification, if the complication is not clearly documented.

⇨ I-10 ALERT

Like other chapters within ICD-10-CM related to specific body systems, the genitourinary chapter contains a section at the end that contains many common postoperative and postprocedural complications. The complication categories within the specific chapters of ICD-10-CM provide much detail and are tailored to the types of complications typically encountered for that type of disease process.

Description of Condition

Postprocedural (acute) (chronic) kidney failure (N99.Ø)

Clinical Tip

Postoperative acute renal failure (ARF) is a serious complication resulting in a prolonged acute care stay and high mortality. An increase in the intra-abdominal pressure above 20 mm Hg is associated with an increase in the incidence of postop ARF and the only proven management strategies for prevention are adequate volume expansion and avoidance of hypovolemia.

Key Terms

Key terms found in the documentation for postprocedural (acute) (chronic) kidney failure may include:

Post-op acute renal failure

Post-op chronic renal failure

⇨ I-10 ALERT

If either acute or chronic postoperative or postprocedural kidney failure is documented, assign an additional code to identify the specific type of kidney disease/failure.

Clinician Note

Ensure that all related conditions are coded, particularly those related to underlying kidney disease.

Postprocedural urethral stricture (N99.1-)

Clinical Tip
Urethral stricture is an abnormal narrowing of the urethra that occurs in male patients more often than in females, due to the longer urethral structure. The condition is the most common late complication of transurethral prostatectomy (TURP), but patient predisposing factors include previous trauma or infection or presence of a long-term urinary catheter.

Key Terms
Key terms found in the documentation for postprocedural urethral stricture may include:

Postcatheterization urethral stricture

Clinician Note
Ensure that all related conditions are coded, particularly those related to underlying urinary system disease.

I-10 ALERT

Because the condition occurs much more frequently in the male population, there are four codes related to male postprocedural urethral stricture, differentiated by type:

Meatal: Occurring at the opening of the urethra at the external meatus

Membranous: Occurs in up to 6 percent of patients who undergo transurethral resection of the prostate (TURP). The scar tissue is caused by the trauma of using too large a resectoscope/catheter or from overly aggressive distal prostate resection.

Anterior: The bulbar and penile urethra, fossa navicularis, and meatus together represent the anterior urethra

Unspecified: Strictural process that is not specified as any of the remaining types above.

Postprocedural adhesions of vagina (N99.2)

Clinical Tip
Adhesions form when there is damage to the visceral or parietal peritoneum and the basement membrane of the mesothelial layer is exposed to the surroundings. Adhesion formation at the vaginal cuff and pelvic sidewall frequently involves bowel, omentum, and adnexa.

Clinician Note
Ensure that all related conditions are coded, particularly those related to underlying female genital system disease.

CDI ALERT

Review medical record documentation for any indication of urinary incontinence and, if present, report separately.

Prolapse of vaginal vault after hysterectomy (N99.3)

Clinical Tip
Vaginal vault prolapse involves a descent of the vaginal cuff below a point that is 2 cm less than the total vaginal length above the plane of the hymen. It occurs when the upper vagina bulges into or outside the vagina. The condition is a common complication following vaginal hysterectomy and pre-existing pelvic floor defect prior to hysterectomy is the single most important risk factor for vault prolapse.

Clinician Note
Ensure that all related conditions are coded, particularly those related to underlying female genital system disease.

Postprocedural pelvic peritoneal adhesions (N99.4)

Clinical Tip
Peritoneal adhesions are a consequence of peritoneal irritation by surgical trauma and may be considered as the pathological part of healing following any peritoneal injury, particularly due to abdominal surgery. Postoperative

I-10 ALERT

Ensure proper code selection: code N73.6 is assigned when the pelvic peritoneal adhesions are not specified as postprocedural and code N73.6 is assigned when the adhesions are specified as being postinfective.

peritoneal adhesions are a major cause of morbidity resulting in multiple complications, many of which can manifest several years after the initial surgical procedure. They may cause pelvic or abdominal pain, small bowel obstruction, and infertility.

Clinician Note
Ensure that all related conditions are coded, particularly those related to underlying female genital system disease.

Complications of stoma of urinary tract (N99.5-)

Clinical Tip
For patients with long-term suprapubic catheters (cystostomies), postprocedural complications, particularly related to urinary tract infections, are not uncommon. Duration of catheterization is the leading risk factor for the development of urinary tract infections. Macroscopic hematuria and blockage of catheter are frequent complications as well.

Clinician Note
Ensure that all related conditions are coded, particularly those related to underlying urinary system disease.

Clinician Documentation Checklist

Clinician documentation should indicate the following:

- Postprocedural (acute) (chronic) kidney failure
  - identify type of kidney disease
- Postprocedural urethral stricture
  - includes postcatheterization urethral stricture
  - identify
    - postprocedural urethral stricture, male
      - postprocedural urethral stricture, meatal
      - postprocedural bulbous urethral stricture
      - postprocedural membranous urethral stricture
      - postprocedural anterior urethral stricture
      - postprocedural fossa navicularis urethral stricture
      - unspecified postprocedural urethral stricture
    - postprocedural urethral stricture, female
- Postprocedural adhesions of vagina
- Prolapse of vaginal vault after hysterectomy
- Postprocedural pelvic peritoneal adhesions
- Complications of stoma of urinary tract
  - identify
    - complication of cystostomy
      - cystostomy hemorrhage
      - cystostomy infection

- cystostomy malfunction
- other cystostomy complications
- complication of other external stoma of urinary tract
  - hemorrhage of incontinent external stoma of urinary tract
  - infection of incontinent external stoma of urinary tract
  - malfunction of incontinent external stoma of urinary tract
  - herniation of incontinent stoma of urinary tract
  - stenosis of incontinent stoma of urinary tract
  - other complication of incontinent external stoma of urinary tract
- complication of other stoma of urinary tract
  - hemorrhage of continent stoma of urinary tract
  - infection of continent stoma of urinary tract
  - malfunction of continent stoma of urinary tract
  - herniation of continent stoma of urinary tract
  - stenosis of continent stoma of urinary tract
  - other complication of continent stoma of urinary tract

Malignant Neoplasm of Breast

Note: Each of the subcategories listed below for malignant neoplasm of breast are subdivided based on the following components: sex (female versus male), and laterality (right, left, unspecified).

Code Axes

Malignant neoplasm of nipple and areola	**C50.0--** HCC QPP
Malignant neoplasm of central portion of breast	**C50.1--** HCC QPP
Malignant neoplasm of upper-inner quadrant of breast	**C50.2--** HCC QPP
Malignant neoplasm of lower-inner quadrant of breast	**C50.3--** HCC QPP
Malignant neoplasm of upper-outer quadrant of breast	**C50.4--** HCC QPP
Malignant neoplasm of lower-outer quadrant of breast	**C50.5--** HCC QPP
Malignant neoplasm of axillary tail of breast	**C50.6--** HCC QPP
Malignant neoplasm of overlapping sites of breast	**C50.8--** HCC QPP
Malignant neoplasm of unspecified site of breast	**C50.9--** HCC QPP
Lobular carcinoma in situ of breast	**D05.0--**
Intraductal carcinoma in situ of breast	**D05.1--**
Other specified type of carcinoma in situ of breast	**D05.8--**
Unspecified type of carcinoma in situ of breast	**D05.9--**

Key Terms

Key terms found in the documentation for malignant neoplasm of the breast may include:

- Colloid carcinoma of breast
- Infiltrating lobular carcinoma of the breast
- Inflammatory breast cancer (IBC)
- Invasive cribriform carcinoma of the breast
- Invasive ductal carcinoma (IDC) of breast
- Invasive lobular carcinoma of the breast
- Invasive papillary carcinoma of the breast
- Malignant phyllodes tumors of the breast
- Medullary carcinoma of breast
- Mucinous carcinoma of breast
- Paget's disease of the breast
- Paget's disease of the nipple
- Triple negative breast cancer
- Tubular carcinoma of breast

⇨ I-10 Alert

The number of specific codes for malignant neoplasm of breast has increased to 54 in ICD-10-CM. These codes include sex and laterality indicators and also more specific and all-inclusive body sites. An additional code should be assigned for estrogen receptor status, if available. In addition, there are 12 codes related to carcinoma in situ of breast, still considered to be a malignancy, but the tumor cells are noninvasive and have not spread to any surrounding tissue at the time of diagnosis.

CDI Alert

Documentation of risk factors should be included in the current record:

- Family history of breast history
- Estrogen receptor status
- Genetic susceptibility to malignant neoplasm of breast (BRCA1, BRCA2)
- Personal history of breast cancer
- Personal history of postmenopausal hormone replacement status
- Personal history of radiation therapy
- Postmenopausal status
- Obesity

Key Terms

Key terms found in the documentation for carcinoma in situ of the breast may include:

Ductal carcinoma in situ (DCIS)

Lobular carcinoma in situ (LCIS)

Clinical Findings

The most common symptom of breast cancer is a mass or lump in the breast, while early stage breast cancer may be asymptomatic and discovered during a routine screening exam.

Physical Examination

History and review of systems may include:

- Breast/nipple pain
- Scaling or thickening of breast skin
- Swelling of the breast
- Irritation or dimpling
- Retracted nipple
- Enlarged lymph nodes

Diagnostic Procedures and Services

- Imaging
  - mammogram
  - ultrasound
  - MRI
  - ductogram
  - biopsy

Therapeutic Procedures and Services

- Surgery
- Radiation therapy
- Hormone therapy
- Chemotherapy
- Targeted therapy for certain types

Clincian Note

Prior authorization of treatment is often dependent upon the type of carcinoma, therefore, careful attention to the medical record documentation including pathology reports is crucial.

The provider is responsible for confirming the findings of pathology and radiology reports within their documentation for inpatient records.

The provider should document admissions for screening mammogram or routine mammogram, including risk factors for the patient. If the patient is having a mammogram due to symptoms, report the symptoms as the reason for the encounter.

Clinician Documentation Checklist

Clinician documentation should indicate the following:

- Includes
  - Connective tissue of breast
  - Paget's disease of breast
  - Paget's disease of nipple
- Identification of
  - estrogen receptor status
    - positive
    - negative
  - laterality
    - right
    - left
  - gender
    - male
    - female
  - site
    - nipple and areola
    - central portion
    - quadrant
      - upper-inner
      - lower-inner
      - upper-outer
      - lower-outer
    - axillary tail
    - overlapping sites of breast
    - unspecified

Carcinoma in situ of breast, other and unspecified sites

- Carcinoma in situ of breast
  - type
    - lobular
    - intraductal
    - other
    - unspecified
- Identification of the laterality of breast
  - right
  - left

Malignant Neoplasm of Liver and Intrahepatic Bile Ducts

Code Axes

Liver cell carcinoma	**C22.Ø** HCC
Intrahepatic bile duct carcinoma	**C22.1** HCC
Hepatoblastoma	**C22.2** HCC
Angiosarcoma of liver	**C22.3** HCC
Other sarcomas of liver	**C22.4** HCC
Other specified carcinomas of liver	**C22.7** HCC
Malignant neoplasm of liver, primary, unspecified as to type	**C22.8** HCC
Malignant neoplasm of liver, not specified as primary or secondary	**C22.9** HCC

Description of Condition

Liver cell carcinoma (C22.Ø)

Clinical Tip
Liver cell carcinoma is a primary tumor and is the most common type of malignancy involving the liver. There are two main causes: one is due to a viral hepatitis B or C infection, and the other is due to hepatic cirrhosis, most commonly caused by alcoholism. The tumor involves the hepatocyte cells, which comprise approximately 80 percent of the liver. Prognosis is typically poor with this type of malignancy.

Cholangiocarcinoma with hepatocellular carcinoma, combined, is found in code C22.Ø. Liver cholangiocarcinoma is found in code C22.1.

CDI ALERT

Physicians will be required to document specific forms of liver malignancies under ICD-10-CM. Ensure that they are aware of the eight different classifications available (i.e., hepatocellular, intrahepatic, angiosarcoma, etc.).

Key Terms
Key terms found in the documentation for liver cell carcinoma may include:

HCC
Hepatocellular carcinoma
Hepatoma
Malignant hepatoma
Primary liver carcinoma
Primary liver cell carcinoma

Clinician Note

Because there appears to be a direct correlation to the increased incidence of HCC and alcohol abuse, alcohol dependence, hepatitis B and hepatitis C these conditions should be documented when present and reported separately using the appropriate code.

Intrahepatic bile duct carcinoma (C22.1)

Clinical Tip

A malignancy that invades bile ducts within the liver is called an intrahepatic bile duct carcinoma; only about 10 percent of all bile duct carcinomas are intrahepatic. Prognosis depends on location of the tumor and the extent of spread, or stage.

Key Terms

Key terms found in the documentation for intrahepatic bile duct carcinoma may include:

Adenocarcinoma of intrahepatic bile duct

Cholangiocarcinoma

Intracholangiocarcinoma

CDI ALERT

Manifestations of cancer that are not integral to the cancer (i.e., not one of the clinical indicators for the cancer) should be documented and reported when they meet criteria as an additional diagnosis:

- Anemia in neoplastic disease
- Ascites
- Coagulation defect due to liver disease
- Encephalopathy due to hepatic failure
- Hemorrhage/bleeding (of site)
- Peritonitis

Hepatoblastoma (C22.2)

Clinical Tip

Hepatoblastoma is a rare liver malignancy that typically affects infants and small children, usually no more than three years of age. The tumor originates from immature liver precursor cells, most often involving the right liver lobe. Several genetic conditions can increase a patient's risk for developing hepatoblastoma, including Beckwith-Wiedemann syndrome, hemihypertrophy, and familial adenomatous polyposis.

I-10 ALERT

In ICD-10-CM, hepatocellular carcinomas and hepatoblastomas each have a separate subclassification: C22.Ø for liver cell carcinoma and C22.2 for hepatoblastoma. This should be kept in mind when using mapping processes and reviewing longitudinal clinical data.

Angiosarcoma of liver (C22.3)

Clinical Tip

A liver angiosarcoma is a tumor that arises from the endothelial cells that line the walls of the blood vessels. The portal vein or central and sublobular veins are often involved. The causes of angiosarcoma include toxic exposure to thorium dioxide (Thorotrast), vinyl chloride, and arsenic, which may have occurred 30 or more years previously.

Key Terms

Key terms found in the documentation for angiosarcoma of liver may include:

Hemangioendothelioma

Hepatic angiosarcoma

Kupffer cell sarcoma

Other sarcomas of liver (C22.4)

Clinical Tip

Besides angiosarcoma of the liver (classified above), there are several other forms of liver sarcomas, which include those listed below. Symptoms, treatment, and prognosis depend upon the stage and progression of the tumor at the time of diagnosis.

Key Terms

Key terms found in the documentation for other sarcomas of liver may include:

Epithelioid hemangioendothelioma

Fibrosarcoma

Leiomyosarcoma

Malignant fibrous histiocytoma

Malignant histiocytoma

Primary hepatic sarcoma

Undifferentiated embryonal sarcoma of the liver

Undifferentiated liver sarcoma

Malignant neoplasm of liver, primary, unspecified as to type (C22.8) and Malignant neoplasm of liver, not specified as primary or secondary (C22.9)

Clinical Tip

Secondary liver carcinoma (C78.7) has metastasized from another primary cancer, such as that of the colon, breast, pancreas, stomach, or lung. It occurs much more frequently than primary liver carcinoma. Primary liver cancer (hepatocellular carcinoma) tends to occur in livers damaged by alcoholic cirrhosis, birth defects, or chronic infection with diseases such as hepatitis B and C, or hemochromatosis.

⇨ I-10 ALERT

Codes C22.8 and C22.9 represent residual subcategories for liver tumors that are not well defined. If the malignancy is documented as primary but no type is specified, code C22.8 should be reported. If no indication of primary or secondary tumor is documented, code C22.9 must be reported, although it is preferable that the attending physician be queried as to specific type.

Clinical Findings

Physical Examination

History and review of symptoms may include:

- Weight loss
- Enlarged liver
- Abdominal pain
- Loss of appetite
- Abdominal swelling
- Jaundice (yellowing of skin/eyes)
- Fever
- Nausea and vomiting

Diagnostic Procedures and Services

- Laboratory
  - alpha-fetoprotein levels
  - liver function
  - prothrombin time
  - BUN
  - CBC
  - viral hepatitis
  - blood chemistry (calcium, glucose)
  - cholesterol
- Imaging
  - ultrasound
  - MRI
  - CT scan
  - angiogram
  - bone scan
  - biopsy

Therapeutic Procedures and Services

- Surgery
- Radiation
- Chemotherapy
- Tumor ablation
- Targeted therapy
- Embolization

Clinician Note

Careful review of the medical record documentation is required to prevent incorrect classification. When documentation indicates terms such as extrahepatic or hepatic duct, the condition is more than likely classified elsewhere.

Clinician Documentation Checklist

Clinician documentation should indicate the following:

- Malignant neoplasm of liver and intrahepatic bile ducts
  - identification of
    - alcohol abuse and dependence
    - hepatitis b
    - hepatitis c
  - type
    - liver cell carcinoma
      - hepatocellular carcinoma
      - hepatoma

- intrahepatic bile duct carcinoma
- cholangiocarcinoma

— hepatoblastoma

— angiosarcoma of liver

- Kupffer cell sarcoma

— other sarcoma of liver

— other specified carcinomas of liver

— malignant neoplasm of liver, primary, unspecified as to type

— malignant neoplasm of liver, not specified to primary or secondary

- Malignant neoplasm of gallbladder
- Malignant neoplasm of other and unspecified parts of biliary tract
  - identification of the site

— extrahepatic bile duct

- common bile duct
- cystic duct
- hepatic duct
- biliary duct or passage

— ampulla of vater

— overlapping sites of biliary tract

- malignant neoplasm involving both intrahepatic and extrahepatic bile ducts
- primary malignant neoplasm of two or more contiguous sites of biliary tract

— unspecified

Malignant Neoplasm of Unspecified Site

Code Axes

Secondary malignant neoplasm of unspecified site	**C79.9** HCC QPP
Disseminated malignant neoplasm, unspecified	**C8Ø.Ø** HCC
Malignant (primary) neoplasm, unspecified	**C8Ø.1** HCC
Carcinoma in situ, unspecified	**DØ9.9**

I-10 ALERT

Providing precise classifications for malignancies without specification of site has always presented challenges; therefore, ICD-10-CM provides four separate codes for classification of these neoplasms.

Description of Condition

Secondary malignant neoplasm of unspecified site (C79.9)

Clinical Tip

This condition may be documented as metastatic cancer or metastatic disease, with no further specification. The diagnosis refers to the site to which the primary tumor has spread. In most cases, the site of metastasis should be known, particularly if treatment has been provided. The most common sites of cancer metastasis are the lungs, bones, and liver. Metastatic cancer cells have the same attributes and are similar, if not identical, to the cancer cells of the primary tumor, regardless of differing body sites. If a primary site is not found, clinicians know by the cell type that the tumor is metastatic.

CDI ALERT

ICD-10-CM often requires more specificity regarding the anatomical location of the malignancy and if it does not, the physician should be queried and the documentation updated accordingly. Clinicians should be educated that when documenting a malignant condition, the specific site should be indicated as to whether the malignancy is primary or secondary, and if secondary, the primary site should be indicated.

Key Terms

Key terms found in the documentation for secondary malignant neoplasm of unspecified site may include:

Metastatic cancer

Metastatic disease

Clinician Note

Ensure that all related conditions are coded, particularly neoplasms of other site or pathological fracture.

Disseminated malignant neoplasm, unspecified (C8Ø.Ø)

Clinical Tip

A disseminated malignant neoplasm is defined as one that has widely metastasized and has spread throughout the body. Besides local invasion, whereby the tumor infiltrates and destroys tissues surrounding the original site, there are other ways that a tumor can metastasize:

- Lymphangitic system or lymph nodes
- Hematogenous: through the blood vessels
- Direct seeding, such as spread to the peritoneum from other abdominal sources

Key Terms
Key terms found in the documentation for disseminated malignant neoplasm may include:

Carcinomatosis

Generalized cancer, unspecified site

Generalized malignancy, unspecified site

Clinician Note
Ensure that all related conditions are coded, particularly neoplasms of other sites or pathological fracture.

> **I-10 ALERT**
>
> Official Coding Guideline I.C.2.j indicates that: "Code C80.0 Disseminated malignant neoplasm, unspecified, is for use only in those cases where the patient has advanced metastatic disease and no known primary or secondary sites are specified. It should not be used in place of assigning codes for the primary site and all known secondary sites."

Malignant (primary) neoplasm, unspecified (C80.1)

Clinical Tip
If a patient is diagnosed with metastatic neoplasm and the primary site cannot be determined due to cancer cells too small to be detected or to regression of the disease, the patient is said to have a cancer of unknown primary origin (CUPO).

> **I-10 ALERT**
>
> Official Coding Guideline I.C.2.k indicates that: "Code C80.1 Malignant (primary) neoplasm, unspecified, equates to Cancer, unspecified. This code should only be used when no determination can be made as to the primary site of a malignancy."

Key Terms
Key terms found in the documentation for malignant (primary) neoplasm, unspecified may include:

Cancer NOS

Cancer unspecified site (primary)

Carcinoma unspecified site (primary)

Malignancy unspecified site (primary)

Clinician Note
Ensure that all related conditions are coded, particularly neoplasms of other sites or pathological fracture.

> **I-10 ALERT**
>
> In most cases, the site of the carcinoma in-situ is known and a code from category range D00–D09 should be assigned.

Carcinoma in situ, unspecified (D09.9)

Clinical Tip
Carcinoma in-situ (CIS) cells do not penetrate the tissue barriers around them and are not considered invasive. Although CIS cells are growing in the characteristic disorganized way that identifies the tumor as a cancer, they do not have the ability to metastasize or have not gained access to the blood or lymph stream to spread to other parts of the body. Although not immediately life threatening, CIS cases should be treated (typically via surgical removal) because they can transform into invasive malignant tumors if left untreated.

CDI Alert

For an encounter in which both the primary site and a metastatic site(s) are initially diagnosed and (equally) treated during the admission, apply the OCG on Selection of Principal Diagnosis for two or more diagnoses that equally meet the definition of principal diagnosis.

Key Terms

Key terms found in the documentation for carcinoma in situ, unspecified may include:

Bowen's disease

Erythroplasia

Grade III intraepithelial neoplasia

Queyrat's erythroplasia

Clinician Note

Review the clinical documentation to ensure that all related conditions are coded, particularly neoplasms of other sites or pathological fracture.

Clinical Tip

Pulmonary lymphangitic spread refers to the small lymph vessels within the lungs and does not mean lymph node metastasis. When documented, it would be reported as metastasis to the lung (C78.Ø-).

Clinician Documentation Checklist

Clinician documentation should indicate the following:

- Carcinoma in situ of breast
  - Type
    - unspecified
- Carcinoma in situ of other and unspecified sites
  - identification of the site
    - urinary organs
      - unspecified
    - other
    - unspecified

Malnutrition

Code Axes

Kwashiorkor	**E4Ø** HCC
Nutritional marasmus	**E41** HCC
Marasmic kwashiorkor	**E42** HCC
Unspecified severe protein-calorie nutrition	**E43** HCC
Moderate protein-calorie malnutrition	**E44.Ø** HCC
Mild protein-calorie malnutrition	**E44.1** HCC
Retarded development following protein-calorie malnutrition	**E45** HCC
Unspecified protein-calorie malnutrition	**E46** HCC

Description of Condition

Malnutrition, also known as protein-energy undernutrition and protein-calorie malnutrition, is an energy (calorie) deficit due to a chronic deficiency of nutrients. There are ranges of severity and several causes, including but not limited to, an unbalanced diet, GI disorders, AIDS, malignancy, anorexia, depression, and systemic infection. Malnutrition may result from complications of these other diseases because these illnesses impair the body's ability to absorb or use nutrients.

CDI ALERT

Body mass index (BMI) may be reported based on documentation by nurses, dietitians, etc., who are not the patient's provider. However, a diagnosis of malnutrition must be based on clinician documentation.

Kwashiorkor (E4Ø)

A form of severe malnutrition that may develop from a diet low in protein and high in carbohydrates, the characteristics of this type of malnutrition include nutritional edema, distended abdomen, hepatomegaly, and dyspigmentation of skin and hair. This form of severe malnutrition is very rarely seen in the U.S. except among the elderly and children who may be victims of abuse or neglect.

Nutritional Marasmus (E41)

Nutritional marasmus is a form of severe malnutrition that is caused by a lack of total nutrition in the diet and is characterized by energy deficiency, peeling skin, and hair discoloration. Marasmus is more common in the U.S. than Kwashiorkor but usually only affects very young children.

Marasmic kwashiorkor (E42)

This form of malnutrition is considered an intermediate form of severe protein-calorie malnutrition with signs of both kwashiorkor and marasmus.

Unspecified severe protein-calorie nutrition (E43)

Key Terms

Key terms found in the documentation may include:

- BMI <16
- Cachexia
- Dehydration
- Diminished functional status
- Feeding tube
- Hepatomegaly
- IV nutrition
- Normocytic anemia
- Nutritional edema
- Periorbital edema
- Protein-calorie malnutrition
- Severe malnutrition
- Severe muscle mass loss
- Starvation edema
- Subcutaneous fat loss
- Undernutrition

Moderate protein-calorie malnutrition (E44.Ø)

The moderate form of malnutrition involves more intense symptoms and intracellular changes.

Mild protein-calorie malnutrition (E44.1)

Mild malnutrition may have little if any symptoms.

Unspecified protein-calorie malnutrition (E46)

Conditions are caused by not getting enough calories or the right amount of key nutrients, such as vitamins and minerals that are needed for health. Malnutrition may occur when there is a lack of nutrients in the diet or when the body cannot absorb nutrients from food.

Clinical Tip

Malnutrition or protein-energy undernutrition can be primary or secondary. Primary malnutrition results from a diet with insufficient nutrient intake. Secondary malnutrition is more common in the U.S. and occurs as a result of other disease/disorders (e.g., GI disorders, malignancy, AIDS, alcoholism, anorexia nervosa), or drugs that interfere with nutrient use.

Providers must assess the following six characteristics in the context of an acute illness or injury, a chronic illness, or social or environmental circumstances to determine if malnutrition is present and whether it is severe or nonsevere (moderate): Insufficient energy intake, weight loss, loss of muscle mass, loss of subcutaneous fat, localized/generalized fluid accumulation (edema), and diminished functional status (hand grip strength).

Key Terms

Key terms found in the documentation may include:

BMI <16-18.9

Dehydration

Diminished functional status

Fluid accumulation

Malnutrition

Mild malnutrition

Moderate malnutrition

Muscle mass loss

Subcutaneous fat loss

Weight loss

Clinical Findings

This disease occurs in stages over a period of time, starting with low levels of nutrients within the blood and tissues that progress to changes in the intracellular function and structure. Once these changes are severe, signs and symptoms appear. Signs and symptoms of protein calorie malnutrition vary greatly and affect multiple body parts and organ systems.

Physical Examination

History and review of symptoms may include:

- Weight loss
- Fluid accumulation (edema)
- Muscle mass loss (severity based on degree of malnutrition)
- Insufficient energy intake
- Loss of subcutaneous fat
- Diminished functional status (hand grip strength)
- BMI <19
- Apathy
- Weakness
- Dizziness
- Lethargy
- Cachexia
- Swollen/bleeding gums
- Tooth decay
- Pale conjunctiva
- Periorbital edema
- Developmental delay
- Loss of knee reflexes

- Impaired cognition
- Bradycardia
- Tachycardia
- Hypotension
- Impaired wound healing
- Brittle/thin hair
- Dry/thin/inelastic skin
- Pallor
- Skin hypopigmentation
- Anemia
- Dehydration
- Enlarged liver
- Renal impairment
- Decreased respiratory rate

Diagnostic Procedures and Services

- Laboratory
  - CBC
  - serum albumin
  - serum electrolytes
  - total lymphocyte count
  - CD4+ T lymphocytes
  - transferrin
  - response to skin antigens
  - BUN
  - glucose
- Imaging
  - decreased bone mineralization
- Other
  - swallow function study

Clinician Note

Protein calorie malnutrition is classified by the extent of progression, from mild to severe. Mild malnutrition has little, if any symptoms and may be described as grade 1. Moderate malnutrition involves additional intracellular changes along with more symptoms and may be described as grade 2. In severe malnutrition the patient clearly exhibits several symptoms and may be described as grade 3.

Severe malnutrition is further subdivided by type such as kwashiorkor and marasmus. Kwashiorkor is a lack of protein in the diet and is characterized by more severe manifestations such as edema, distended abdomen, ulcerating dermatoses, and hepatomegaly. Kwashiorkor is also very rare in the U.S. and should not be routinely reported. Marasmus is more common in the U.S., usually only affects very young children and is characterized by energy deficiency, hair discoloration, growth retardation, and peeling skin.

Clinician Documentation Checklist

Clinician documentation should indicate the following:

- History including dietary intake relevant to the encounter
- Procedures performed (CT, MRI, laboratory, cardiovascular, swallow testing, etc.)

Clinical guidelines have been established to appropriately code mild to severe malnutrition. At least two of the following six conditions should be present and documented before assigning an ICD-10-CM code for malnutrition/undernutrition.

- Insufficient energy (calorie) intake
- Weight loss
- Loss of muscle mass
- Loss of subcutaneous fat
- Localized/generalized fluid accumulation that may mask weight loss (edema)
- Diminished functional status (measured by hand grip strength)

In order to report severe malnutrition such as marasmus or kwashiorkor, more severe symptoms outlined in the physical examination section must be present and documented in addition to those bulleted above.

In addition, the following clinical values commonly used to confirm if protein calorie malnutrition is present and the severity of malnutrition should be documented when indicated:

Measurement	Normal	Mild Malnutrition	Moderate Malnutrition	Severe Malnutrition
% Normal body weight	90–110%	85–90%	75–85%	<75%
Body mass index (BMI)	19–24	18–18.9	16–17.9	<16
Serum albumin (g/dL)	3.5–5.0	3.1–3.4	2.4–3.0	<2.4
Serum transferrin (mg/dL)	220–400	201–219	150–200	<150
Total Lymphocyte count (per µL)	2000–3500	1501–1999	800–1500	<800

I-10 ALERT

When "emaciated" or "emaciation" is documented in the medical record, but no indication of whether or not the patient is suffering from malnutrition is documented, assign code E41 Nutritional marasmus.

Mastectomy

Code Axes

Mastectomy for gynecomastia	**19300**
Mastectomy, partial	**19301-19302**
Mastectomy, simple, complete	**19303**
Mastectomy, subcutaneous	**19304**
Mastectomy, radical	**19305-19306**
Mastectomy, modified radical	**19307**

CPT ALERT

For procedures 19301–19307, the intraoperative placement of clip[s] is included and is not separately reportable.

Description of Condition

Mastectomy is the surgical removal of the breast and the most common treatment for breast cancer. The tumor size, location, type, age of patient, cancer stage and lymph node involvement are the main factors in determining the appropriate type of mastectomy performed. Mastectomies are usually performed for breast malignancies, but may also be performed for other reasons, for example, a mastectomy done for prophylactic removal of a breast due to a personal or family history of breast cancer.

Mastectomy, partial (e.g., lumpectomy, tylectomy, quadrantectomy, segmentectomy) (19301)

Mastectomy, partial (e.g., lumpectomy, tylectomy, quadrantectomy, segmentectomy); with axillary lymphadenectomy (19302)

CPT ALERT

A lumpectomy with attention to surgical margins, with a separate incision in the right axillary, with removal of two superficial sentinel lymph nodes, would be reported with 19301 for the lumpectomy, along with 38500 for the sentinel node excision. Code 19302 is not appropriate in this case as it requires complete axillary dissection.

Clinical Tip

A partial mastectomy may be done for breast cancer treatment where the tumors are small, possibly described as stage I or II, and where no other pathologic indicators that predispose recurrence are present. The tumor is excised along with a section of healthy tissue. Some of the lining over the chest muscles below the tumor may also be removed. This procedure may also be referred to as a lumpectomy.

Key Terms

Key terms found in the documentation may include:

- Axillary lymphadenectomy
- Lumpectomy
- Partial mastectomy
- Quadrantectomy
- Segmentectomy
- Subtotal
- Tylectomy

Mastectomy, simple, complete (19303)

All subcutaneous breast tissue is removed, with or without nipple and skin. The entire breast is removed but the lymph nodes and surrounding muscle are left intact. In a modification of the simple mastectomy, skin and nipple may be spared, but all subcutaneous breast tissue is removed.

Mastectomy, subcutaneous (19304)

The physician performs a subcutaneous mastectomy. The physician makes an incision in the inframammary crease. The breast is dissected from the pectoral fascia and from the skin. The breast tissue is removed, but the skin and pectoral fascia remain.

Mastectomy, radical, including pectoral muscles, axillary lymph nodes (19305)

The breast along with overlying skin, axillary lymph nodes, and pectoralis major and minor muscles are removed. This procedure may be done when the cancer cells have invaded the chest wall.

Mastectomy, radical, including pectoral muscles, axillary and internal mammary lymph nodes (Urban type operation) (19306)

The breast tissue, skin, and pectoral muscles are removed along will all tissue within the parameters of the sternum, the rectus fascia, the latissimus dorsi muscle, and the clavicle, including the axillary and internal mammary lymph nodes.

Mastectomy, modified radical, including axillary lymph nodes, with or without pectoralis minor muscle, but excluding pectoralis major muscle (19307)

The breast tissue and skin are dissected from the pectoral fascia; the pectoralis minor muscle may also be resected but the pectoralis major muscle is left intact.

Clinical Tip

Following radical mastectomy, patients with insufficient skin for coverage may require skin grafts or myocutaneous flaps.

Clinician Documentation Checklist

Clinician documentation should indicate the following:

- Identify
  - type of mastectomy performed
  - laterality
  - intraoperative lymph node identification
  - pathological findings
  - delayed closure, if applicable

CPT ALERT

When a modified radical mastectomy with sentinel node biopsy is performed, a frozen section of the nodes is obtained and the axilla is dissected if the nodes are positive. Code 19307 for modified radical mastectomy is reported along with add-on code 38900 Intraoperative identification (e.g., mapping) of sentinel lymph node(s) includes injection of non-radioactive dye, when performed (List separately in addition to code for primary procedure). It would not be appropriate to report the axillary node biopsy separately from the axillary dissection.

Migraine

CDI ALERT

Migraine as adverse effect of medication: documentation must link the nature of the adverse effect as the type of migraine and state the drug or classification, when known.

Code Axes

Migraine without aura	**G43.Ø-** QPP
Migraine with aura	**G43.1-** QPP
Hemiplegic migraine	**G43.4-** QPP
Persistent migraine aura without cerebral infarction	**G43.5-** QPP
Persistent migraine aura with cerebral infarction	**G43.6-**
Chronic migraine without aura	**G43.7-** QPP
Cyclical vomiting	**G43.A-**
Ophthalmoplegic migraine	**G43.B-** QPP
Periodic headache syndromes in child or adult	**G43.C-** QPP
Abdominal migraine	**G43.D-**
Other migraine	**G43.8-** QPP
Migraine, unspecified	**G43.9-** QPP

Clinical Tip

Migraine is defined as a moderate to severe headache that is intermittent, lasts four to 72 hours, and is throbbing in quality. Some patients experience nausea and become sensitive to lights and noise, in association with the headache. Migraine mechanisms are believed to involve chemical substances such as serotonin, increased stickiness of blood platelets, alterations in cerebral blood flow, and increased irritability of the nerve cells in the brain.

The following definitions should be used for all subclassifications related to migraine:

Intractable migraine: Sustained and severe migraine headaches, along with their manifestations, that are not adequately controlled by standard outpatient treatments. Other terms may include: pharmacoresistant, pharmacologically resistant, treatment resistant, medically refractory, or poorly controlled.

Status migrainosus: A debilitating migraine headache lasting more than 72 hours.

Migraine with aura: A less common type of migraine that includes symptoms or feelings that occur immediately preceding a migraine headache. The symptoms are also called a prodrome, which may last for five to 20 minutes, or may continue with the headache. Some of the most common prodromes include the following:

- Blind spots or scotomas
- Weakness
- Hallucinations

- Blindness in half of the visual field in one or both eyes (hemianopsia)
- Seeing zigzag patterns (fortification)
- Seeing flashing lights (scintilla)
- Feeling prickling skin (paresthesia)

Description of Condition

Migraine without and with aura (G43.Ø-, G43.1-)

Clinical Tip

Migraine is defined as a moderate to severe headache that it is intermittent, lasts four to 72 hours, and is throbbing in quality. Some patients experience nausea and become sensitive to lights and noise, in association with the headache. Migraine mechanisms are believed to involve chemical substances such as serotonin, increased stickiness of blood platelets, alterations in cerebral blood flow and increased irritability of the nerve cells in the brain. A migraine with aura is a less common type of migraine that includes symptoms or feelings that occur immediately preceding a migraine headache. The symptoms are also called a prodrome, which may last for five to 20 minutes, or may continue with the headache.

Key Terms

Key terms found in the documentation may include:

Basilar migraine
Classical migraine
Common migraine
Migraine equivalents
Migraine preceded or accompanied by transient focal neurological phenomena
Migraine triggered seizures
Migraine with acute-onset aura
Migraine with aura without headache (migraine equivalents)
Migraine with prolonged aura
Migraine with typical aura
Retinal migraine
Without aura

Clinician Note

Ensure that all related conditions are coded appropriately, particularly if seizure activity is documented.

CDI ALERT

Ensure that not only are conditions related to intractability and status migrainosus clearly documented, but if any associated seizure activity is present, it should be documented and classified separately.

Hemiplegic migraine (G43.4-)

CDI Alert

If hemiplegia or a related condition is documented on a record with a migraine, ensure that the physician links the conditions before assigning codes from this subcategory.

Clinical Tip

Hemiplegic migraine is a rare, neurological disease that is characterized by a migraine with aura accompanied by motor weakness. The patient may experience visual disturbances, sensory loss, weakness to paralysis on one side of the body, confusion, speech difficulty, impaired consciousness, coma, or memory loss. Familial hemiplegic migraine (FHM) is a variation of hemiplegic migraine where at least one first-degree or second-degree relative also has hemiplegic migraine.

Key Terms

Key terms found in the documentation may include:

Familial migraine
Sporadic migraine

I-10 Alert

If a patient has a persistent migraine aura with a cerebral infarction, a separate code should be assigned to classify the type of cerebral infarction (I63.-).

Clinician Note

Ensure that all related conditions are coded appropriately, particularly if seizure activity is documented.

Persistent migraine aura without and with cerebral infarction (G43.5-, G43.6-)

CDI Alert

If a cerebral infarction or a related condition is documented on a record with a migraine, ensure that the physician links the conditions before assigning codes from this subcategory.

Clinical Tip

Persistent migraine aura without infarction (PAWOI) is a relatively rare condition that can cause neurological symptoms such as loss of vision, visual snow, increased afterimages, or tinnitus. The condition is typically diagnosed when there are aura symptoms lasting more than a week without evidence of cerebral infarction. A 2006 study published in the Journal of the American Medical Association indicated that active migraines with aura in women were associated with an increased risk of vascular disease, including cerebral infarction, although the overall occurrence of a stroke during or immediately following a migraine attack is fortunately a rare event.

Clinician Note

Telephone transmission of electroencephalograms (EEG) is considered medically necessary for the diagnosis of certain types of migraines. For this reason, careful attention to the medical record documentation is crucial to correct code assignment and, therefore, substantiating the medical necessity of the procedure.

I-10 Alert

Codes in subcategory G43.7- Chronic migraine without aura, are differentiated from codes in subcategory G43.Ø- Migraine without aura, by the frequency of the migraines, as defined above.

Chronic migraine without aura (G43.7-)

Clinical Tip

A chronic migraine is defined as a headache that occurs 15 or more days a month with headache lasting four hours or longer for at least three consecutive months in patients with current or prior diagnosis of migraine.

Key Terms
Key terms found in the documentation may include:

Chronic migraine without aura, without refractory migraine

Chronic migraine without aura, with refractory migraine

Transformed migraine

Clinician Note
Ensure that all related conditions are coded appropriately, particularly if seizure activity is documented.

Cyclical vomiting (G43.A-)

Clinical Tip
Cyclical vomiting syndrome is a condition whose symptoms are recurring attacks of intense nausea, vomiting, and sometimes abdominal pain in the setting of migraine headaches. There are three criteria used to diagnose the condition:

- A history of three or more periods of acute, intense nausea with unrelenting vomiting and sometimes pain lasting hours to days; in some cases several months duration has been reported.
- Intervening symptom-free intervals, which can last weeks to months.
- Diagnostic workup that excludes metabolic, gastrointestinal, or central nervous system structural or biochemical disease.

Clinician Note
Ensure that all related conditions are coded appropriately, particularly if seizure activity is documented.

⇨ I-10 ALERT

The codes in subcategory G43.A- include those related to the presence of intractability. Ensure that this is clearly documented in the medical record.

Ophthalmoplegic migraine (G43.B-)

Clinical Tip
An ophthalmoplegic migraine is a very rare eye disorder that is also classified as a cranial neuralgia. Symptoms include headaches and a weakening of muscles around the eye, oculomotor nerve palsy. In some cases, these headaches commonly precede episodes of partial paralysis of one or more ocular nerve (most commonly the third cranial nerve), drooping of the eyelid, double vision, and dilation of pupils. Onset is typically in infancy or early childhood. The exact etiology is unknown.

Key Terms
Key terms found in the documentation may include:

Acephalgic migraine

Basilar migraine

Ocular migraine

Ophthalmic migraine

Silent migraine

⇨ I-10 ALERT

The codes in subcategory G43.B- include those related to the presence of intractability. Ensure that this is clearly documented in the medical record.

Clinician Note
Ensure that all related conditions are coded appropriately, particularly if seizure activity is documented.

⇨ I-10 ALERT

The codes in subcategory G43.C- include those related to the presence of intractability. Ensure that this is clearly documented in the medical record.

Periodic headache syndromes in child or adult (G43.C-)

Clinical Tip
The childhood periodic syndromes include cyclical vomiting syndrome (CVS), abdominal migraine (AM), and benign paroxysmal vertigo of childhood (BPVC) as migraine precursors. It is also widely believed that periodic syndrome is a common childhood precursor of adult migraine.

Clinician Note
Ensure that all related conditions are coded appropriately, particularly if seizure activity is documented.

⇨ I-10 ALERT

The codes in subcategory G43.D- include those related to the presence of intractability. Ensure that this is clearly documented in the medical record.

Abdominal migraine (G43.D-)

Clinical Tip
A variant of classical migraine headaches, abdominal migraines involve abdominal pain, usually near the midline or navel. Children with abdominal migraines typically develop migraine headaches as they age. Diagnosis of the condition requires ruling out other causes of the pain, particularly of GI origin.

Clinician Note
Ensure that all related conditions are coded appropriately, particularly if seizure activity is documented.

⇨ I-10 ALERT

The codes in subcategory G43.8- include those related to the presence of intractability. Ensure that this is clearly documented in the medical record.

Menstrual migraine (G43.82-, G43.83-)

Clinical Tip
There are two subsets of menstrual migraines. The first, menstrually related migraine without aura, must have an onset during the perimenstrual time period (two days before to three days after the onset of menstruation) and this relationship must be confirmed in two to three of menstrual cycles, regardless of whether attacks occur at other times of the menstrual cycle. Symptoms of the second type, pure menstrual migraine without aura, are similar to the above criteria except that migraine headaches are strictly limited to the perimenstrual time period and do not occur at other times of the month. Estrogen and serotonin levels and interactions are thought to be the underlying cause of the condition.

Key Terms

Key terms found in the documentation may include:

Menstrual headache

Menstrually related migraine

Premenstrual headache

Premenstrual migraine

Pure menstrual migraine

Clinical Findings

Recurrent moderate to severe headaches are most commonly caused by a migraine. There are many possible triggers for migraines including: head trauma, neck pain, fluctuating estrogen levels, skipping meals, weather changes, stress, sleep deprivation, specific foods, etc. Migraine pain may be unilateral or bilateral and may last from four hours to several days.

Physical Examination

History and review of systems may include:

- Moderate to severe headache
- Nausea
- Sensitivity to light and certain sounds
- Fifteen or more days with a headache per month
- Vertigo
- Imbalance
- Speech disturbance
- Visual disturbance
- Sensory disturbance
- Focal weakness
- Complete neurological examination

Diagnostic Procedures and Services

- Laboratory
  - blood tests
- Imaging
  - MRI or CT

Therapeutic Procedures and Services

- IV fluid

Medication List

- Analgesics containing opioids, caffeine, or butalbital
- Antiemetics
- Ergot
  - ergotamine (Ergomar, Migergot)
- Glucocorticoids
- Opioids

- Pain relievers
  - acetaminophen
  - ibuprofen
  - NSAIDs
- Preventive medication
  - antidepressants
    - amitriptyline (Vanatrip, Elavil)
  - antiseizure medication
    - divalproex (Depakote)
  - beta blockers
    - atenolol (Tenormin)
    - metoprolol (Lopressor, Toprol)
    - nadolol (Corgard)
    - propranolol (Inderal)
  - calcium channel blockers
  - naproxen
  - onabotulinumtoxinA
    - topiramate (Topamax)
    - verapamil (Calan, Verelan)
- Triptans
  - almotriptan (Axert)
  - eletriptan (Relpax)
  - frovatriptan (Frova)
  - rizatriptan (Maxalt)
  - zolmitriptan (Zomig)

Clinician Note

Ensure that all related conditions are coded appropriately, particularly if seizure activity is documented.

Clinician Documentation Checklist

Clinician documentation should indicate the following:

- Drug, if responsible
- Type
  - migraine without aura
    - common migraine
  - migraine with aura
    - identify any associated seizure
    - includes
      - basilar migraine
      - classical migraine
      - migraine equivalents

        - migraine preceded or accompanied by transient focal neurological phenomena
        - migraine triggered seizures
        - migraine with acute-onset aura
        - migraine with aura without headache
        - migraine with prolonged aura
        - migraine with typical aura
        - retinal migraine
  - hemiplegic migraine
    - includes
      - familial migraine
      - sporadic migraine
  - Persistent migraine aura without cerebral infarction
  - Persistent migraine aura with cerebral infarction
    - document type of cerebral infarction
  - Chronic migraine without aura
    - includes
      - transformed migraine
  - cyclical vomiting
  - ophthalmoplegic migraine
  - periodic headache syndromes in adult or child
  - abdominal migraine
  - other migraine
    - other specified migraine
    - menstrual migraine
      - identify associated premenstrual tension syndrome
      - includes
        - menstrual headache
        - menstrual migraine
        - menstrually related migraine
        - premenstrual headache
        - premenstrual migraine
        - pure menstrual migraine
  - unspecified migraine
- Document each type of migraine as:
  - not intractable
  - intractable
    - includes
      - pharmacoresistant (pharmacologically resistant)
      - treatment resistant
      - refractory (medically)
      - poorly controlled
  - with status epilepticus
  - without status epilepticus

Nerve Blocks

Code Axes

Introduction/injection of anesthetic agent (nerve block), diagnostic or therapeutic	**64400–64530**

Description of Procedure

These services are for the injection of an anesthetic agent or other substance and are most frequently used for the treatment of chronic pain. These codes are not used to report anesthesia services.

Introduction/injection of anesthetic agent (nerve block), diagnostic or therapeutic, somatic nerves (64400–64489)

Key Terms

Key terms found in the documentation may include:

Block

Inj

Injection

TAP block

Clinical Tip

Somatic nerves are a part of the peripheral nervous system and are associated with the voluntary control of body movements through the skeletal muscles.

Documentation for nerve blocks of the somatic nerves should include:

- The specific nerve(s) injected
- The substance administered
- The strength and amount of the substance

Documentation should also include the reason for the nerve block and the response of prior treatment if any.

Introduction/injection of anesthetic agent (nerve block), diagnostic or therapeutic, paravertebral spinal nerves (64490–64495)

Facet joint injections should be reported using the appropriate codes from range 64490–64495. Correct code selection is dependent upon:

- Level of the spine injected
- Number of levels reported
- Whether the service was performed unilaterally or bilaterally

Single level: A single level injection occurs when the physician administers one or more substances to a level using one or more needles. A physician may insert a needle and attach a small tube through which the first substance is administered via a syringe. The physician may then change out the syringe and administer a second substance. However, only one needle puncture is performed.

In another method, the physician inserts the needle, administers a substance, and then removes the needle and makes a second puncture with a new needle and syringe to administer an additional substance. Despite the fact that there are two puncture sites, only a single level is being treated.

Multiple levels: When the physician documentation clearly indicates that multiple levels of the spine were injected, add-on codes 64491–64492 and 64494–64495, respectively, are reported.

Bilateral injections: Modifier 50 should be appended when the documentation states that injections were made on the same level but on different sides. Add-on codes 64491–64492 or 64494–64495 are not appropriate when the documentation indicates that the injections were performed bilaterally.

Anesthetic/steroids: Examine the documentation for the name and dosage of the anesthetic agent and/or steroid agent administered. List the appropriate HCPCS Level II code separately.

Clinician Note

Documentation must indicate if the procedure was performed unilaterally or bilaterally. This supports the use of modifier 50 when documentation indicates that the injection was performed bilaterally.

Clinical Tip

Medicare considers facet joint blocks to be reasonable and necessary for chronic pain (persistent pain for three (3) months or greater) suspected to originate from the facet joint. Facet joint block is one of the methods used to document/confirm suspicions of posterior element biomechanical pain of the spine. Hallmarks of posterior element biomechanical pain are as follows:

- The pain does not have a strong radicular component
- There is no associated neurological deficit and the pain is aggravated by hyperextension, rotation, or lateral bending of the spine, depending on the orientation of the facet joint at that level
- A paravertebral facet joint represents the articulation of the posterior elements of one vertebra with its neighboring vertebrae; it is further noted that there are two (2) facet joints at each level, left and right

During a paravertebral facet joint block procedure, a needle is placed in the facet joint or along the medial branches that innervate the joints under fluoroscopic guidance and a local anesthetic and/or steroid is injected. After the injection(s) has been performed, the patient is asked to indulge in the activities that usually aggravate his/her pain and to record his/her impressions of the effect of the procedure. Temporary or prolonged abolition of the pain suggests that the facet joints are the source of the symptoms and appropriate treatment may be prescribed in the future. Some patients have long-lasting relief with local anesthetic and steroid; others require a denervation procedure for more permanent relief. Before proceeding to a denervation treatment, the patient should experience at least a 50 percent reduction in symptoms for the duration of the local anesthetic effect.

Diagnostic or therapeutic injections/nerve blocks may be required for the management of chronic pain. It may take multiple nerve blocks targeting different anatomic structures to establish the etiology of the chronic pain in a given patient. It is standard medical practice to use the modality most likely to establish the diagnosis or treat the presumptive diagnosis. If the first set of procedures fails to produce the desired effect or to rule out the diagnosis, the provider should proceed to the next logical test or treatment indicated. For the purpose of this paravertebral facet joint block, an anatomic region is defined per the CPT manual as cervical/thoracic (64490, 64491, 64492) or lumbar/sacral (64493, 64494, 64495).

Introduction/injection of anesthetic agent (nerve block), diagnostic or therapeutic, autonomic nerves (64505–64530)

The autonomic nervous system is a part of the peripheral nervous system and controls visceral functions, which occur below the level of consciousness. It can be further subdivided into the parasympathetic nervous system and the sympathetic nervous system.

Key Terms

Key terms found in the documentation may include:

ANS

PSNS

SNS

Documentation Tip

Documentation for nerve blocks of the autonomic nerves should include:

- The specific nerve(s) injected
- The substance administered
- The strength and amount of the substance

Documentation should also include the reason for the nerve block and the response of prior treatment if any.

Clinician Documentation Checklist

Clinician documentation should indicate the following:

- Medical condition being treated
- Reason for the nerve block
- Patient response to prior pain treatment
- Nerves injected
- Substance administered
  - strength administered
  - amount administered
- Facet joint injections

- Anatomic region
  - cervical/thoracic
  - lumbar/sacral
  - number of levels reported
    - single level
    - second level
    - third or additional levels
  - bilateral injections
  - anesthetic/steroids
- Contrast used
  - fluoroscopy
  - CT

Nicotine Dependence (Cigarettes, Chewing Tobacco, Other Tobacco Product)

Code Axes

Nicotine dependence, unspecified, uncomplicated	**F17.2ØØ**
Nicotine dependence, unspecified, in remission	**F17.2Ø1**
Nicotine dependence unspecified, withdrawal	**F17.2Ø3**
Nicotine dependence, unspecified, with other nicotine-induced disorders	**F17.2Ø8**
Nicotine dependence, unspecified, with unspecified nicotine-induced disorders	**F17.2Ø9**
Nicotine dependence, cigarettes, uncomplicated	**F17.21Ø**
Nicotine dependence, cigarettes, in remission	**F17.211**
Nicotine dependence, cigarettes, with withdrawal	**F17.213**
Nicotine dependence, cigarettes, with other nicotine-induced disorders	**F17.218**
Nicotine dependence, cigarettes, with unspecified nicotine-induced disorders	**F17.219**
Nicotine dependence, chewing tobacco, uncomplicated	**F17.22Ø**
Nicotine dependence, chewing tobacco, in remission	**F17.221**
Nicotine dependence, chewing tobacco, with withdrawal	**F17.223**
Nicotine dependence, chewing tobacco, with other nicotine-induced disorders	**F17.228**
Nicotine dependence, chewing tobacco, with unspecified nicotine-induced disorders	**F17.229**
Nicotine dependence, other tobacco product, uncomplicated	**F17.29Ø**
Nicotine dependence, other tobacco product, in remission	**F17.291**
Nicotine dependence, other tobacco product, with withdrawal	**F17.293**
Nicotine dependence, other tobacco product, with other nicotine-induced disorders	**F17.298**
Nicotine dependence, other tobacco product, with unspecified nicotine-induced disorders	**F17.299**

Description of Condition

Nicotine dependence (F17)

Nicotine dependence, the most common chemical dependence, is a chronic disorder characterized by use of high quantities of or frequent use of nicotine products in which the individual becomes physically and mentally dependent upon to function. Long-term consequences are physical, psychological, and behavioral. Some of the physical consequences of nicotine use are emphysema, heart disease, stroke, and cancer. Criterion denoting dependence is increased tolerance and continued use despite impairment of health and social life. Cessation results in withdrawal symptoms. Nicotine dependence without negative consequences documented (e.g., uncomplicated) is reported with subcategory F17.200.

Key Terms

Key terms found in the documentation may include:

Smoker (current usage)

Smoker under treatment for tobacco dependence

Tobacco dependence

Clinical Findings

Physical Examination

History and review of systems may include some of the following criteria over the past 12 months:

- Increased heart rate
- Elevated BP
- Weight loss
- Respiratory bronchitis
- Larger amounts of tobacco used
- Constant need or unsuccessful attempts to stop or cutback
- Strong craving to use tobacco
- Considerable time spent on activities needed to obtain tobacco
- Tobacco use that conflicts with work or school performance
- Continued use despite tobacco causing persistent social and interpersonal issues
- Smoking in situations that may be hazardous (e.g., in bed)
- Continued use despite persistent physical and psychological problems related to tobacco
- Use of tobacco to avoid or relieve withdrawal symptoms

Withdrawal symptoms may include:

- Nervousness
- Weight gain
- Headache

- Decreased heart rate
- Irritability
- Difficulty concentrating
- Insomnia

Therapeutic Procedures and Services

- Smoking cessation counseling
  - individual or group counseling
- Nicotine replacement therapy
- Hypnosis

Medication List

- Antidepressant
- Bupropion (Wellbutrin, Zyban)
- Varenicline (Chantix)
- Nortriptyline
- Clonidine (Catapres)

Clinician Note

Documentation of smoking status should indicate the frequency and amount used and identifies the type of nicotine product. If dependency is not indicated, report as tobacco use. Note in the medical record when smoking cessation counseling was provided (Z71.6). A periodic update of smoking status should be performed. The providers' clinical judgment is required for the documentation of "in remission."

Clinician Documentation Checklist

Clinician documentation should indicate the following:

- Exposure to environmental tobacco smoke
- History of tobacco use
- Occupational exposure to environmental tobacco smoke
- Tobacco dependence (e.g., current regular cigarette smoker)
- Tobacco use (e.g., unknown usage of cigarettes)

Obstetrical Package

When documenting obstetrical care, it is important to understand the global obstetrical care package. The concept is similar to the global surgical package. The global obstetrical package includes all the services normally provided during an uncomplicated pregnancy including the antepartum (during pregnancy), delivery, and postpartum (puerperium). The following definitions apply:

Antepartum care: This includes the initial prenatal history and physical examination as well as the history and physical examination (including weight, blood pressure, fetal heart tone, and routine chemical urinalysis) performed during the monthly visits up to 28 weeks gestation; biweekly visits up to 36 weeks gestation, and weekly visits until the time of delivery.

Delivery: The delivery portion of the global obstetrical package includes admission to the hospital or birthing center including the admission history and physical examination, the management of uncomplicated labor and either vaginal or cesarean delivery. Vaginal delivery includes episiotomy and forceps. Also included is any postdelivery management such as discharge services.

Postpartum care: This includes all routine services required up to six weeks postdelivery.

Any services provided outside of those listed above should be documented and reported separately. For example, if a patient has a pregnancy complicated by hyperemesis and therefore needs additional evaluation and management services during the first trimester, these additional E/M services are reported using the appropriate code from the Evaluation and Management section of the CPT manual.

Vaginal delivery, antepartum and postpartum care (59400–59430)

The provider uses these codes to report routine obstetrical care including all antepartum, delivery, and postpartum care or a portion of the global surgical package. Codes from this section should not be used to report the vaginal delivery when the patient has had a previous cesarean delivery (vaginal birth after cesarean or VBAC). In those instances, a code from the 59610–59622 range is used. Correct code assignment is dependent upon the services rendered. For example, if only the vaginal delivery and postpartum care are provided, code 59410 would be reported. However, if the provider managed the entire pregnancy, delivery, and postpartum care, code 59400 is reported.

Also within this section are codes used to report antepartum care only (59425–59426). Correct code selection is dependent upon the number of visits provided. Likewise, code 59430 is used to report only postpartum care.

External cephalic version (59412) is performed by manipulating the fetus from the outside of the abdominal wall, turning the fetus from a breech position to a cephalic position. The clinician places both hands on the patient's abdomen and locates each pole of the fetus by palpation. The fetus is shifted so that the breech or rear end of the fetus is moved upward and the head downward. The physician may elect to use tocolytic drug therapy to suppress uterine contractions during the manipulation. This code may be used for manipulation prior to or during delivery. It may be reported in addition to any of the delivery codes. This includes the cesarean delivery as the physician may attempt to perform the external cephalic version but is unable to manipulate the fetus to a normal cephalic presentation and, therefore, must deliver the infant by cesarean delivery.

Cesarean delivery (59510–59525)

Codes within this range are used to report all or a portion of the global obstetrical package when the delivery is by cesarean section. As with the vaginal delivery codes, correct code selection is dependent upon what portions of the global obstetrical package are provided.

Also within this section is code 59525. This code is used to report a subtotal or total hysterectomy that is performed at the same surgical encounter as the cesarean delivery. Note that this is an add-on code and is listed in addition to the cesarean delivery code.

For those patients who have had a previous cesarean delivery, are expecting to deliver vaginally but require a cesarean delivery, a code from the 59620–59622 range is reported. Again, correct code assignment is dependent upon the level of care provided.

Delivery after previous cesarean (59610–59622)

As mentioned above, there are times when a patient has had a previous cesarean birth and presents with the expectation of delivering vaginally (VBAC). Because previous cesarean delivery can complicate the vaginal delivery and may require a cesarean delivery, separate codes have been developed to report these services.

Codes 59610–59614 are used to report a vaginal delivery after previous cesarean delivery. Correct code selection is dependent upon how much of the global obstetrical package was provided.

Codes 59618–59622 are reported when a vaginal delivery was attempted but delivery had to be by cesarean section after a previous cesarean delivery.

Clinician Documentation Checklist

Clinician documentation should indicate the following:

- Antepartum care
  - prenatal history
  - physical exam
  - weight
  - blood pressure
  - fetal heart tone
  - urinalysis
- Delivery
  - management of labor
  - vaginal delivery w no prior Cesarean

  - cesarean
    - classical
    - low
  - delivery after previous cesarean
- Postpartum
  - weight
  - blood pressure
  - urinalysis

Other Specified Disorders of Kidney and Ureter

Code Axes

Hypertrophy of kidney	**N28.81**
Megaloureter	**N28.82**
Nephroptosis	**N28.83**
Pyelitis cystica	**N28.84**
Pyeloureteritis cystica	**N28.85**
Ureteritis cystica	**N28.86**
Other specified disorders of kidney and ureter	**N28.89**

CDI ALERT

Ensure that documentation is complete for these conditions and that they are not classified inappropriately as unspecified disorders of kidney and ureter.

Description of Condition

Hypertrophy of kidney (N28.81)

CDI ALERT

Although the term hypertrophy is often used to indicate enlargement, documentation stating enlarged kidney should not be assumed to mean hypertrophy of kidney. There are many other conditions that may cause enlargement of the kidney such as polycystic kidney disease or hydronephrosis. Query the physician to determine the exact nature of the condition.

Clinical Tip
Kidney hypertrophy is a general increase in the size of the kidney due to an increase in cell volume, but not due to tumor formation, or to an increase in the number of cells. If the other kidney has been surgically removed, compensatory kidney hypertrophy is a result and the remaining kidney takes on the work previously performed by both kidneys.

Key Terms
Key terms found in the documentation for hypertrophy of kidney may include:

Compensatory kidney hypertrophy

Clinician Note
Ensure that all related conditions are coded, particularly those related to underlying kidney function.

Megaloureter (N28.82)

Clinical Tip
Megaloureter is a descriptive term that represents a ureter that is dilated out of proportion to the remainder of the urinary tract. The condition may be congenital or acquired, in some cases caused by infection or obstruction. It is normally surgically repaired, because retrograde flow of urine can result.

Key Terms

Key terms found in the documentation for megaloureter may include:

- Idiopathic megaureter
- Megaureter
- Nonreflux megaureter
- Obstructed ureter
- Reflux megaureter

Clinician Note

Ensure that all related conditions are coded, particularly those related to underlying ureter obstruction or malfunction.

Nephroptosis (N28.83)

Clinical Tip

Nephroptosis is a condition in which the kidney descends more than two vertebral bodies (or > 5 cm) during a position change from supine to upright. The condition affects generally more female than male patients and is often asymptomatic but can be treated with nephropexy, a surgical procedure that secures the floating kidney to the retroperitoneum. It is thought to be due to a deficiency in the supporting perirenal fascia.

Key Terms

Key terms found in the documentation for nephroptosis may include:

- Floating kidney
- Renal ptosis

Clinician Note

Ensure that all related conditions are coded, particularly those related to underlying kidney disorder.

Pyelitis cystica (N28.84)

Clinical Tip

This condition consists of small subepithelial cysts which elevate the mucous membrane of the renal pelvis and appear as round radiolucent areas on urographic studies. It is related to chronic irritation of the urinary collecting system and recurring urinary tract infections, most frequently due to a stone or infection.

Key Terms

Key terms found in the documentation for pyelitis cystica may include:

- Ureteritis cystica

Pyeloureteritis cystica (N28.85)

Clinical Tip

This condition is similar to pyelitis cystica (above) but the cysts extend into the ureter as well. It is related to chronic irritation of the urinary collecting system and recurring urinary tract infections, most frequently due to a stone or infection.

Clinician Note

Intravenous pyelography and/or retrograde urography are the gold standard for diagnosis and support code assignment. Findings reveal small and multiple filling defects of the ureter and pelvis. Ureteroscopy can provide pathological confirmation of the benign diagnosis. Differential diagnosis to ureteritis cystica includes tumors of the ureters and pelvis, nonopaque calculi, blood clots and iatrogenically induced air-bubbles.

Ureteritis cystica (N28.86)

CDI ALERT

Carefully examine the clinical documentation as ureteritis cystica (UC) can mimic other conditions such as transitional cell carcinoma, blood clots, air bubbles, radiolucent stones, fibroepithelial polyps, and sloughed renal papillae. Do not report ureteritis cystica unless confirmed by the clinician's documentation.

Clinical Tip

This condition is similar to pyelitis cystica (above) but the cysts involve only the ureter. It is related to chronic irritation of the urinary collecting system and recurring urinary tract infections, most frequently due to a stone or infection.

Clinician Note

Intravenous pyelography and/or retrograde urography are the gold standard for diagnosis and support code assignment. Findings reveal small and multiple filling defects of the ureter and pelvis. Ureteroscopy can provide pathological confirmation of the benign diagnosis. Differential diagnosis to ureteritis cystica includes tumors of the ureters and pelvis, nonopaque calculi, blood clots and iatrogenically induced air-bubbles.

Clinician Documentation Checklist

Clinician documentation should indicate the following:

- Other disorders of kidney and ureter
  - type
    - cyst of kidney, acquired
      - cyst (multiple) (solitary) of kidney, acquired
    - other specified disorders of kidney and ureter
      - hypertrophy of kidney
      - megaloureter
      - nephroptosis
      - pyelitis cystica
      - pyeloureteritis cystica
      - ureteritis cystica
      - other disorders of kidney and ureter
      - unspecified disorder of kidney and ureter

- nephropathy
- renal disease (acute)
- renal insufficiency (acute)

- Other disorders of kidney and ureter in diseases
  - identify underlying disease, such as
    - amyloidosis
    - nephrocalcinosis
    - schistosomiasis

Other Symptoms and Signs Involving Cognitive Functions and Awareness

Code Axes

Age-related cognitive decline	R41.81
Altered mental status, unspecified	R41.82
Borderline intellectual functioning	R41.83
Attention and concentration deficit	R41.840
Cognitive communication deficit	R41.841
Visuospatial deficit	R41.842
Psychomotor deficit	R41.843
Frontal lobe and executive function deficit	R41.844
Other and unspecified symptoms and signs involving cognitive functions and awareness	R41.89, R41.9

Clinician Note
Many payers, including Medicare, have quality measures in place to determine that quality and cost effective care is provided to the patient. It is imperative that the results of cognitive screening and any associated conditions be documented in the medical record.

Description of Condition

Age-related cognitive decline (R41.81)

Clinical Tip
Normal aging is associated with a decline in abilities related to numeric/arithmetic and processing speed, memory, reasoning, verbal ability, and visuoperceptual skills. Patients for whom response and skills are worse than expected for the current age are difficult to clearly diagnose. Research is currently being conducted to determine where normal aging stops and pathology begins.

Key Terms
Key terms found in the documentation for age-related cognitive decline may include:

Senility

Clinician Note
Many payers will not provide coverage of psychotherapy services for age-related cognitive decline unless the medical record documentation can indicate that an improvement in the patients status is expected.

Altered mental status, unspecified (R41.82)

Clinical Tip

Altered mental status is a very general term that refers to general changes in brain function, such as confusion, amnesia (memory loss), loss of alertness, loss of orientation (not cognizant of self, time, or place), defects in judgment or thought, poor regulation of emotions, and disruptions in perception, psychomotor skills, and behavior. Other medical conditions and trauma must be ruled out before a full neurological work-up is performed.

Key Terms

Key terms found in the documentation for altered mental status, unspecified may include:

Change in mental status

Clinician Note

Many payers will not provide coverage of psychotherapy services for altered mental status unless the medical record documentation can indicate that an improvement in the patients status is expected.

Borderline intellectual functioning (R41.83)

Clinical Tip

This condition is broadly defined as a person with an IQ stated to be between 71 and 84. The designation is meant to differentiate these patients from those in the "intellectual disabilities" categories. Research has shown that borderline intellectual functioning is developmental, can be present in both children and adults, and can be a factor associated with relatively poor outcomes in psychiatric disorders.

CDI ALERT

If the specific IQ score is not documented, clarify whether a patient would be classified in the intellectual disabilities category or more appropriately in the borderline intellectual functioning category.

Attention and concentration deficit (R41.840)

Clinical Tip

A variety of environmental factors can negatively affect attention and concentration. Some of these include caffeine, some antidepressant medications, sleep disorders, heavy metal poisoning, and traumatic brain injury, just to name a few. Problems with attention and concentration may also be due to deficiencies in magnesium, thyroid, B-12, or iron levels. Patients undergoing work up for attention or concentration problems should not be classified with ADHD.

Clinician Note

Ensure that all other related diagnoses are coded appropriately, particularly that for underlying neurological disorders.

I-10 ALERT

This particular code, being in the symptoms and signs chapter of ICD-10-CM, is not intended to be assigned for patients who have been diagnosed with one of the attention-deficit hyperactivity disorders (ADHD) (refer to category F90). The code is intended to be reported either when a patient suffers from these symptoms temporarily or as the initial symptom code when being worked up for ADHD.

Cognitive communication deficit (R41.841)

Clinical Tip

This condition involves the breakdown of applied communication skills. Cognitive-communication assessment refers to appraisal of thought processes, including attention, orientation, organization/sequencing, recall and problem solving, insight, processing speed, and pragmatics.

Clinician Note

Ensure that all other related diagnoses are coded appropriately, particularly that for underlying neurological disorders.

Visuospatial deficit (R41.842)

Clinical Tip

The condition involves an inability or deterioration in the ability to comprehend and conceptualize visual representations and spatial relationships in learning and performing a task. The two components of visual processing are: locating an object in space (where?) and determining the identity of an object (what?).

Clinician Note

Ensure that all other related diagnoses are coded appropriately, particularly that for underlying neurological disorders.

Psychomotor deficit (R41.843)

Clinical Tip

This condition involves relating the psychologic processes associated with muscular movement to the production of voluntary movements. Examples include decreased rate of speech, decreased energy, decreased libido and anhedonia (an absence of pleasure from the performance of acts that would ordinarily be pleasurable).

Clinician Note

Ensure that all other related diagnoses are coded appropriately, particularly that for underlying neurological disorders.

Coverage may be provided for occupational therapy and/or activities of daily living for this condition when documentation also indicates that the patient's status is likely to improve.

Frontal lobe and executive function deficit (R41.844)

Clinical Tip

Executive function describes a set of cognitive abilities that control and regulate other abilities and behaviors and are necessary for goal-directed behavior. They include the ability to initiate and stop actions, to monitor and change behavior as needed, and to plan future behavior when faced with novel tasks and situations. Patients with this deficit are unable or hindered in their ability to anticipate outcomes and adapt to changing situations. The ability to form concepts and think abstractly is often affected.

Clinician Note

Ensure that all other related diagnoses are coded appropriately, particularly that for underlying neurological disorders.

Pacemakers and Implantable Defibrillators

Code Axes

Pacemaker or implantable defibrillators	**33202–33249** QPP **33262–33264** **33270–33273**

Description of Procedure

A pacemaker may be either permanent or temporary. A permanent pacemaker is used to maintain cardiac stability and a normal sinus rhythm. A temporary pacemaker is used to treat transient bradycardia that may be due to conditions such as acute myocardial infarction or drug toxicity and may be followed by the insertion of a permanent pacemaker.

CPT Alert

Note that the insertion of a temporary pacemaker is considered an integral part of critical care and is not reported separately.

An implantable cardio-defibrillator monitors heart rhythms and if a potentially dangerous rhythm is sensed it delivers a shock to restore normal rhythm.

Both systems have two major components, an operating system and electrodes. Either of these components may need to be removed and replaced at some point.

Documentation should provide the following information:

What type of system?

Is the device permanent or temporary?

How many leads are placed?

Are any components being removed without replacement?

Are components being replaced and if so which components?

Is the system being converted to a biventricular system (additional lead being placed)?

Clinical Tip

There is a new, experimental technology called a leadless cardiac pacemaker. This system includes a pulse generator with built-in battery and electrode for implantation in a cardiac chamber via transcatheter approach. Documentation will indicate that the physician made a small puncture in the groin and using a transcatheter placed the pacemaker into the heart. There will be no documentation indicating a lead placement. Services related to the leadless pacemaker are reported with the appropriate code from 0387T–0391T.

Key Terms

Dual lead pacemaker

Dual lead defibrillator

Leadless pacemaker

Multiple lead defibrillator

Permanent pacemaker

Temporary pacemaker

Clinician Documentation Checklist

Clinician documentation should indicate the following:

- Approach
  - open
  - endoscopic
  - transvenous
  - atrial
  - ventricular
- Purpose of the procedure
  - insertion
  - replacement
  - revision
  - repair
- Type of system inserted
  - single chamber
  - dual chamber
- Device expected length of service
  - permanent
  - temporary
- How many leads are placed
- Identification of
  - components being removed without replacement
  - components being replaced
- System conversion to biventricular system

Preventive Services — Prostate Cancer Screening

Code Axes

Prostate cancer screening; digital rectal examination	**G0102**
Prostate cancer screening; prostate specific antigen test (PSA)	**G0103**

Description of Procedure

For Medicare and many other third-party payers, coverage of prostate cancer screening tests includes the following procedures furnished to an individual for the early detection of prostate cancer:

- Screening digital rectal examination
- Screening prostate specific antigen blood test

⇨ I-10 ALERT

When reporting prostate cancer screening, digital rectal examinations, and screening prostate-specific antigen (PSA) blood tests, diagnosis code Z12.5 Encounter for screening for malignant neoplasm of prostate, must be used to indicate the screening nature of the service.

Prostate cancer screening; digital rectal examination (G0102)

Screening digital rectal examinations are covered at a frequency of once every 12 months for men who have attained age 50 (at least 11 months have passed following the month in which the last Medicare-covered screening digital rectal examination was performed). Documentation will indicate that the health care provider performed an examination of an individual's prostate for nodules or other abnormalities of the prostate.

Key Terms

DRE

Clinician Note

The size and any abnormalities should be noted in the medical record as well as any changes from previous examinations.

Prostate cancer screening; prostate specific antigen test (PSA) (G0103)

Screening prostate specific antigen (PSA) tests are performed to detect the marker for adenocarcinoma of prostate. PSA is a reliable immunocytochemical marker for primary and metastatic adenocarcinoma of prostate. Documentation supporting this service will include a laboratory result.

Prostatectomy

Code Axes

Prostatectomy **55801–55866**

Description of Procedure

Excision of the prostate, other than by transurethral methods, is reported with the appropriate code from range 55801–55845, 55866. Documentation should be carefully reviewed to determine:

- The approach
  - perineal
  - retropubic
  - laparoscopic
- The extent
  - total
  - subtotal
- The method
  - one stage
  - two stage
- If lymphadenectomy was performed

Prostatectomy, perineal, subtotal (including control of postoperative bleeding, vasectomy, meatotomy, urethral calibration and/or dilation, and internal urethrotomy) (55801)

Documentation supporting a subtotal perineal radical prostatectomy will indicate that the prostate was removed through an incision made in the perineum. The bladder outlet is revised; however, the seminal vesicles remain intact.

Key Terms

Key terms found in the documentation may include:

Subtotal radical prostatectomy

Prostatectomy, perineal, radical (55810)

Documentation for this service will indicate that the seminal vesicles and vas deferens are also removed. When documentation indicates that local lymph nodes were removed for analysis, code 55812 is supported. When a separate incision is made and all lymph nodes are removed from the back wall of the pelvis, code 55815 is supported.

CDI ALERT

Terms such as "biopsy," "lymphadenectomy," "perineal," "retropubic," "radical," "subtotal," or "nerve sparing" provide the guidance needed to ensure correct code assignment.

Prostatectomy (including control of postoperative bleeding, vasectomy, meatotomy, urethral calibration and/or dilation, and internal urethrotomy); suprapubic, subtotal, stages 1 or 2 (55821)

Prostatectomy (including control of postoperative bleeding, vasectomy, meatotomy, urethral calibration and/or dilation, and internal urethrotomy); retropubic, subtotal (55831)

Prostatectomy retropubic radical, with or without nerve sparing (55840)

When documentation indicates that an incision was made in the lower abdomen just above the pubic area, a suprapubic approach is performed. However, when the documentation indicates that the incision was made in the lower abdomen and the physician approached the prostate by going behind the pubic bone, a retropubic prostatectomy was performed. Note that if the seminal vesicles are not removed, a subtotal prostatectomy was performed. Documentation supporting a retropubic radical prostatectomy states that the seminal glands and vas deferens were also removed.

Clinician Documentation Checklist

Clinician documentation should indicate the following:

- Medical condition being treated
- Approach
  - perineal
  - retropubic
  - laparoscopic
- Extent
  - total
  - subtotal
- Method
  - one stage
  - two stages
- Other services
  - radiation application
  - lymph node biopsy

Respiratory Distress of Newborn

Code Axes

Respiratory distress syndrome of newborn	**P22.Ø**
Transient tachypnea of newborn	**P22.1**
Other respiratory distress of newborn	**P22.8**
Respiratory distress of newborn, unspecified	**P22.9**

Description of Condition

Respiratory distress syndrome of newborn (P22.Ø)

Respiratory distress syndrome (RDS) is a breathing disorder that affects newborns. RDS rarely occurs in full-term infants. Respiratory distress syndrome is the most common disorder of the premature infant, generally less than 34 weeks gestation. The incidence and severity increase with decreasing gestational age. RDS is more common in premature infants because their lungs are unable to produce enough surfactant.

Key Terms

Key terms found in the documentation may include:

Cardiorespiratory distress syndrome of newborn

Hyaline membrane disease

Idiopathic respiratory distress syndrome [IRDS or RDS] of newborn

Pulmonary hypoperfusion syndrome

Respiratory distress syndrome, type I

Clinical Findings

RDS is caused by pulmonary surfactant deficiency in the lungs and risk increases with the degree of prematurity.

Physical Examination

The following symptoms will occur immediately or within a few hours of delivery.

- Nasal flaring
- Rapid and labored breathing
- Grunting respirations
- Use of accessory muscles
- Cyanosis
- Apnea
- Lethargy
- Decreased breath sounds

CDI ALERT

Documentation should include prematurity or documentation of other deficiency of surfactant, progressively more severe respiratory distress after birth, as well as findings of cyanosis, grunting, nasal flaring, intercostal and subcostal retractions and tachypnea. Chest x-rays frequently have a ground-glass appearance. Oxygen requirements progressively increase over the first few hours after birth. There may also be documentation of apnea and refractory hypoxemia and acidosis.

Treatments include endotracheal intubation, positive pressure ventilation, continuous positive airway pressure (CPAP), supplementary oxygen, and surfactant placement via ET tube.

- Diagnostic Procedures and Services
- Laboratory
  - arterial blood gas
  - blood cultures
  - tracheal aspirate cultures
  - cerebrospinal fluid culture
- Imaging
  - chest x-ray
- Other
  - transcutaneous CO_2 monitor

Therapeutic Procedures and Services

- Surfactant therapy
- Mechanical ventilation
- Supplementary oxygen

Transient tachypnea of newborn (P22.1)

Transient tachypnea of the newborn (TTN) is the most common respiratory disorder of the mature newborn and is self-limited, due to the inability to absorb fetal lung fluid. Infants with transient tachypnea of newborn present within the first few hours of life with tachypnea, increased oxygen requirement, and ABGs negative for carbon dioxide retention.

Treatment is generally close observation and symptomatic care with low flow supplemental oxygen.

Key Terms

Key terms found in the documentation may include:

Idiopathic tachypnea of newborn

Respiratory distress syndrome, type II

Wet lung syndrome

Other respiratory distress of newborn (P22.8)

Documentation Tip

Codes are not assigned for respiratory distress syndrome (RDS type I) or transitory tachypnea of newborn (RDS type II) unless the provider specifically documents these conditions. Code P22.8 would be assigned if the provider has documented a specific type of respiratory distress syndrome in the newborn that is not coded elsewhere.

Respiratory distress of newborn, unspecified (P22.9)

Documentation Tip

If the provider indicates "respiratory distress of newborn" without further documentation code P22.9 is assigned.

Clinician Documentation Checklist

Clinician documentation should indicate the following:

- Conditions acquired in utero, during birth, or during the first 28 days after birth
- Type of disorder
  - metabolic acidemia
    - before onset of labor
    - during labor
    - at birth
- Respiratory distress
  - respiratory distress syndrome of newborn
    - cardiorespiratory distress syndrome
    - hyaline membrane disease
    - pulmonary hypoperfusion syndrome
  - transient tachypnea
    - idiopathic tachypnea
    - respiratory distress type II
    - wet lung syndrome
- Congenital pneumonia
  - specify the organism
  - pneumonia due to
    - viral agent
    - *Chlamydia*
    - *Staphylococcus*
    - *Streptococcus*
    - *Escherichia coli*
    - pseudomonas
    - bacterial agent
- Neonatal aspiration
  - specify with or without respiratory symptoms
  - specify any pulmonary hypertension
  - due to
    - meconium
    - amniotic fluid and mucus
    - blood
    - milk and food
- Interstitial emphysema
  - interstitial
  - pneumothorax
  - pneumomediastinum
  - pneumopericardium

- Pulmonary hemorrhage
  - tracheobronchial hemorrhage
  - massive pulmonary hemorrhage
- Chronic respiratory disease
  - Wilson-Mikity syndrome
  - bronchopulmonary dysplasia
  - congenital pulmonary fibrosis
  - ventilator lung
- Other respiratory perinatal conditions
  - primary atelectasis
    - primary failure to expand terminal respiratory units
    - pulmonary hypoplasia associated with short gestation
    - pulmonary immaturity
  - atelectasis
  - resorption atelectasis without respiratory distress syndrome
  - cyanotic attacks
  - primary sleep apnea
  - apnea of prematurity
  - obstructive apnea of newborn
  - respiratory failure
  - respiratory arrest
  - respiratory depression
  - laryngeal stridor
  - sniffles
  - snuffles

Respiratory Failure

Code Axes

Note: All four subcategories of respiratory failure contain fifth characters that represent the following code classification axes: unspecified whether with hypoxia or hypercapnia; with hypoxia: defined as a condition in which the body is deprived of an adequate oxygen supply, regardless of whether the body has an adequate perfusion by blood; with hypercapnia: defined as an increased level of carbon dioxide in the blood, usually exhaled during regular breathing.

Acute respiratory failure	**J96.Ø-** HCC
Chronic respiratory failure	**J96.1-** HCC
Acute and chronic respiratory failure	**J96.2-** HCC
Respiratory failure, unspecified	**J96.9-** HCC
Acute respiratory distress syndrome	**J8Ø** HCC
Postprocedural respiratory failure	**J95.82-** HCC

I-10 ALERT

Understanding the differences between hypoxia and hypercapnia is essential for appropriate classification of respiratory failure in ICD-10-CM.

Description of Condition

Acute respiratory failure (J96.Ø-)

Clinical Tip

Acute respiratory failure may be life-threatening and involve the most abnormal arterial blood gas measurements, but the two types (hypoxic and hypercapnic) are very different. Hypoxemic is the most common form and can be associated with most lung diseases, representing a lower than normal arterial oxygen level. Hypercapnic respiratory failure, with a high level of carbon dioxide ($PaCO_2$) is most often associated with drug overdoses, severe airway disorders, or neuromuscular diseases. Acute RF develops within minutes or hours.

CDI ALERT

Ensure that the documentation is adequate and can differentiate between acute respiratory failure and acute respiratory distress syndrome, which is classified to category J8Ø.

Clinician Note

Note that a documentation of respiratory insufficiency does not support the assignment of an acute respiratory failure code.

Chronic respiratory failure (J96.1-)

Chronic or long-term respiratory failure is most often caused by various types of chronic obstructive pulmonary diseases (COPD), neuromuscular diseases (e.g., myasthenia gravis), cystic fibrosis, and even morbid obesity. Chronic RF develops over days or longer, worsens over time, and triggers should be identified, which are most commonly related to a superimposed infection. Although chronic in presentation, this condition is sufficiently severe and may cause major complications, such as organ failure or dysfunction, acute myocardial infarction (AMI), respiratory arrest, or shock.

CDI ALERT

If chronic respiratory failure is documented, ensure that there is no superimposed acute component as well. Acute on chronic respiratory failure is a common condition in this patient group.

I-10 ALERT

For ICD-10-CM the word "adult" was changed to "acute" in the "respiratory distress syndrome" terminology. It is now understood that the disease process can occur in either an adult or a pediatric patient. However, be aware that a separate classification category exists for respiratory distress syndrome of the newborn (P22.Ø).

I-10 ALERT

Codes in subcategory J95.82 are differentiated by severity; code J95.821 represents acute postprocedural respiratory failure and code J95.822 represents the acute and chronic form of the condition.

CDI ALERT

The documentation for postprocedural respiratory failure must clearly make the cause-and-effect relationship between the condition and the fact that it was a result of the procedure or surgery in order to assign a code from this subcategory.

Acute and chronic respiratory failure (J96.2-)

Acute and rapid deterioration of a patient with chronic respiratory failure is known as acute on chronic respiratory failure. These are typically COPD patients or those with neuromuscular disease or chest wall disorders. Patients with this condition may require long-term mechanical ventilation.

Acute respiratory distress syndrome (ARDS) (J8Ø)

Acute respiratory distress syndrome is considered the most acute form of acute lung injury (ALI) (nontraumatic). The syndrome is defined by the ratio of the partial pressure of oxygen in the patient's arterial blood (PaO_2) to the fraction of oxygen in the inspired air (FIO_2). In ARDS, the PaO_2/FIO_2 ratio is less than 200, and in ALI, it is less than 300. Patients with ARDS typically have pulmonary edema, as the alveolar space fills with fluid. Many patients also develop pulmonary hypertension, which usually resolves as the syndrome resolves.

Key Terms

Key terms found in the documentation may include:

Adult hyaline membrane disease

Postprocedural respiratory failure (J95.82-)

Postoperative respiratory failure is the need for ventilation for more than 48 hours after surgery or reintubation with mechanical ventilation post extubation. Comorbid conditions that are risk factors are obstructive sleep apnea, COPD, CHF, advanced age, ASA class ≥ 2 and pulmonary hypertension. Patients who have had surgery of the aortic, thoracic, and upper abdomen areas have higher odds of developing postoperative respiratory failure.

Clinician Note

Differentiate between *expected* respiratory requirements postsurgery and a condition or complication requiring additional ventilation time or reintubation. Identify the causative condition when known (aspiration, exacerbation of COPD, pneumonia, etc.).

Clinical Findings

Conditions or diseases that may lead to respiratory failure are disorders that affect the nerves, muscles, tissues, or bones that support breathing or have a direct effect on the lungs. Examples include: muscular dystrophy, spinal cord injuries, chest injury that damages the tissues and ribs around the lungs, scoliosis, COPD, pneumonia, and ARDS.

Physical Examination

History and review of systems may include:

- Shortness of breath
- A feeling of the inability to breath in enough air
- Rapid breathing
- Abnormal lung sounds (crackling)

- Arrhythmia
- Asterixis
- Cyanosis
- Dyspnea
- Confusion
- Severe sleepiness
- Cor pulmonale—may be present with chronic respiratory failure
- Hypotension
- Gastric distention
- Diarrhea

Diagnostic Procedures and Services

- Laboratory
  - arterial blood gas
  - CBC
  - chemistry panel
  - serum creatinine
  - TSH—in chronic respiratory failure
- Imaging
  - chest x-ray
- Other
  - pulse oximetry
  - EKG
  - PFT—in evaluation of chronic respiratory failure

Therapeutic Procedures and Services

Treatment will depend on severity, if the condition is acute or chronic and the underlying cause.

- Oxygen therapy
- Mechanical ventilation
- Tracheostomy
- IV fluids
- CPAP—useful with chronic respiratory failure
- Medications may be given to treat the underlying cause

Clinician Documentation Checklist

Clinician documentation should indicate the following:

- Respiratory failure
  - with hypoxia
  - with hypercapnia
  - unspecified whether with hypoxia or hypercapnia
- Type
  - acute

- chronic
- acute and chronic
  - acute on chronic respiratory failure
- unspecified

Respiratory Diseases Affecting Interstitium

- Acute respiratory distress syndrome
  - in adult or child
  - adult hyaline membrane disease
- Pulmonary edema
  - identify
    - exposure to environmental tobacco smoke
    - history of tobacco use
    - occupational exposure to environmental tobacco smoke
    - tobacco dependence
    - tobacco use
  - type
    - acute
      - acute edema of lung
    - chronic
      - pulmonary congestion (chronic) (passive)
      - pulmonary edema
- Pulmonary eosinophilia
  - includes
    - allergic pneumonia
    - eosinophilic asthma
    - eosinophilic pneumonia
    - Loffler's pneumonia
    - tropical (pulmonary) eosinophilia

Intraoperative and Postprocedural Complications, Disorders of Respiratory System

- Procedure that was performed
- Specific part of respiratory tract that was involved
- Complications that occurred were
  - during procedure (intraoperative)
  - after procedure (postprocedural)
- Type of complications
  - tracheostomy complications
    - hemorrhage from tracheostomy stroma
    - infection of tracheostomy stroma
      - identify type of infection such as:
        - cellulitis

- ❖ sepsis
- — malfunction of tracheostomy stroma
  - ♦ tracheal stenosis due to tracheostomy
  - ♦ obstruction of tracheostomy airway
  - ♦ mechanical complication
- — tracheoesophageal fistula following tracheostomy
- — other
- — unspecified

- acute pulmonary insufficiency following
  - — thoracic surgery
  - — nonthoracic surgery
- chronic pulmonary insufficiency following
  - — surgery
- chemical pneumonitis due to anesthesia
  - — identify
    - ♦ Mendelson's syndrome
    - ♦ postprocedural aspiration pneumonia
    - ♦ the drug, if responsible
- postprocedural subglottic stenosis
- intraoperative hemorrhage and hematoma of respiratory system organ complicating a procedure
  - — respiratory system procedure
  - — other procedure
- postprocedural hematoma or hemorrhage of respiratory organ following a procedure
  - — respiratory system procedure
  - — other procedure
- accidental puncture and laceration during a procedure
  - — respiratory system procedure
  - — other procedure
- postprocedural pneumothorax
- postprocedural airleak
- postprocedural respiratory failure
  - — acute
  - — acute and chronic
- transfusion-related acute lung injury
- complication of respirator (ventilator)
  - — mechanical complication
  - — ventilator associated pneumonia
    - ♦ identification of the causal organism
  - — other

- other complications and disorders
  - intraoperative
  - postprocedural
    - identification of disorders such as
      - aspiration pneumonia
      - bacterial or viral pneumonia

Rhythm and Conduction Disorders

Code Axes

Atrioventricular and left bundle-branch block	**I44.Ø–I44.7** HCC
Other and unspecified conduction disorders	**I45.Ø–I45.9**
Atrial fibrillation and flutter	**I48.Ø–I48.9-** HCC QPP
Other cardiac arrhythmias	**I49.Ø–I49.9** HCC

Clinical Tip

Mobitz I and Mobitz II AV blocks are both classified as second degree AV blocks, and are based on electrocardiographic (ECG) patterns, not on location. Even though slightly different, both are classified to code I44.1

Key Terms

Key terms found in the documentation for conduction disorders may include:

Accelerated atrioventricular conduction
Accessory atrioventricular conduction
A-fib
Anomalous atrioventricular excitation
Atrial fibrillation
Atrial flutter
Atrioventricular (AV) block, type I and II
Atrioventricular (AV) dissociation
Bifascicular block
Complete heart block Mobitz block, type I and II
Fascicular block
Interference dissociation
Isorhythmic dissociation
Left bundle branch block (LBBB)
Left bundle-branch hemiblock
Lown-Ganong-Levine syndrome
Nonparoxysmal AV nodal tachycardia
Pre-excitation atrioventricular conduction
Right bundle branch block (RBBB)
Sick sinus syndrome (SSS)
Sinoatrial block
Sinoauricular block
Stokes-Adams syndrome
Third degree AV block
Trifascicular block

⇨ I-10 ALERT

ICD-10-CM codes for cardiac arrhythmia conditions provide code options for paroxysmal, persistent, chronic, typical, and atypical forms of atrial fibrillation and flutter.

Ventricular fibrillation

Ventricular flutter

Wenckebach's block

Wolff-Parkinson-White (WPW) syndrome

Clinician Note

Many of the conduction disorders support the medical necessity of pacemaker insertion, cardioverter-defibrillator insertion, and intracardiac electrophysiologic procedures. Physician documentation should be examined to determine if there are other underlying conditions which should be reported separately.

Clinical Tip

Atrial fibrillation may be classified into one of three categories:

Paroxysmal: These episodes end spontaneously within seven days and most episodes last less than 24 hours

Persistent: These episodes last more than seven days and may require electrical or pharmacologic intervention

Permanent (chronic): This atrial fibrillation has lasted more than one year, regardless of whether cardioversion has been attempted and has failed or has never been attempted

Atrial flutter is classified into two categories, Type I and Type II:

Type I: Typical (common) atrial flutter has an atrial rate of 240 to 340 beats/minute

Type II: Atypical atrial flutter follows a significantly different re-entry pathway than Type I and is faster; usually 340 to 440 beats/minute

Ensure that documentation is consistent when involving the different types of atrial fibrillation and flutter.

Clinical Findings

Bundle branch and fascicular blocks are generally asymptomatic and are diagnosed by ECG. Atrioventricular (AV) blocks may be asymptomatic or exhibit mild to severe symptoms including bradycardia, fatigue, light-headedness, presyncope, syncope, or heart failure. AV blocks are diagnosed by ECG and may be treated with medication or often require a pacemaker.

Atrial fibrillation affects nearly 2.3 million adults in the U.S. and is the most common type of irregular heartbeat.

Physical Examination

A-fib may be asymptomatic or the patient history or current symptoms may include one or more of the following:

- Irregularly irregular pulse
- Rapid and irregular heartbeat
- Weakness
- Light-headedness

- Dyspnea
- Fatigue
- Fluttering in the chest
- Vague chest discomfort/pain
- Palpitations
- Shortness of breath
- Swollen feet or legs

Diagnostic Procedures and Services

- Laboratory
  - TFTs
- Imaging
  - chest x-ray
  - echocardiography
- Other
  - ECG
  - Holter monitor

Therapeutic Procedures and Services

- Procedures
  - electrical cardioversion
  - ablation
  - pacemaker

Medications List

- Blood clot prevention
  - antiplatelets
  - anticoagulants
- Heart rate/rhythm control
  - antiarrhythmic drugs
  - beta blockers
  - calcium channel blockers
  - digitalis

Clinician Documentation Checklist

Clinician documentation should indicate the following:

- Heart blocks
  - atrioventricular block
    - first degree
    - second degree (Mobitz type I and II, Wenckebach)
    - third degree (complete NOS)
    - other
    - unspecified
  - left anterior fascicular block

- left posterior fascicular block
- other (left bundle branch hemiblock NOS)
- unspecified (other fascicular block)

- Other conduction disorders
  - right fascicular block
  - other and unspecified right bundle branch block
  - bifascicular block
  - trifascicular block
  - nonspecific intraventricular block
  - other specified heart block (sinoatrial block, sinoauricular block)
  - pre-excitation syndrome
  - accelerated atrioventricular conduction
  - accessory atrioventricular conduction
  - anomalous atrioventricular excitation
  - Lown-Ganong-Levine syndrome
  - pre-excitation atrioventricular conduction
  - Wolff-Parkinson-White syndrome
  - other
    - long qt syndrome
    - other specified conduction disorder
    - AV dissociation
    - interference dissociation
  - unspecified
- Cardiac arrest
  - due to underlying cardiac condition
  - due to other underlying condition
  - cause unspecified

Cardiac Arrhythmias

- Tachycardia
  - re-entry ventricular
  - supraventricular
  - atrioventricular
  - atrioventricular re-entrant (nodal)
  - junctional
  - ventricular
  - unspecified (paroxysmal)
- Atrial fibrillation and flutter
  - paroxysmal
  - persistent
  - chronic
  - typical
  - atypical

- unspecified
- Other cardiac arrhythmias
  - ventricular fibrillation
  - ventricular flutter
  - atrial premature depolarization
  - junctional premature depolarization
  - ventricular premature depolarization
  - premature beats NOS
  - other premature depolarization
  - sick sinus syndrome
  - other specified cardiac arrhythmias
  - unspecified cardiac arrhythmias

Sepsis (Systemic, Generalized, Complication)

Code Axes

The majority of the ICD-10-CM sepsis codes are in categories A4Ø and A41:

Streptococcal sepsis	**A4Ø.Ø–A4Ø.9** HCC
Sepsis due to Staphylococcus aureus	**A41.Ø1–A41.4** HCC QPP
Sepsis due to other Gram-negative organisms	**A41.5Ø–A41.59** HCC
Other and unspecified sepsis	**A41.81, A41.89** HCC

Description of Condition

Clinical Tip

Sepsis is a life-threatening systemic infection of the bloodstream, most typically originating in the urinary tract, lungs, GI systems, or via a surgical wound or infected implanted device. Symptoms may progress to shock or organ failure, and the condition may be fatal.

Bacteremia is an abnormal finding on blood culture that indicates bacteria in the blood and does not represent an infectious state. Bacteremia elicits an immune response which can exhibit as fever. If bacteremia is stated but clinical evidence supports the presence of sepsis, a systemic infection with features of a more severe immune response, query the provider for clarification.

Documentation Tip

Physician documentation must demonstrate the severity of the illness through the history and physical, progress notes, review and comment on all consults, and review and comment on ancillary test results indicating either the improvement or worsening of the patient status.

CDI ALERT

Negative or inclusive blood cultures do not preclude a diagnosis of sepsis. The presence of one or more risk factors, the appropriate clinical presentation, and specific treatment in conjunction with physician confirmation validates the diagnosis.

Streptococcal sepsis (A4Ø), including codes for sepsis due to strep, group A (A4Ø.Ø), group B (A4Ø.1), strep pneumoniae (A4Ø.3), and other and unspecified strep (A4Ø.8, A4Ø.9)

ICD-10-CM contains multiple codes in this category, including those for group A, group B, strep pneumoniae, and other and unspecified forms of the disease. Group B is most commonly responsible for infections in the pediatric population and also in pregnant patients.

Key Terms

Key terms found in the documentation may include:

- Bloodstream infection (although necessary to differentiate from bacteremia)
- Septicemia
- Septic intoxication
- Septic syndrome
- Severe sepsis
- Severe sepsis with organ failure
- Toxemia
- Urosepsis (antiquated term; necessary to differentiate from UTI)

Documentation Tip

The diagnosis of sepsis cannot be made based solely on laboratory or blood work findings. The physician must document the systemic infection.

Sepsis due to Staphylococcus aureus, including codes and for methicillin susceptible Staphylococcus aureus (MSSA) (A41.Ø1), for methicillin resistant Staphylococcus aureus (MRSA) (A41.Ø2)

ICD-10-CM diagnosis codes representing staph sepsis conditions mirror those in ICD-9-CM, with specific codes for MRSA and MSSA.

Key Terms

Key terms found in the documentation may include:

- Bloodstream infection (although necessary to differentiate from bacteremia)
- MRSA sepsis
- MSSA sepsis
- Septicemia
- Septic intoxication
- Septic syndrome
- Severe sepsis
- Toxemia
- Urosepsis (antiquated term; necessary to differentiate from UTI)

Sepsis due to Hemophilus influenzae is (A41.3) and sepsis due to anaerobes is (A41.4) which would include Clostridium and Bacteroides.

ICD-10-CM diagnosis codes representing Gram-negative *Haemophilus influenzae* and anaerobic sepsis mirror those in ICD-9-CM. While the code for *Haemophilus influenzae* is specific, code A41.4 includes any (gram positive or negative) anaerobic organism, classified as such but for which there is no assigned index entry (unlike actinomycosis which is A42.7).

CDI ALERT

In some cases skin bacteria contaminates the blood sample, which is another reason physician correlation and clarification of diagnosis is essential before code assignment.

Sepsis due to other Gram-negative organisms (A41.5-), including specific codes for sepsis due to Escherichia coli (A41.51), Pseudomonas(A41.52), Serratia (A41.53), and other and unspecified Gram-negative sepsis (A41.59, A41.5Ø)

ICD-10-CM diagnosis codes representing Gram-negative sepsis conditions mirror those in ICD-9-CM, with specific codes for sepsis due to E. coli, Pseudomonas, Serratia, and infections due to other Gram-negative organisms such as *Acinetobacter baumanni, Klebsiella pneumoniae.* Gram-negative sepsis is an increasingly common disorder and, with problems due to multiple drug resistance, the symptoms can lead to such serious complications as shock, adult respiratory distress syndrome, and disseminated intravascular coagulation.

CDI ALERT

Colonization is the presence of an organism without current disease. It should be documented when confirmed or suspected as it has potential risks for both patient and care-givers; colonization is reported as "carrier" from category Z22.

Key Terms

Key terms found in the documentation may include:

Bloodstream infection (although necessary to differentiate from bacteremia)

Septicemia

Septic intoxication

Severe sepsis

Toxemia

Urosepsis (antiquated term; necessary to differentiate from UTI)

Other specified sepsis (A41.89), includes sepsis due to Enterococcus (Strep group D) (A41.81).

Enterococcus faecalis and *Enterococcus faecium* are the most common of these pathogens. *Enterococcus* species are important nosocomial pathogens because of their resistance to antibiotics; *E. faecium* represents most vancomycin-resistant *Enterococcus* (VRE).

CDI ALERT

When the documentation indicates that the patient has severe sepsis, sepsis with acute organ dysfunction, sepsis with multiple organ dysfunction, or systemic inflammatory response syndrome (SIRS) due to infectious process with acute organ dysfunction, the appropriate code from R65.2- should also be assigned.

Viral sepsis (A41 and B97)

Viral sepsis, other than disseminated herpesviral disease, will require two codes. Sepsis will be identified by A41.89 when the organism is specified, or A41.9 when unspecified, in addition to a code from category B97 to identify the viral organism or a code to identify the localized infection.

Candidal sepsis (B37.7)

Candidiasis is a yeast fungal (mycosis) infection. Disseminated or invasive candidiasis is considered sepsis, also known as candidemia. Fungemia NOS (B49) is a fungal sepsis due to an unspecified mycosis. Treatment is by antifungals, such as fluconazole and amphotericin.

ICD-10-CM sepsis codes in chapter 1 but not in categories A4Ø or A41 are found in the following table.

Code	Description
A42.7	Actinomycotic sepsis

Code	Description
A22.7	Anthrax sepsis
B37.7	Candidal sepsis
A26.7	Erysipelothrix sepsis
A28.2	Extraintestinal yersiniosis (sepsis)
A54.86	Gonococcal sepsis
BØØ.7	Disseminated herpesviral disease (sepsis)
A32.7	Listerial sepsis
A24.1	Acute and fulminating melioidosis (sepsis)
A39.2–A39.4	Acute, chronic, or unspecified meningococcemia (sepsis)
AØ2.1	Salmonella sepsis
A2Ø.7	Septicemic plague
A21.7	Generalized tularemia (sepsis)

ICD-10-CM sepsis codes related to the pregnant patient are found in the following table.

Code	Description
OØ3.37	Sepsis following incomplete spontaneous abortion
OØ3.87	Sepsis following complete or unspecified spontaneous abortion
OØ4.87	Sepsis following (induced) termination of pregnancy
OØ7.37	Sepsis following failed attempted termination of pregnancy
OØ8.82	Sepsis following ectopic and molar pregnancy
O75.3	Other infection during labor (sepsis)
O85	Puerperal sepsis

ICD-10-CM sepsis codes in chapter 19 and represent postprocedural complications are found in the following table.

Code	Description
J95.Ø2	Infection of tracheostomy stoma
T8Ø.211	Bloodstream infection due to central venous catheter
T8Ø.22- T8Ø.29-	Acute infection following transfusion, infusion, or injection of blood and blood products; infection following other infusion, transfusion and therapeutic injection
T81.4-	Infection following a procedure (sepsis)
T82.6- T82.7-	Infection and inflammatory reaction due to cardiac valve prosthesis; infection and inflammatory reaction due to other cardiac and vascular devices, implants and grafts
T83.5- T83.6-	Infection and inflammatory reaction due to prosthetic device, implant and graft in urinary system; infection and inflammatory reaction due to prosthetic device, implant and graft in genital tract

CDI Alert

Vasopressors, such as norepinephrine, dopamine, and epinephrine are used to reverse hypoperfusion, increase cardiac output, and facilitate oxygen delivery in severe sepsis or septic shock that fails fluid resuscitation or as an adjunct to fluid resuscitation. A central catheter line is needed for delivery. The procedure of introduction of vasopressor in central vein would be reported.

Code	Description
T84.5- T84.6- T84.7-	Infection and inflammatory reaction due to internal joint prosthesis; infection and inflammatory reaction due to internal fixation device; infection and inflammatory reaction due to other internal orthopedic prosthetic devices, implants and grafts
T85.7-	Infection and inflammatory reaction due to other internal prosthetic devices, implants and grafts (peritoneal dialysis catheter; insulin pump; other)
T86.-	Transplanted organ infection
T88.Ø-	Infection following immunization (sepsis)

Clinician Note

Physician documentation must provide the cause and effect relationship between the procedure and the postprocedural sepsis.

Clinical Findings

Sepsis is a systemic response to bacterial infection in which chemicals released in the bloodstream to fight the infection cause an inflammatory state throughout the body.

Physical Examination

History and review of symptoms may include:

- Fever
- Tachycardia
- Rapid respiratory rate
- Mental status change
- Difficulty breathing
- Chills
- Major decrease in urine output
- Diaphoresis
- Decreased BP
- Organ dysfunction

Diagnostic Procedures and Services

- Laboratory
  - blood culture
  - electrolyte panel
  - urinalysis
  - procalcitonin levels
  - arterial blood gas
  - CBC
  - liver and renal function
- Imaging
  - chest x-ray
  - CT

- MRI
- ultrasound
- Other
  - pulse oximetry

Therapeutic Procedures and Services

- IV antibiotics
- Oxygen therapy
- Therapy to support any organ dysfunction
- Infection control
  - Surgery

Clinician Documentation Checklist

Clinician documentation should indicate the following:

Streptococcal

- Group a
- Group b
- Pneumonia
  - pneumococcal

Other sepsis

- *Staphylococcus aureus*
  - methicillin susceptible
  - methicillin resistant
  - *Haemophilus influenzae*
  - anaerobes
  - coagulase negative staphylococcus sepsis
- Gram-negative organisms
  - *Escherichia coli*
  - *Pseudomonas*
  - *Serratia*
- Other specified sepsis
  - *Enterococcus*

Shoulder Disorders

I-10 ALERT

There are several more specific ICD-10-CM codes available for shoulder lesions; the other classification axis that provides additional codes is that related to laterality. These codes specify that the condition is nontraumatic.

CDI ALERT

Ensure that laterality (right, left) is specified in the documentation for any of the musculoskeletal disorders that occur on paired body sites.

Code Axes

Adhesive capsulitis of shoulder	**M75.Ø-**
Rotator cuff tear or rupture, not specified as traumatic	**M75.1-**
Tendinitis (bicipital or calcific)	**M75.2-, M75.3-**
Impingement syndrome of shoulder	**M75.4-**
Bursitis of shoulder	**M75.5-**
Other and unspecified shoulder lesions	**M75.8-, M75.9-**

Description of Condition

Adhesive capsulitis of shoulder (M75.Ø-)

Clinical Tip

Adhesive capsulitis is a very common shoulder disorder and is caused by shoulder joint capsule inflammation. Symptoms include pain, stiffness, and loss of motion.

Key Terms

Key terms found in the documentation for adhesive capsulitis may include:

Frozen shoulder

Periarthritis of shoulder

Clinician Note

Ensure that all related conditions are coded appropriately.

Rotator cuff tear or rupture, not specified as traumatic (M75.1-)

Clinical Tip

Rotator cuff tears affect the shoulder tendons and most commonly involve the supraspinatus tendon. Many rotator cuff tears are chronic in nature and occur due to age degeneration. The tears can be classified as incomplete (partial thickness) or complete (full thickness), the latter involving through-and-through tears.

Key Terms

Key terms found in the documentation for rotator cuff tear may include:

Rotator cuff syndrome

Supraspinatus syndrome

Supraspinatus tear or rupture, not specified as traumatic

Clinical Findings

Physical Examination

History and review of systems may include:

- Shoulder pain-mild to severe
- Increased pain with abduction or flexion
- Decreased range of motion
- Shoulder weakness
- Palpation
- Neck
- Assessment of:
  - supraspinatus
  - infraspinatus
  - teres minor
  - subscapularis
- Neer test
- Hawkins test
- Apley scratch test

Diagnostic Procedures and Services

- Imaging
  - MRI
  - x-rays
  - ultrasound

Therapeutic Procedures and Services

- NSAID
- Strengthening exercises
- Surgery

Clinician Note

Ensure that all related conditions are coded appropriately and that if the tear is traumatic, category S46.Ø1- is referenced.

Tendinitis (bicipital or calcific) (M75.2-, M75.3-)

Clinical Tip

Calcific tendinitis is a condition that causes small 1 to 2 cm calcium deposits in the tendinous areas of the shoulder's rotator cuff. It may also be documented as calcified bursa of the shoulder. Bicipital tendinitis is an inflammation of the long head of biceps tendon, which can be due to instability of the tendon, bone spurs on the biceps tendon, or as a result of a previous injury.

Clinician Note

Ensure that all related conditions are coded appropriately and that if the tendinitis is due to a traumatic injury, that a code from the injuries chapter is referenced.

⇨ I-10 ALERT

ICD-10-CM includes a specific subcategory for impingement syndrome of the shoulder.

Impingement syndrome of shoulder (M75.4-)

Clinical Tip

When the tendons of the rotator cuff muscles become irritated and inflamed as they pass through the subacromial space, an impingement syndrome may result. There are many potential causes, including subacromial bone spurs, osteoarthritic spurs on the acromioclavicular (AC) joint, and variations in the shape of the acromion. Documentation may include information related to the three stages of impingement syndrome:

Stage I: Hemorrhage and edema are present, with palpable tenderness over the greater tuberosity at supraspinatus insertion

Stage II: Fibrosis and thickening of supraspinatus, biceps, and subacromial bursa due to chronic inflammation or repeated episodes of impingement

Stage III: Prolonged history of refractory tendinitis, significant tendon degeneration, and associated rotator cuff tears, biceps ruptures, and bone changes.

Key Terms

Key terms found in the documentation for shoulder impingement syndrome may include:

Painful arc syndrome

Supraspinatus syndrome

Swimmer's shoulder

Thrower's shoulder

Clinician Note

Ensure that all related conditions are coded appropriately and that if the impingement is due to a traumatic injury, that a code from the injuries chapter is referenced.

Bursitis of shoulder (M75.5-)

Clinical Tip

There are several bursae in the shoulder region: the subacromial, the subdeltoid, the subcoracoid, and the subscapular and their main function is to facilitate the gliding of soft tissue structures over bony surfaces. Any of the above bursae can become irritated, inflamed, and painful as a result of overuse of or trauma to the shoulder region, but the subacromial bursa is most commonly the culprit in this condition.

Clinician Note

Ensure that all related conditions are coded appropriately and that if bursitis is due to a traumatic injury, that a code from the injuries chapter is referenced.

Clinician Documentation Checklist

Clinician documentation should indicate the following:

- Type
  - due to use, overuse, pressure
  - gonococcal
  - infective
  - rheumatoid
  - syphilitic
  - other specified
    - adhesive
    - idiopathic
    - gouty
- Anatomic site

Skin Lesions — Removal of

Code Axes

Paring or cutting	**11055–11057**
Removal of skin tags	**11200–11201**
Shaving of epidermal or dermal lesions	**11300–11313**
Excision—benign lesions	**11400–11471**
Excision—malignant lesions	**11600–11646**

Description of Procedure

There are many methods that may be utilized to treat skin lesions and often the method employed is determined by the type of lesion being treated. There are a number of components that should be recorded in the documentation regardless of the methodology used:

- Anatomical location
- Preoperative diagnosis
- Postoperative diagnosis
- Size of the lesion
- Number of lesions
- Methodology used
- Type of closure is required
- Any complications

Paring or cutting of benign hyperkeratotic lesion (e.g., corn or callus) (11055–11057)

Documentation will indicate that the provider removed tissue by cutting away the edge or surface of the lesion. A hyperkeratotic lesion refers to an overgrowth of skin. The number of lesions treated should be clearly identified in the documentation. Each lesion should be described separately in terms of location and physical characteristics. Although not required for coding, it is advisable to also include the size of the lesion.

Key Terms

Key terms found in the documentation may include:

Cutting

Incision

Paring

Removal of skin tags, multiple fibrocutaneous tags, any area; up to and including 15 lesions (11200)

Removal of skin tags, multiple fibrocutaneous tags, any area; each additional ten lesions, or part thereof (List separately in addition to code for primary procedure) (11201)

Skin or fibrocutaneous tags are benign growths thought to be caused by friction and often are numerous when present. They may be removed by various methods including scissor excision, scalpel, ligature strangulation, and electrosurgical destruction.

Documentation should include the method used, the anatomical location, the size, and the number of lesions removed.

Key Terms
Key terms found in the documentation may include:

Cutting

Electrodessication

Sharp dissection

Skin tags

Shaving of epidermal or dermal lesion, single lesion, trunk, arms or legs (11300–11303)

Shaving of epidermal or dermal lesion, scalp, neck, hands, feet, genitalia (11305–11308)

Shaving of epidermal or dermal lesion, single lesion, face, ears, eyelids, nose, lips, mucous membrane (11310–11313)

Shaving is the sharp removal by transverse incision or horizontal slicing. It is different from excision in that it does not include a full thickness dermal excision and, therefore, does not require suture closure. If documentation notes that suturing is required, the lesion is not shaved but rather excised.

Examine the documentation to determine the site of the lesion as well as the size.

Key Terms
Key terms found in the documentation may include:

Cautery

Horizontal

Shaving

Excision, benign lesion including margins, except skin tag (unless listed elsewhere) trunk, arms or legs (11400–11406)

Excision, benign lesion including margins, except skin tag (unless listed elsewhere) scalp, neck, hand, feet, genitalia (11420–11426)

Excision, benign lesion including margins, except skin tag (unless listed elsewhere) face, ears, eyelids, nose, lips, mucous membrane (11440–11446)

Documentation supporting this code assignment will include a pathology report indicating that the lesion is benign, the size of the lesion, the size of the margin, and the anatomical site. Excision of lesions requires a full thickness, through the dermis incision, and may require a suture closure.

> **CPT ALERT**
>
> Simple closure when performed is included in the removal and should not be reported separately.

Excision, malignant lesion, including margins, trunk, arms or legs (11600–11606)

Excision, malignant lesion, including margins, scalp, neck, hands, feet, genitalia (11620–11626)

Excision, malignant lesion, including margins, face, ears, eyelids, nose, lips (11640–11646)

Documentation supporting this code assignment will include a pathology report indicating that the lesion is malignant, the size of the lesion, the size of the margin, and the anatomical site. Excision of lesions requires a full thickness, through the dermis incision, and may require a suture closure.

> **CPT ALERT**
>
> When a closure other than simple is required, it may be reported separately.

Clinician Documentation Checklist

Clinician documentation should indicate the following:

- Preoperative diagnosis
- Postoperative diagnosis
- Type of lesion
  - benign
  - malignant
  - skin tags
- Anatomical location
- Techniques
  - paring or cutting
  - chemical destruction
  - electrocauterization
  - electrosurgical destruction
  - ligature strangulation
  - removal with anesthesia

- removal without anesthesia
- sharp excision or scissoring
- shaving
- Size of lesion
- Number of lesions
- Type of closure
- Complications

Spinal Disc Disorders (Dorsopathies)

> **I-10 ALERT**
>
> ICD-10-CM contains several codes for spinal dorsopathies with varying classification axes. In some cases, all cervical conditions are together and then all thoracic conditions and then all lumbosacral conditions. Laterality is included, where appropriate; some combination codes are available as well.

Code Axes

Cervical disc disorders **M5Ø.[Ø-3,8,9]-**

Includes subcategories for myelopathy, radiculopathy, disc displacement, disc degeneration, and other and unspecified disc disorders

Thoracic, thoracolumbar, and lumbosacral intervertebral disc disorders **M51.[Ø-4,8]-,9]**

Includes subcategories for myelopathy, radiculopathy, disc displacement, disc degeneration, Schmorl's nodes, and other and unspecified disc disorders

Spinal instabilities **M53.2X-**

Includes subcategories for spinal regions

Radiculopathy **M54.1-**

Includes subcategories for spinal regions

Sciatica **M54.3-, M54.4-**

Includes subcategories for laterality

> **CDI ALERT**
>
> Not only does the general site of the dorsopathy have to be documented, but the specific vertebral level as well. For example, instead of merely documenting "cervical disc displacement," the information should include one of the following specific areas: occipito-atlanto-axial region, mid-cervical region, cervicothoracic region. The definitions above may also be documented.

Clinical Tip

The spinal regions may be defined as follows:

Occipito-atlanto-axial region: C0-C1-C2

Mid-cervical region: C4-C5-C6-C7

Cervicothoracic region: C7-T1

Thoracic region: T1-T12

Thoracolumbar region: T9-L2

Lumbar region: L1-L5

Lumbosacral region: L1-L5 and S1-S5

Sacral and sacrococcygeal region: S1-S5 and coccyx

Description of Condition

> **I-10 ALERT**
>
> There are six different subcategories with various types of cervical disc disorders, each differentiated by the three different cervical regions.

Cervical disc disorders (M5Ø.-)

Includes subcategories for myelopathy, radiculopathy, disc displacement, disc degeneration, and other and unspecified disc disorders

Clinical Tip

The most common cervical disc disorders include the following:

Myelopathy: Most often found with spinal stenosis and involves pinching of the affecting vertebral segment of the spinal cord. It causes a compromise of coordination of the extremities.

Radiculopathy: When the pinched nerve of myelopathy progresses and involves pain, weakness, numbness, and a "pins and needles" sensation in the arm, it has progressed to radiculopathy.

Disc displacement: Displacement of a cervical intervertebral disc refers to protrusion or herniation of the disc between two adjacent bones (vertebrae) of the cervical spine. The protrusion or herniation may compress the spinal cord or other nerves, causing pain, and changes in sensory, motor, and reflex functions.

Disc degeneration: Refers to a breakdown of the normal architecture of the various components of the spine. The disc no longer provides adequate cushioning between the vertebrae and the bones then come closer and closer together, in some cases impinging on the spinal cord or other nerves.

Key Terms

Key terms found in the documentation for cervical disc disorders may include:

Cervical degenerative disc disease with radiculopathy

Cervical DJD with radiculopathy

Cervical DJD with myelopathy

Cervical myelopathy

Cervical radiculopathy

Cervicothoracic disc disorders with cervicalgia

Cervicothoracic disorders

Clinician Note

Review documentation to determine the site of the disc(s) affected as well as associated disorders such as myelopathy, radiculopathy, or displacement. Coding to the highest specificity may be necessary to get preauthorization for treatments such as physical therapy.

Thoracic, thoracolumbar, and lumbosacral intervertebral disc disorders (M51.-)

Includes subcategories for myelopathy, radiculopathy, disc displacement, disc degeneration, Schmorl's nodes, and other and unspecified disc disorders

Clinical Tip

The most common spinal disc disorders include the following:

Myelopathy: Most often found with spinal stenosis and involves pinching of the affecting vertebral segment of the spinal cord. It causes a compromise of coordination of the extremities.

Radiculopathy: When the pinched nerve of myelopathy progresses and involves pain, weakness, numbness, and a "pins and needles" sensation in the leg, it has progressed to radiculopathy.

Disc displacement: Displacement of a cervical intervertebral disc refers to protrusion or herniation of the disc between two adjacent bones (vertebrae) of the spine. The protrusion or herniation may compress the spinal cord or other nerves, causing pain, and changes in sensory, motor, and reflex functions.

Disc degeneration: Refers to a breakdown of the normal architecture of the various components of the spine. The disc no longer provides adequate cushioning between the vertebrae and the bones then come closer and closer together, in some cases impinging on the spinal cord or other nerves.

Key Terms

Key terms found in the documentation for thoracic, thoracolumbar, and lumbosacral disc disorders may include:

Lumbago due to displacement of intervertebral disc

Sciatica due to intervertebral disc disorder

Clinician Note

Review documentation to determine the site of the disc(s) affected as well as associated disorders such as myelopathy, radiculopathy, or displacement. Coding to the highest specificity may be necessary to get preauthorization for treatments such as physical therapy.

⇨ I-10 ALERT

In the subcategory for spinal instabilities, there are nine codes, differentiated by spinal region, that represent various instability conditions.

Spinal instabilities (M53.2X-)

Clinical Tip

The term spinal instabilities refers to abnormal movement between one vertebra and another. Disc degeneration may cause loss of the tension or "turgor," which allows the disc to bulge and increases movements between the vertebrae. The loss of disc height causes displacement of the facet joints, which then override beyond their correct congruent alignment. In some cases, this abnormal slipping and overriding of the facet joints induces arthritic overgrowth of the joints and also produces bone spurs around the joint margins.

Clinician Note

Review documentation to determine the site of the disc(s) affected as well as associated disorders such as myelopathy, radiculopathy, or displacement. Coding to the highest specificity may be necessary to get preauthorization for treatments such as physical therapy.

Radiculopathy (M54.1-)

Clinical Tip

The term radiculopathy refers to an abnormally inflamed or pinched nerve, most often involving the nerve root near the spine. Although many radiculopathy conditions are due to an intervertebral disc disorder, some may be caused by other structures in the spinal column, or by an inadequate vascular supply. Most radiculopathy cases involve the cervical (affecting the arm) and lumbar (affecting the leg) spinal regions.

Key Terms

Key terms found in the documentation for radiculopathy may include:

Brachial neuritis or radiculitis

Lumbar neuritis or radiculitis

Lumbosacral neuritis or radiculitis

Radiculitis

Thoracic neuritis or radiculitis

Clinician Note

Review documentation to determine the site of the disc(s) affected as well as associated disorders such as myelopathy or displacement. Coding to the highest specificity may be necessary to get preauthorization for treatments such as physical therapy.

Sciatica (M54.3-, M54.4-)

Clinical Tip

Sciatica refers to a set of symptoms that may include pain, weakness, numbness, or tingling in the leg, referred from an impingement on the sciatic nerve in the lumbar spine. This nerve runs down the back of the leg and controls the muscles on the back of the knee and lower leg and also provides sensation for the back of the thigh, part of the lower leg, and the sole of the foot. It most often affects only one side.

Clinician Note

Ensure that all related conditions (e.g., disc disorders with myelopathy) are documented appropriately.

Clinician Documentation Checklist

Clinician documentation should indicate the following:

- Type
  - degeneration
  - displacement
  - pain
  - panniculitis
  - other specified
  - unspecified
- Severity
  - with myelopathy
  - with radiculopathy
- Anatomic sites
  - cervical
    - C4-C5
    - C5-C6
    - C6-C7

- cervicobrachial
- cervicocranial
- occipito-atlanto-axial
- thoracic
- thoracolumbar
- lumbosacral
- lumbar
- sacral
- sacrococcygeal
- multiple sites (specify sites involved)

Spinal Injection, Drainage, or Aspiration

Code Axes

Spinal puncture, lumbar, diagnostic	**62270**
Spinal puncture, therapeutic, for drainage of cerebrospinal fluid (by needle or catheter)	**62272**

Description of Procedure

Documentation indicating a diagnostic service will specify that a biopsy needle is inserted, fluid is drawn through the needle, and the sample is sent for testing. After the procedure is completed, the wound is dressed.

This is differentiated from a therapeutic service in that for the therapeutic service the L3 and L4 vertebrae are located and local anesthesia is administered. The lumbar puncture needle is inserted. In some cases, spinal fluid is drawn through the needle as in a lumbar puncture test. In other cases, a catheter is inserted and the fluid empties into a reservoir. Pressure reading is performed with a manometer. When the procedure is completed, the needle is removed and the wound is dressed.

Key Terms

Key terms found in the documentation may include:

Spinal tap

Injection(s) of diagnostic or therapeutic substance(s) (including anesthetic, antispasmodic, opioid, steroid, other solution), not including neurolytic substances, including needle or catheter placement, interlaminar epidural or subarachnoid; without imaging guidance (62320, 62322)

Documentation will indicate that once the patient is placed in the appropriate position a needle is inserted into the vertebral interspace. Contrast media may be injected to confirm proper needle placement under fluoroscopy. Once location has been confirmed, a solution, other than a neurolytic agent is injected. Documentation may indicate that more than one substance, such as an anesthetic and a steroid, is injected. This procedure is commonly performed to manage chronic pain or to treat chronic spinal conditions.

Key Terms

Key terms found in the documentation may include:

Chronic pain

Epidural injection

Clinician Documentation Checklist

Clinician documentation should indicate the following:

- Medical condition being investigated or treated
  - diagnostic
  - therapeutic
- Anatomical
  - identification of vertebrae
- Anesthesia
- Fluid drawn
- Catheter inserted
- Pressure reading with manometer
- Contrast media used
- Fluoroscopy guidance
- Substance injected

Transient Ischemic Attack

Code Axes

Transient cerebral ischemic attacks and related syndromes G45.-

Description of Condition

Transient ischemic attack (TIA) is a focal cerebral neurologic deficit of sudden onset and brief duration, typically lasts less than one hour that typically leave no residual effects. Otherwise known as warning mini-strokes, a TIA can indicate high probability of cerebral infarction/hemorrhage occurring that may result in permanent disability or death. The flow of blood to the brain is temporarily interrupted because of stenosis, stricture, embolism, spasm or occlusion of the arteries, or the creation of a thrombus.

Vertebro-basilar artery syndrome (G45.Ø)

VBS affects the posterior circulation of the brain including the brainstem, cerebellum, and occipital cortex.

Carotid artery syndrome(hemispheric) (G45.1)

This syndrome affects the frontal circulation of the brain, the frontal two-thirds of the cerebral hemisphere, including the deep white matter and the basal ganglia.

Multiple and bilateral precerebral artery syndromes (G45.2)

Clinical Tip

These syndromes represent arterial insufficiency or ischemia of the specified arteries. The insufficiencies that cause the interrupted flow of blood include atherosclerosis, sudden orthostasis, or internal or external forces that exacerbate or occlude the arteries.

Key Terms

Key terms found in the documentation may include:

Transient ischemic attack

TIA

Cerebral artery spasm

Cerebral ischemic syndrome

Hemispheric carotid syndrome

Internal carotid artery syndrome

Mini-stroke

Vertebral artery syndrome

Vertebral steal syndrome

Amaurosis fugax (G45.3)

AF caused by retinal artery ischemia can result in sudden, transient monocular partial or total vision loss. AF is also seen when carotid artery plaque breaks free and moves to the retinal artery causing decreased blood to the retina and temporary loss of vision.

⇨ I-10 ALERT

If the TIA or syndrome is due to precerebral artery or cerebral artery atherosclerosis, thrombosis, embolism, obstruction, stenosis, or occlusion, not resulting in a cerebral infarction, see category I65 and/or I66.

Clinical Findings

Physical Examination

History and review of systems may include sudden onset of:

- Aphasia
- Ataxia
- Blindness in one or both eyes
- Confusion
- Double vision
- Dizziness
- Loss of balance
- Memory loss
- Numbness or paralysis of face, arm or leg, typically unilateral
- Slurred speech
- Stiff neck/pain
- Sudden, severe headache
- Weakness

Diagnostic Procedures and Services

- Laboratory
  - blood glucose
  - CBC
  - erythrocyte sedimentation rate
  - HDL and total cholesterol
  - homocysteine
  - lipid profile
  - platelet count
  - prothrombin time test (PT)
- Imaging
  - angiography
  - arteriography
  - carotid duplex ultrasonography
  - computerized tomography (CT)
  - computerized tomography angiography (CTA)
  - ECG
  - echocardiography
  - gradient echo MRI
  - MRI
  - toxicology screening

Therapeutic Procedures and Services

Therapies are directed at addressing any underlying risk factors, treating co-existing conditions and preventing the occurrence of further attacks or a cerebrovascular accident.

Possible procedures include:

- Arterial angioplasty and stenting
- Carotid endarterectomy

Medication List

- Anticoagulation
  - dabigatran (Pradaxa)
  - heparin
  - warfarin (Coumadin, Jantoven)
- Antiplatelet and statins
  - clopidogrel (Plavix)
  - dipyridamole (Aggrenox)
- Thrombolytic agent
  - alteplase (Activase)

Clinician Documentation Checklist

Clinician documentation should indicate the following:

Specific Type:

- Vertebro-basilar artery syndrome
  - vertebral steal syndrome
- Carotid artery syndrome (hemispheric) (internal)
- Multiple and bilateral precerebral syndromes
- Amaurosis fugax
- Transient global amnesia
- Other transient cerebral ischemic attacks and related syndromes
  - recurrent focal cerebral ischemia
- Unspecified transient cerebral ischemic attack
  - Includes:
    - — intermittent cerebral ischemia
    - — spasm of cerebral artery
    - — transient cerebral ischemia
    - — transient ischemic attack (TIA)

Trigger Point Injections

Code Axes

Injection(s); single or multiple trigger point(s), 1-2 muscle(s)	**20552**
Injection(s); single or multiple trigger point(s), 3 or more muscle(s)	**20553**

Description of Procedure

Trigger points are focal, discrete spots of hypersensitive irritability identified within bands of muscle. These points cause local or referred pain. Trigger points may be formed by acute or repetitive trauma to the muscle tissue, which puts too much stress on the fibers.

These services are often performed for the following conditions:

- Cervicalgia
- Fasciitis
- Myalgia and myositis
- Muscle spasm
- Sciatica
- Tendinitis

CDI ALERT

Documentation should include details that support the medical necessity in addition to the number of muscles treated and therapies tried prior to this procedure.

Documentation will state that the physician identifies the trigger point injection site by palpation or radiographic imaging and marks the injection site. The needle is inserted and the medicine is injected into the trigger point. The injection may be done under separately reportable image guidance. After withdrawing the needle, the patient is monitored for reactions to the therapeutic agent. The injection procedure is repeated at the other trigger points for multiple sites.

Key Terms

Trigger point

CDI ALERT

Supplies used when providing this procedure should be clearly documented and may be reported with the appropriate HCPCS Level II code. Check with the specific payer to determine coverage.

Clinician Documentation Checklist

Clinician documentation should indicate the following:

- The medical condition being treated
- Therapies prior to this procedure
- Site of injection
  - single
  - multiple
- Use of image guidance
- Therapeutic agents administered
- Number of muscles treated
- Patient reaction to therapeutic agent

Ulcer — Nonpressure

Code Axes

Non-pressure chronic ulcer of thigh	**L97.1-** HCC
Non-pressure chronic ulcer of calf	**L97.2-** HCC
Non-pressure chronic ulcer of ankle	**L97.3-** HCC
Non-pressure chronic ulcer of heel and midfoot	**L97.4-** HCC
Non-pressure chronic ulcer of other part of foot	**L97.5-** HCC
Non-pressure chronic ulcer of other part of lower leg	**L97.8-** HCC
Non-pressure chronic ulcer of unspecified part of lower leg	**L97.9-** HCC
Non-pressure chronic ulcer of skin, not elsewhere classified	**L98.4-** HCC
Non-pressure chronic ulcer of buttock	**L98.41-** HCC
Non-pressure chronic ulcer of back	**L98.42-** HCC
Non-pressure chronic ulcer of skin of other sites	**L98.49-** HCC

Description of Condition

Clinical Tip

Chronic skin ulcers initially affect superficial tissues and, depending on the state of the patient's health and other circumstances, may progress to affect muscle and bone. Patients at risk for development of skin ulcers include chronic, debilitating disease with impairment of sensation or impaired immune systems, and delayed healing after injury or trauma. Intrinsic loss of pain and pressure sensations due to nerve damage, poor circulation, and infection contribute to the formation and progression of chronic skin ulcers. In the early stages, with prompt, effective treatment, skin ulcers are reversible. If left untreated or inadequately treated, poorly-healing skin lesions can become extensively infected, necrotic, and ultimately, irreversible.

Key Terms

Key terms found in the documentation include:

Mal perforans ulcer

Nonhealing ulcer of skin

Noninfected sinus of skin

Trophic ulcer

Tropical ulcer

⇨ I-10 Alert

ICD-10-CM classifies non-pressure skin ulcer by anatomic site, laterality and severity. Paired sites are classified as right, left, or of unspecified laterality.

For example, pressure ulcer of the left ankle with breakdown of skin is classified by site (ankle), by laterality (left), and severity as documented in the record:

L97.321 Non-pressure chronic ulcer of left ankle limited to breakdown of skin

Underlying conditions should be documented and reported first. Skin ulcers due to atherosclerosis (I7Ø.-), diabetes (EØ8.62, EØ9.62, E1Ø.62, E11.62-. E13.62-), varicose ulcers (I83.-), or other causal pathology should be linked appropriately in the documentation to support complete and accurate reporting.

Gangrene (I96.-) is classified separately. When documented with chronic skin ulcer, sequence I96 Gangrene, first to accurately represent severity of condition.

Unlike pressure ulcer (L89), which is reported by stage, chronic non-pressure ulcer of the skin (L97–L98) is reported by severity as documented in the record. For each anatomic site (and laterality), the hierarchy of disease progression is classified as follows in order of progression from mild to severe:

Chronic ulcer:

- Limited to breakdown of skin
- Fat layer exposed
- Necrosis of muscle
- Necrosis of bone

CDI Alert

Clinicians (i.e., physicians and other qualified health care practitioners) should document the severity and extent of ulcer as clearly and thoroughly as possible in the record, including any changes in ulcer status or complications associated with the healing process. Although the physician is responsible for documenting the associated diagnoses, nonprovider clinicians should document the depth of non-pressure ulcers and any changes in healing status for each ulcer, by anatomic site.

I-10 Alert

Categories L97 and L98 include valid codes that are six characters in length. These codes include both the site and stage of the ulcer. The following axes of classification describe:

Fourth character:
- Anatomic site or region (skin NEC)

Fifth character:
- Anatomic site
- Anatomic site with laterality

Sixth character:
- Stage (severity, progression status) of ulcer

Do not report unspecified ulcer stage (sixth character 9) if the severity or progression of ulcer is documented in the medical record. Unspecified ulcer (sixth character 9) is only reported when there is **no documentation** regarding the stage, severity, or progression of skin ulcer.

Clinician Note

Document the specific anatomic site and laterality. For multiple skin ulcers, document the specific ulcer depth of each ulcer site, whether a new or (old) healing ulcer.

Document any complications with healing, overlapping sites or other changes in the status or nature of the ulcer.

Specify the ulcer depth accurately and thoroughly for each ulcer. For each anatomic site (and laterality), the hierarchy of disease progression is classified as follows in ICD-10-CM in order of progression from mild to severe:

Chronic skin ulcer:

- Bone involvement without necrosis
- Limited to breakdown of skin
- Fat layer exposed
- Muscle involvement without necrosis
- Necrosis of muscle
- Necrosis of bone

Document any change in skin ulcer severity, depth, or healing status during an admission or encounter. For example, if a skin ulcer worsens during an admission, from an exposed fat layer to necrosis of muscle, note the depth progression accordingly.

Clinician Documentation Checklist

Clinician documentation should indicate the following:

- Includes
  - chronic ulcer of skin of lower limb
  - nonhealing ulcer of skin
  - noninfected sinus of skin
  - trophic ulcer
  - tropical ulcer
  - ulcer of skin of lower limb
- Identification of
  - any associated underlying condition
    - atherosclerosis of lower extremities
    - chronic venous hypertension
    - diabetic ulcers
    - postphlebitic syndrome
    - postthrombotic syndrome
    - varicose ulcer
  - any associated gangrene
  - site
    - thigh

  - calf
  - ankle
  - heel and midfoot
    - plantar surface of midfoot
  - other parts of foot
    - toe
  - other part of lower leg
  - unspecified part of lower leg
- Laterality of thigh, calf, ankle, heel and midfoot, foot and leg
  - right
  - left
- extent of nonpressure ulcer
  - limited to breakdown of skin
  - with bone involvement
  - with fat layer exposed
  - with muscle involvement
  - with necrosis of muscle
  - with necrosis of bone
  - unspecified severity

Other Disorders of Skin and Subcutaneous Tissue

- Pyogenic granuloma
- Factitial dermatitis
  - neurotic excoriation
- Febrile neutrophilic dermatosis (sweet)
- Eosinophilic cellulitis (wells)
- Nonpressure chronic ulcer of skin
  - identify
    - site
      - buttock
      - back
      - skin of other sites
        - unspecified
    - extent of nonpressure ulcer
      - limited to breakdown of skin
      - with fat layer exposed
      - with necrosis of muscle
      - with necrosis of bone
      - with unspecified severity

- Mucinosis of skin
  - focal mucinosis
  - lichen myxedematosus
  - reticular erythematous mucinosis
- Other infiltrative disorders of skin and subcutaneous tissue
- Other specified disorders of skin and subcutaneous tissue
- Unspecified disorders of skin and subcutaneous tissue

Ulcer — Pressure

Code Axes

Pressure ulcer of elbow	**L89.Ø-** HCC
Pressure ulcer of back	**L89.1-** HCC
Pressure ulcer of hip	**L89.2-** HCC
Pressure ulcer of buttock	**L89.3-** HCC
Pressure ulcer of contiguous sites of back, buttock and hip	**L89.4-** HCC
Pressure ulcer of ankle	**L89.5-** HCC
Pressure ulcer of heel	**L89.6-** HCC
Pressure ulcer of other site	**L89.8-** HCC
Pressure ulcer of unspecified site	**L89.9-** HCC

Description of Condition

Clinical Tip

Pressure ulcers initially affect superficial tissues and, depending on the state of the patient's health and other circumstances, may progress to affect muscle and bone. Patients at risk for development of pressure ulcers include the bedridden, unconscious, or immobile such as stroke patients or those with paralysis and limited motion. Intrinsic loss of pain and pressure sensations, disuse atrophy, malnutrition, anemia, and infection contribute to the formation and progression of decubitus ulcers. In the early stages, the condition is reversible, but left untended, the decubitus ulcer can become extensively infected, necrotic, and ultimately, irreversible.

The National Pressure Ulcer Advisor Panel (NPUAP) has recently updated the definition and staging of pressure ulcers. A pressure ulcer is now defined as a "localized injury to the skin and/or underlying tissue, usually over a bony prominence, as a result of pressure, or pressure in combination with shear and/or friction."

Pressure ulcers are classified by location, shape, depth, and healing status. The depth of the lesion or stage of ulcer is the most important element in clinical measurement:

Unstageable/unspecified stage: lesion inaccessible for evaluation due to nonremovable dressings, eschar, sterile blister, and suspected deep injury in evolution. Deep tissue injury may be difficult to detect in individuals with dark skin tones and, as such, evolution of the wound may progress rapidly. Suspected deep tissue injury may be characterized by purple or maroon discoloration of the skin with or without blistering. Affected tissue may be painful and variant in temperature and texture from surrounding normal tissue.

⇨ I-10 Alert

ICD-10-CM classifies pressure ulcer by anatomic site, laterality, and stage. Paired sites are classified as right, left, or of unspecified laterality. Large areas, such as the back, are further divided into lower and upper regions.

For example, pressure ulcer of the back is divided first by main site (back), by laterality (unspecified, right or left), and subregion (upper, lower):

L89.121 Pressure ulcer of left upper back, stage 1

Category L89 excludes nonpressure ulcers (L97.-), diabetic ulcers (EØ8.62, EØ9.62, E1Ø.62, E11.62-. E13.62-), and varicose ulcers (I83.-). Code and report these conditions separately.

Gangrene (I96.-) is classified separately. When documented with pressure ulcer, sequence I96 Gangrene, first to accurately represent severity of condition.

CDI Alert

These classifications are differentiated by anatomic site, laterality, and severity (stage). Ensure documentation is specific regarding extent or progression of ulcer to avoid misrepresentation of severity.

Ensure documentation of site and laterality is thorough and specific to avoid reporting unspecified codes.

Code I96 should be reported and sequenced first to report gangrene documented with pressure ulcer. Gangrene is an additional severity indicator that poses significant risk for potentially fatal serious systemic infection (sepsis) requiring aggressive treatment.

Documentation should specify any underlying cause, pathology, chronic disease, or disability to explain the patient's immobile or bedridden status.

Stage 1 (I): Non-blanching erythema (a reddened area on the skin).

Stage 2 (II): Abrasion, blister, shallow open crater, or other partial thickness skin loss.

Stage 3 (III): Full thickness skin loss involving damage or necrosis into subcutaneous soft tissues.

Stage 4 (IV): Full thickness skin loss with necrosis of soft tissues through to the muscle, tendons, or tissues around underlying bone.

Key Terms

Key terms found in the documentation include:

Bed sore

Decubitus ulcer

Plaster ulcer

Pressure area

Pressure sore

Clinician Note

Specify the ulcer stage accurately in the diagnosis. Document the specific anatomic site and laterality. For example, the back is separated into upper and lower, right and left quadrants. For paired anatomic sites, specify laterality (right or left).

For example:

L89.131 Pressure ulcer of the right lower back, stage 1

L89.141 Pressure ulcer of the left lower back, stage 1

Document contiguous, overlapping ulcer sites if present.

Document the appropriate clinical stage for "healing" ulcers that accurately reflects the stage of the ulcer during the healing process. For multiple pressure ulcers, document the specific pressure ulcer stage of each ulcer site, whether a new or (old) healing ulcer.

Document any change in pressure ulcer stage (severity or progression) during an admission or encounter. For example, if a pressure ulcer worsens during an admission, from a stage 2 ulcer to stage 3 ulcer, the coder should note the progression in severity accordingly.

Clinician Documentation Checklist

Clinician documentation should indicate the following:

- Includes
  - bed sore
  - decubitus ulcer
  - plaster ulcer
  - pressure area
  - pressure sore

⇨ I-10 ALERT

Category L89 Pressure ulcer, includes valid combination codes that are five or six characters in length. These codes include both the site and stage of the ulcer. The following axes of classification describe:

Fourth character:
  Anatomic region
Fifth character:
  Anatomic site (specified to subregion or laterality)
Sixth character:
  Stage (severity, progression status) of ulcer

Do not confuse unstageable ulcer (sixth character 0) with unspecified ulcer stage (sixth character 9). Unstageable ulcer (sixth character 0) is reported when the stage, severity or progression of ulcer cannot be clinically determined. Unspecified ulcer (sixth character 9) is reported when there is **no documentation** regarding the stage, severity, or progression of pressure ulcer.

CDI ALERT

Clinicians (physicians and other qualified health care practitioners) should document the pressure ulcer stage as clearly and thoroughly as possible in the record, including any changes in ulcer status or complications associated with the healing process. Although the physician is responsible for documenting the associated diagnoses, nonprovider clinicians should document the stage of ulcer, and any changes in healing status for each ulcer, by anatomic site.

- Identification of
  - pressure ulcer described as healing
  - any associated gangrene
  - site
    - elbow
    - back
      - upper
        - shoulder blade
      - lower
      - unspecified
    - sacral region
      - coccyx
      - tailbone
    - hip
    - buttock
    - contiguous site of back, buttock and hip
    - ankle
    - heel
    - other sites
      - head
        - face
      - other site
    - unspecified site
  - laterality of elbow, hip, buttock, back, ankle and heel
    - right
    - left
  - stage
    - stage 1: pressure pre-ulcer changes limited to persistent focal edema
    - stage 2: pressure ulcer with abrasion, blister, partial thickness skin loss involving epidermis and/or dermis
    - stage 3: pressure ulcer with full thickness skin loss involving damage or necrosis of subcutaneous tissues
    - stage 4: pressure ulcer with necrosis of soft tissues through to underlying muscle, tendon, or bone
    - unspecified stage
    - unstageable: pressure ulcers whose stage cannot be clinically determined
      - ulcer covered by eschar or treated with skin or muscle graft
      - pressure ulcers documented as deep tissue injury and not due to trauma

⇨ I-10 ALERT

ICD-10-CM codes for ulcerative colitis are similar to Crohn's disease codes and represent those conditions that include rectal bleeding, intestinal obstruction, fistula, abscess, and other and unspecified complications.

Ulcerative Colitis

Code Axes

Note: Sixth characters for subcategories K51.Ø1, K51.21, K51.31, K51.41, K51.51, K51.81, and K51.91 are used to indicate any complications that may be present including rectal bleeding, intestinal obstruction, fistula, abscess, other, and unspecified complications.

Ulcerative (chronic) pancolitis without complications	**K51.ØØ** HCC
Ulcerative (chronic) pancolitis with complications	**K51.Ø1-** HCC
Ulcerative (chronic) proctitis without complications	**K51.2Ø** HCC
Ulcerative (chronic) proctitis with complications	**K51.21-** HCC
Ulcerative (chronic) rectosigmoiditis without complications	**K51.3Ø** HCC
Ulcerative (chronic) rectosigmoiditis with complications	**K51.31-** HCC
Inflammatory polyps of colon without complications	**K51.4Ø** HCC
Inflammatory polyps of colon with complications	**K51.41-** HCC
Left-sided colitis without complications	**K51.5Ø** HCC
Left-sided colitis with complications	**K51.51-** HCC
Other ulcerative colitis without complications	**K51.8Ø** HCC
Other ulcerative colitis with complications	**K51.81-** HCC
Ulcerative colitis, unspecified, without complications	**K51.9Ø** HCC
Ulcerative colitis, unspecified, with complications	**K51.91-** HCC

Description of Condition

Clinical Tip

Differentiating ulcerative colitis from Crohn's disease involving the colon is important in these cases because treatment and complications vary significantly between them. Some of the components that help distinguish ulcerative colitis are as follows:

- Nearly always involves the rectum
- Common symptoms are bloody diarrhea, rectal urgency, and tenesmus
- Endoscopy reveals loss of the typical vascular pattern, friability, exudates, ulcerations, and granularity in a continuous, circumferential pattern
- Only the mucosal layer of the bowel is involved
- Fistulae and sinus tracks are rare (they are common in Crohn's disease)

Key Terms
Key terms found in the documentation may include:

- Backwash ileitis
- Distal ulcerative colitis
- Left-sided ulcerative colitis
- UC
- Ulcerative pancolitis
- Ulcerative proctitis
- Ulcerative rectosigmoiditis

Clinician Note
Unlike ulcerative colitis, irritable bowel syndrome does not usually cause inflammation of the intestinal mucosa. A code indicating ulcerative colitis should be assigned only when there is documentation substantiating this condition.

CDI ALERT

Ensure that if any of the following complications are present they are clearly documented in the medical record: rectal bleeding, intestinal obstruction, fistula, or abscess. Any other complications that are indicated as being due to ulcerative colitis should also be documented.

Inflammatory polyps of colon without complications (K51.40)

Inflammatory polyps of colon with complications (K51.41-)

Note: Sixth characters for subcategory K51.41 include that for rectal bleeding, intestinal obstruction, fistula, abscess, other and unspecified complications.

Clinical Tip
Inflammatory polyps may be referred to as "pseudopolyps" because in a sense, they are not true polyps, but are reactions to the chronic inflammation in the colon.

Clinician Note
The ICD-10-CM system differentiates between inflammatory and noninflammatory polyps. Documentation should be carefully reviewed to determine appropriate code assignment.

⇨ I-10 ALERT

The identification of the type of polyp is essential for accurate classification in ICD-10-CM. If a polyp is specified as adenomatous, category D12 in the benign neoplasms section of the neoplasms chapter should be reviewed. Polyps for which no specific identification is provided should be classified to code K63.5 Polyp of colon. Inflammatory polyps, which are typically found in inflammatory bowel diseases, are classified in the ulcerative colitis category (K51).

Review endoscopy and pathology reports to ascertain which type of polyp was found.

Left-sided colitis without complications (K51.50)

Left-sided colitis with complications (K51.51-)

Note: Sixth characters for subcategory K51.51 include that for rectal bleeding, intestinal obstruction, fistula, abscess, other and unspecified complications.

Clinical Tip
The vast majority of cases of ulcerative colitis involve the rectum. From there, the inflammation extends up through the sigmoid and descending colon, which are located in the upper left part of the abdomen. When this is the extent of the disease process, it may be referred to as left-sided colitis or left hemicolitis.

Clinician Documentation Checklist

Clinician documentation should indicate the following:

- Identification of manifestation such as pyoderma gangrenosum:
- Type
  - ulcerative (chronic) pancolitis
    - backwash ileitis
  - ulcerative (chronic) proctitis
  - ulcerative (chronic) rectosigmoiditis
  - inflammatory polyps of colon
  - left-sided colitis
    - left hemicolitis
  - other ulcerative colitis
  - unspecified ulcerative colitis
- Associated
  - without complication
  - with complication
    - rectal bleeding
    - intestinal obstruction
    - fistula
    - abscess
    - other complication
    - unspecified complications

Urinary Tract Infection (UTI)

Code Axes

Other disorders of urinary system **N39.-**

Description of Condition

Microbial infection, usually bacterial, of unspecified part of the urinary tract, can involve the parenchyma of the kidney, the renal pelvis, the ureter, the bladder, the urethra or combinations of these organs. The most common organism causing such infection is *Escherichia coli*.

Urinary tract infection, site not specified (N39.Ø)

Clinical Tip

Predisposing factors for urinary tract infection include calculi or other urinary tract obstruction, foreign bodies such as stents or catheters, congenital urinary anomalies, pregnancy, diabetes mellitus, and neurogenic bladder. Women are approximately four times more likely to develop a urinary tract infection than men.

Key Terms

Key terms found in the documentation may include:

Bacteriuria

E. coli

Urinary tract infection, site not specified

UTI

Clinical Tip

When there is evidence that the site of the UTI can be further specified as cystitis, urethritis, etc., query the provider for specificity. If a specific site is confirmed, report the code for the specific site instead of N39.0. For example:

- For cystitis see N30–N30.91
- For urethritis see N34–N34.3

Clinical Findings

Physical Examination

History and review of systems may include:

- Back pain
- Burning or pain when urinating
- Chills
- Cloudy or reddish urine
- Dysuria

I-10 ALERT

Urinary tract infections related to urinary catheters or others devices are coded in subcategory T83.5-.

CDI ALERT

The term "urosepsis" must be queried as to the condition it represents, either a UTI or sepsis with UTI.

⇨ I-10 ALERT

To identify the infectious agent, use an additional code (B95–B97).

- Fever
- Flank pain
- Foul smelling urine
- Increased urinary frequency
- Increased urinary urgency
- Malaise
- Nausea
- Polyuria
- Pressure in the lower belly

Diagnostic Procedures and Services

- Laboratory
  - CBC
  - urinalysis
  - urine culture
- Imaging
  - cystoscopy
  - cystourethrogram

Therapeutic Procedures and Services

- Cranberry juice
- Increase total fluid intake

Medication List

- Antibiotics
  - azithromycin (Zithromax, Zmax)
  - ceftriaxone (Rocephin)
  - cephalexin (Keflex)
  - ciprofloxacin (Cipro)
  - doxycycline (Monodox, Vibramycin)
  - fosfomycin (Monurol)
  - levofloxacin (Levaquin)
  - nitrofurantoin (Macrodantin, Macrobid)
  - trimethoprim (Bactrim, Septra)

Clinician Documentation Checklist

Clinician documentation should indicate the following:

- Specific type:
  - Urinary tract infection, site not specified
    - identify infectious organism (bacterial, viral)

Wound Exploration

Code Axes

Wound exploration—trauma (e.g., penetrating gunshot, stab wound) **20100–20103**

Description of Procedure

Documentation will indicate that the physician explores a penetrating wound such as a gunshot, stab wound, or impaling by a foreign body in the operating room. Because code assignment is dependent upon anatomical location, it is critical that the documentation be carefully read to determine the exact site. Documentation will indicate that nerve, organ, and blood vessel integrity was assessed. Enlargement of the wound in order to make this assessment may be recorded.

During the procedure the physician may record that the wound was debrided, that foreign bodies were removed, and the ligation or coagulation of minor blood vessels in the subcutaneous tissues, fascia, and muscle were performed. The wound may be closed or packed open when contaminated by the penetrating body.

Key Terms

Key terms found in the documentation may include:

Assaulted

Gun shot

Knife wound

Stabbing

Clinician Documentation Checklist

Clinician documentation should indicate the following:

- Site(s) of wound(s)
  - neck
  - chest
  - abdomen/flank/back
  - extremity
- Procedures performed
  - debridement
  - expanded dissection of wound for exploration
  - extraction of foreign material
  - open examination
  - tying or coagulation of small vessels

Wound Repair

Code Axes

Repair—simple	**12001–12018**
Repair—intermediate	**12031–12057**
Repair—complex	**13100–13153**

Description of Procedure

Simple wound repair is defined as the closure of wounds involving the epidermis or dermis and may include the subcutaneous tissues without involvement of the deeper tissues. Simple wounds require one layer closure.

An intermediate repair is defined as a wound that requires layered closure of one or more of the deeper layers of subcutaneous tissues and nonmuscular fascia. A heavily contaminated wound that requires extensive cleaning but only single layer closure is also classified as an intermediate repair.

Complex repair is defined as one that requires more than a single layer closure, debridement, undermining, stents, or retention sutures. Documentation will indicate that the physician debrides the wound by removing foreign material or damaged tissue. Irrigation of the wound is performed and antimicrobial solutions are used to decontaminate and cleanse the wound. The physician may trim skin margins with a scalpel or scissors to allow for proper closure. The wound is closed in layers. The physician may perform scar revision, which creates a complex defect requiring repair. Stents or retention sutures may also be used in complex repair of a wound.

Documentation must include the anatomical location, size of wound, depth of wound, and any procedures such as debridement or decontamination when performed. Instrumentation such as the type of suture or glue that was used to accomplish the closure should also be noted.

CPT Alert

Reconstructive procedures, such as utilization of local flaps, may be required and are reported separately when complex wound closure is performed.

Key Terms

Key terms found in the documentation may include:

- Fascia
- Multiple layers
- Single layer
- Subfascial

Clinician Documentation Checklist

Clinician documentation should indicate the following:

- Type of wound(s)
  - superficial
  - intermediate
  - complicated
- Site(s) of wound(s)
  - wound size
  - length of wound(s)
- Complications
  - dehiscence
- Anesthesia
- Debridement
- Decontamination
- Removal of foreign materials
- Ligation
- Materials
  - sutures
  - staples
  - tissue adhesives
  - stents

Section 4: Terminology Translator

To use the table below, find the term used in the medical record documentation in column one. Column two indicates the term(s) used in the ICD-10-CM system for that condition.

Medical Record Terminology	ICD-10-CM Terminology
Abscess of lung	Gangrene and necrosis of lung
Achalasia and cardiospasm	Achalasia of cardia
Acute coronary occlusion without MI	Acute coronary thrombosis not resulting in MI
Acute infective polyneuritis	Guillain-Barré syndrome
Acute pyelonephritis w/ or w/o lesion of medullary necrosis	Acute tubulo-interstitial nephritis
Acute respiratory failure following trauma and surgery	Postprocedural respiratory failure
Adenocarcinoma of intrahepatic bile duct	Intrahepatic bile duct carcinoma
After-cataract	Other secondary cataract
Allergic alveolitis and pneumonitis	Hypersensitivity pneumonitis (due to: cause)
Allergic rhinitis cause unspecified	Vasomotor rhinitis
Angina decubitus	Other forms of angina pectoris
Asbestosis	Pneumoconiosis due to asbestos and other mineral fibers
Asiderotic anemia	Anemia secondary to blood loss
Atrial flutter	Persistent/Atypical/Typical atrial flutter
Atrophic gastritis	Chronic superficial gastritis
Attacks without alteration of consciousness	Localization-related epilepsy
Autoimmune/Non-autoimmune hemolytic anemias	Drug-induced autoimmune hemolytic anemia
Avian Influenza virus (pneumonia, other resp infection)	Identified novel influenza A virus (with manifestation: pneumonia, other respiratory)
Backwash ileitis	Ulcerative colitis
Bacterial colitis	Bacterial intestinal infection, unspecified
Basilar migraine	Juvenile myoclonic epilepsy
Bed sore	Pressure ulcer
Benign childhood epilepsy with centrotemporal EEG spikes	Localization-related epilepsy
Biliary cirrhosis	Primary biliary cirrhosis Secondary biliary cirrhosis
Blood in stool	Melena
Bloodstream infection [although necessary to differentiate from bacteremia]	Septicemia due to (organism)
Bowen's disease	Carcinoma in situ site unspecified

Medical Record Terminology	ICD-10-CM Terminology
Brachial neuritis or radiculitis	Radiculopathy
Brittle diabetes	Type I diabetes mellitus
C. difficile colitis	Enterocolitis due to Clostridium difficile
Cancrum oris	Necrotizing ulcerative stomatitis
Cataracta brunescens	Age-related cataract
Cataracta complicate	Complicated cataract
Cerebrospinal fluid rhinorrhea	Cerebral spinal fluid leak
Cervical degenerative disc disease with radiculopathy	Cervical disc disorder
Cervical DJD with myelopathy	Cervical disc disorder
Cervical DJD with radiculopathy	Cervical disc disorder
Cervical myelopathy	Cervical disc disorder
Cervical radiculopathy	Cervical disc disorder
Cervical spondylosis with myelopathy	Vertebral artery compression syndromes
Cervicothoracic disc disorders with cervicalgia	Cervical disc disorder
Cervicothoracic disorders	Cervical disc disorder
Cheyne-Stokes respiration	Periodic breathing
Childhood epilepsy with occipital EEG paroxysms	Localization-related epilepsy
Chlorosis	Anemia secondary to blood loss
Cholangiocarcinoma	Liver cell carcinoma
Chronic airway obstruction, NEC	Chronic obstructive pulmonary disease
Chronic cold hemagglutinin disease	Other autoimmune hemolytic anemia
Chronic hypotension	Idiopathic hypotension
Chronic lymphadenitis	Chronic lymphadenitis, except mesenteric
Chronic nonalcoholic liver disease	Nonalcoholic steatohepatitis (NASH) Fatty liver, NEC
Classical migraine	Juvenile myoclonic epilepsy
Coccidiosis	Isosporiasis
Cold agglutinin disease	Other autoimmune hemolytic anemia
Cold agglutinin hemoglobinuria	Other autoimmune hemolytic anemia
Cold type (secondary) (symptomatic) hemolytic anemia	Other autoimmune hemolytic anemia
Collapsed vertebra NOS	Collapsed vertebra
Colloid carcinoma of breast	Malignant neoplasm of breast
Complications of surgical and medical care, not elsewhere classified	Complications of surgical and medical care, not elsewhere classified
Compression fracture	Collapsed vertebra
Condyloma acuminatum	Anogenital (venereal) warts
Congenital factor (VII/IX/XI) deficiency	Hereditary factor VII deficiency Hereditary factor IX deficiency Hereditary factor XI deficiency
Congestive heart failure, unspecified	Heart failure, unspecified

Medical Record Terminology	ICD-10-CM Terminology
Coronary atherosclerosis of (native) (bypass) (transplant) vessel	Atherosclerotic heart disease of (native) (bypass) (transplant) with or w/o angina (type)
Coronary cataract	Age-related cataract
Coronary slow flow syndrome	Angina
Cranial neuritis	Other neurologic disorders in Lyme disease
Cyst of thyroid	Nontoxic single thyroid nodule
Decubitus ulcer	Pressure ulcer
Defibrination syndrome	Disseminated intravascular coagulation
Degenerative cataract	Complicated cataract
Diabetes due to autoimmune process	Type I diabetes mellitus
Diabetes due to immune mediated pancreatic islet beta-cell destruction	Type I diabetes mellitus
Diabetes due to insulin secretory defect	Type II diabetes mellitus
Diabetes mellitus due to genetic defects in insulin action	Other specified diabetes
Diabetes mellitus due to genetic defects of beta-cell function	Other specified diabetes
Diabetes NOS	Type II diabetes mellitus
Diabetes w/o complication type I (juvenile) controlled	Type 1 diabetes mellitus without complications
Diabetes w/o complication type I (juvenile) uncontrolled	Type 1 diabetes with hyperglycemia
Diabetes w/o complication type II controlled	Type 2 diabetes mellitus without complications Other specified diabetes mellitus without complications
Diabetes w/o complications type II uncontrolled	Type 2 diabetes mellitus with hyperglycemia
Diffusely adherent E. coli	Escherichia coli, enteropathogenic
Ductal carcinoma in situ	Carcinoma in situ of breast
E. coli O157:H7	Enterohemorrhagic Escherichia coli infections
Empyema	Pyothorax (with or without: fistula)
Epilepsia partialis continua [Kozhevnikov]	Localization-related epilepsy
Epithelioid hemangioendothelioma	Other sarcomas of liver
Erythema chronicum migrans	Lyme disease
Erythroplasia	Carcinoma in situ site unspecified
External hemorrhoids without complication	Residual hemorrhoidal skin tags
External thrombosed hemorrhoids	Perianal venous thrombosis
Extracapillary glomerulonephritis	Recurrent and persistent hematuria
Familial migraine	Hemiplegic migraine
Fibrosarcoma	Other sarcomas of liver
Flatulence eructation and gas pain	Abdominal distension (gaseous)
Focal epilepsy	Intractable epilepsy

Medical Record Terminology	ICD-10-CM Terminology
Food poisoning (due to organism)	Foodborne (organism) intoxication
Foot and mouth disease	Other viral infections with skin and mucous membrane lesions
Frozen shoulder	Adhesive capsulitis
Glaucoma: Use additional code for stage	Glaucoma: [Diagnoses specify type/laterality] Stage included in seventh character
Glaucomatous flecks	Complicated cataract
Glaukomflecken	Complicated cataract
Glomerulonephritis – mesangial proliferative	Recurrent and persistent hematuria
Grade III intraepithelial neoplasia	Carcinoma in situ site unspecified
Granulomatous colitis	Crohn's disease
HCC	Intrahepatic bile duct carcinoma
Hemangioendothelioma	Angiosarcoma of liver
Hemoglobinuria due to hemolysis from external causes	Paroxysmal nocturnal hemoglobinuria
Hemophagocytic syndromes	Hemophagocytic lymphohistiocytosis
Hepatic angiosarcoma	Angiosarcoma of liver
Hepatitis (unspecified)	[Diagnosis includes type, causal factors and complications:] Toxic liver disease (specify complications) Nonspecific reactive hepatitis Peliosis hepatitis
Hepatocellular carcinoma	Liver cell carcinoma
Hepatoma	Intrahepatic bile duct carcinoma
Hereditary peripheral neuropathy	Hereditary motor and sensory neuropathy
Herpangina	Enteroviral vesicular pharyngitis
Hypermature cataract	Age-related cataract
Hyperpotassemia	
Hypertrophy of prostate	Enlarged prostate
Hypochromic anemia	Anemia secondary to blood loss
Hypochromic microcytic anemia	Anemia secondary to blood loss
Hypochromic or microcytic anemia	Anemia secondary to blood loss
Hypoferric anemia	Anemia secondary to blood loss
Hypoparathyroidism	Idiopathic hypoparathyroidism Other hypoparathyroidism Hypoparathyroidism, unspecified Postprocedural hypoparathyroidism
Hypopotassemia	Hyperkalemia
Iatrogenic thyroiditis	Drug-induced thyroiditis
Idiopathic diabetes	Type I diabetes mellitus
Idiopathic myocarditis	Isolated myocarditis
Idiopathic osteoporosis with current pathological fracture	Drug-induced osteoporosis
Immature cataract	Age-related cataract

Medical Record Terminology	ICD-10-CM Terminology
Immune complex hemolytic anemia	Other autoimmune hemolytic anemia
Immunohemolytic anemia	Other autoimmune hemolytic anemia
Incipient cataract	Age-related cataract
Inclusion conjunctivitis	Chlamydial conjunctivitis
Indolent cataract	Age-related cataract
Infiltrating lobular carcinoma of the breast	Malignant neoplasm of breast
Inflammatory breast cancer (IBC)	Malignant neoplasm of breast
Inflammatory cataract	Complicated cataract
Insulin resistant diabetes	Type II diabetes mellitus
Intermediate coronary syndrome	Angina
Intermediate coronary syndrome	Unstable angina
Intracholangiocarcinoma	Liver cell carcinoma
Invasive cribriform carcinoma of the breast	Malignant neoplasm of breast
Invasive ductal carcinoma (IDC) of breast	Malignant neoplasm of breast
Invasive lobular carcinoma of the breast	Malignant neoplasm of breast
Invasive papillary carcinoma of the breast	Malignant neoplasm of breast
Involutional osteoporosis with current pathological fracture	Age-related osteoporosis
Iodine hypothyroidism	Hypothyroidism due to meds and other exogenous substances
Ischemic chest pain	Angina
Janz syndrome	Juvenile myoclonic epilepsy
Juvenile onset diabetes	Type I diabetes mellitus
Kelly-Paterson syndrome	Anemia secondary to blood loss
Ketosis-prone diabetes	Type I diabetes mellitus
Kupffer cell sarcoma	Angiosarcoma of liver
Left bundle branch hemiblock	Left anterior fascicular block Left posterior fascicular block Other/unspecified fascicular block
Left heart failure	Left ventricular failure
Leiomyosarcoma	Other sarcomas of liver
Letterer-Siwe disease	Malignant mast cell tumor
Leukemic reticuloendotheliosis	Hairy cell leukemia
Leukocytopenia unspecified	Decreased white blood cell count, unspecified
Lobular carcinoma in situ (LCIS)	Carcinoma in situ of breast
Localization-related idiopathic epilepsy and epileptic syndromes with seizures of localized onset	Localization-related epilepsy
Lown-Ganong-Levine syndrome	Pre-excitation syndrome
Lumbago due to displacement of intervertebral disc	Lumbar disc disorder Lumbosacral disc disorder
Lumbar neuritis or radiculitis	Radiculopathy
Lumbosacral neuritis or radiculitis	Radiculopathy

Medical Record Terminology	ICD-10-CM Terminology
Lupus erythematosus (non-systemic)	Discoid lupus erythematosus Subacute cutaneous lupus erythematosus Other local lupus erythematosus
Lyme disease meningoencephalitis	Other neurologic disorders in Lyme disease
Lyme disease myopericarditis	Other conditions associated with Lyme disease
Lyme disease polyencephalitis	Other neurologic disorders in Lyme disease
Lymphosarcoma	Lymphoblastic lymphoma
Malignant fibrous histiocytoma	Other sarcomas of liver
Malignant hepatoma	Intrahepatic bile duct carcinoma
Malignant histiocytoma	Other sarcomas of liver
Malignant histiocytosis	Histiocytic sarcoma
Malignant neoplasm of other specified sites (of site)	Malignant neoplasm of overlapping sites (of site)
Malignant phyllodes tumors of the breast	Malignant neoplasm of breast
Marginal zone lymphoma	Other non-follicular lymphoma Extranodal marginal zone B-cell lymphoma of mucosa associated lymphatic tissue
Mechanical complication of esophagostomy	[Diagnoses specify type of complication:] Esophagostomy hemorrhage Esophagostomy malfunction
Medullary carcinoma of breast	Malignant neoplasm of breast
Membranous glomerulopathy	Recurrent and persistent hematuria
Membranous nephritis	Recurrent and persistent hematuria
Membranous nephropathy	Recurrent and persistent hematuria
Meningitis due to coxsackie virus/Echo virus	Enteroviral meningitis
Mesangial proliferative GN	Recurrent and persistent hematuria
Mucinous carcinoma of breast	Malignant neoplasm of breast
Necrosis of artery	Necrotizing vasculopathy
Neovascularization cataract	Complicated cataract
Nodular lymphoma	Follicular lymphoma (specify grade/site) Cutaneous follicle center lymphoma specify grade/site) Other/unspecified follicular lymphoma
Noise-induced hearing loss	Noise effects on (specify laterality) inner ear
Non-healing ulcer of skin	Chronic skin ulcer
Non-infected sinus of skin	Chronic skin ulcer
Nontransmural myocardial infarction	Non nontransmural myocardial infarction
Nuclear cataract, nonsenile	Infantile and juvenile nuclear cataract
Nuclear sclerosis	Age-related cataract
Nuclear sclerosis cataract	Age-related cataract
Occlusion and stenosis (cerebral/precerebral artery) w/Infarction	Cerebral infarction due to (thrombosis, embolism, occlusion)
Osteoporosis NOS with current pathological fracture	Age-related osteoporosis

Medical Record Terminology	ICD-10-CM Terminology
Osteoporosis of disuse with current pathological fracture	Drug-induced osteoporosis
Osteoporosis with current fragility fracture	Age-related osteoporosis
Osteoporotic fracture	Age-related osteoporosis
Paget's disease of the breast	Malignant neoplasm of breast
Paget's disease of the nipple	Malignant neoplasm of breast
Pain in or around eye	Ocular pain
Painful arc syndrome	Shoulder impingement syndrome
Painful respiration	Chest pain on breathing Pleurodynia
Paralysis agitans	Parkinson's disease Vascular parkinsonism
Paraplegia	Tropical spastic paraplegia Paraplegia unspecified Paraplegia, complete Paraplegia, incomplete
Paroxysmal supraventricular tachycardia	Supraventricular tachycardia Junctional premature depolarization
Paroxysmal ventricular tachycardia	Re-entry ventricular arrhythmia Ventricular tachycardia
Pars planitis	Posterior cyclitis (specify laterality)
Partial tear of rotator cuff	Incomplete rotator cuff tear/rupture of shoulder, nontraumatic (specify laterality)
Periarthritis of shoulder	Adhesive capsulitis
Pernicious anemia	Vitamin B12 deficiency anemia due to intrinsic factor deficiency
Pharmacoresistant (pharmacologically) resistant epilepsy	Intractable epilepsy
Plaster ulcer	Pressure ulcer
Pleurisy w/o effusion	Pyothorax without fistula Pleural plaque (w/ or w/o asbestos) Fibrothorax
Plummer-Vinson syndrome	Anemia secondary to blood loss
Pneumonia due to other virus	Human metapneumovirus pneumonia
Pneumonia in aspergillosis	Invasive pulmonary aspergillosis
Poorly controlled epilepsy	Intractable epilepsy
Post-traumatic osteoporosis with current pathological fracture	Drug-induced osteoporosis
Posthemorrhagic anemia (chronic)	Anemia secondary to blood loss
Postmenopausal osteoporosis with current pathological fracture	Age-related osteoporosis
Postmyocardial infarction syndrome	Dressler's syndrome
Postoophorectomy osteoporosis with current pathological fracture	Drug-induced osteoporosis
Postpancreatectomy diabetes mellitus	Other specified diabetes
Postprocedural diabetes mellitus	Other specified diabetes

Medical Record Terminology	ICD-10-CM Terminology
Postsurgical malabsorption osteoporosis with current pathological fracture	Drug-induced osteoporosis
Preinfarction syndrome	Angina
Pressure area	Pressure ulcer
Pressure sore	Pressure ulcer
Primary hepatic sarcoma	Other sarcomas of liver
Primary hypercoagulable state	Activated protein C resistance Prothrombin gene mutation Other primary thrombophilia Antiphospholipid syndrome Lupus anticoagulant syndrome
Primary liver carcinoma	Intrahepatic bile duct carcinoma
Primary liver cell carcinoma	Intrahepatic bile duct carcinoma
Prinzmetal angina	Angina pectoris with documented spasm
Progressive muscular atrophy	Amyotrophic lateral sclerosis
Pseudomembranous colitis (C. difficile)	Enterocolitis due to Clostridium difficile
Pseudopolyposis	Inflammatory polyps [Combination diagnoses specify assoc. complications:] Inflammatory polyps with rectal bleeding Inflammatory polyps with intestinal obstruction Inflammatory polyps of colon with fistula Inflammatory polyps with abscess
Pulmonary collapse	Atelectasis Other pulmonary collapse
Pulmonary congestion and hypostasis	Hypostatic pneumonia
Punctate cataract	Age-related cataract
Queyrat's erythroplasia	Carcinoma in situ site unspecified
Radiculitis	Radiculopathy
Red cell aplasia acquired adult with thymoma	Acquired pure red cell aplasia (specify as:) acute , chronic, transient
Reflex sympathetic dystrophy (site)	Complex regional pain syndrome (site)
Reflux esophagitis	Gastro-esophageal reflux disease with esophagitis
Refractory (medically) epilepsy	Intractable epilepsy
Regional enteritis	Crohn's disease
Reticulosarcoma	Diffuse large B-cell lymphoma
Retinal migraine	Juvenile myoclonic epilepsy
Right bundle branch block	Right fascicular block Other/unspecified right bundle branch block
Right bundle branch block and (right) (left) (anterior) (posterior) fascicular block	Bifascicular block
Roseola infantum due to human herpesvirus 6	Exanthema subitum [sixth disease] due to human herpesvirus 6
Rotator cuff syndrome	Rotator cuff tear

Medical Record Terminology	ICD-10-CM Terminology
Sciatica due to intervertebral disc disorder	Lumbar disc disorder Lumbosacral disc disorder
Secondary diabetes mellitus NEC	Other specified diabetes
Senile	Age-related
Senile cataract	Age-related cataract
Senile osteoporosis	Age-related osteoporosis w/o current pathological fracture
Senile osteoporosis with current pathological fracture	Age-related osteoporosis
Senility	Age-related cognitive decline
Senility without mention of psychosis	Age-related cognitive decline Age-related physical debility
Septic intoxication	Septicemia due to (organism)
Septic myocarditis	Infective myocarditis
Septic syndrome	Septicemia due to (organism)
Septicemia	Sepsis due to (organism)
Septicemia due to (organism)	Sepsis due to (organism)
Sideropenic dysphagia	Sideropenic dysphagia (iron deficiency anemia)
Simple partial seizures developing into secondarily generalized seizures	Localization-related epilepsy
Sinoatrial node dysfunction	Sick sinus syndrome
Sporadic migraine	Hemiplegic migraine
STEMI	ST elevation myocardial infarction
Stress fracture, spinal	Fatigue fracture of vertebra
Sub capsular flecks	Complicated cataract
Subsequent (refers to episode of care)	Subsequent (refers to consecutive AMIs)
Supraspinatus syndrome	Shoulder impingement syndrome
Supraspinatus syndrome	Rotator cuff tear
Supraspinatus tear or rupture, not specified as traumatic	Rotator cuff tear
Supraventricular premature beats	Atrial premature depolarization
Swimmer's shoulder	Shoulder impingement syndrome
Swyer-James-MacLeod syndrome	Unilateral pulmonary emphysema
Thoracic neuritis or radiculitis	Radiculopathy
Thrower's shoulder	Shoulder impingement syndrome
Tick born fever	Colorado fever
Toxemia	Septicemia due to (organism)
Toxic cataract	Drug-induced cataract
Tracheoesophageal fistula	Pyothorax with fistula
Transmural Q-wave infarction	ST elevation myocardial infarction
Traveler's diarrhea	Other intestinal Escherichia coli infections
Treatment resistant epilepsy	Intractable epilepsy
Trophic ulcer	Chronic skin ulcer

Medical Record Terminology	ICD-10-CM Terminology
Tropical ulcer	Chronic skin ulcer
Tubular carcinoma of breast	Malignant neoplasm of breast
Undifferentiated embryonal sarcoma of the liver	Other sarcomas of liver
Undifferentiated liver sarcoma	Other sarcomas of liver
Unilateral hyperlucent lung syndrome	Unilateral pulmonary emphysema
Unilateral pulmonary artery functional hypoplasia	Unilateral pulmonary emphysema
Unilateral transparency of lung	Unilateral pulmonary emphysema
Universal ulcerative colitis	Ulcerative pancolitis
Unspecified chronic pulmonary heart disease	Cor pulmonale (chronic)
Unspecified sudden hearing loss	Sudden idiopathic hearing loss
Urosepsis [antiquated term; necessary to differentiate from UTI]	Septicemia due to (organism)
Ventilation pneumonitis	Air conditioner and humidifier lung
Warm type (secondary) (symptomatic) hemolytic anemia	Other autoimmune hemolytic anemia
Water clefts	Age-related cataract
Wedging of vertebra NOS	Collapsed vertebra
Word deafness	Auditory processing disorder

Appendix 1: Physician Query Samples

The major purpose of queries is to obtain clarification when documentation in the health record impacts an externally reportable data element and is illegible, incomplete, unclear, inconsistent, or imprecise. As noted earlier in this manual, queries should not be leading by eliciting a specific response, introduce new information not documented elsewhere, be "yes/no" in format, or appear to question a provider's clinical judgment.

The query examples that follow here are intended to provide those actively working with physicians in clinical documentation improvement activities, to encourage accurate and appropriate documentation.

Pressure Ulcer Clarification

Dr. Walker:

You documented a diagnosis of sacral pressure ulcer for this patient, but did not specify the stage of pressure ulcer. A dressing change was performed on 7/5. The nurse noted "breakdown of skin with clean, circumscribed edges." Nursing documentation is unclear whether this indicates a partial (Stage II) or full (Stage III) thickness skin ulcer.

Can this patient's pressure ulcer be specified to The National Pressure Ulcer Advisor Panel (NPUAP) stage as:

- Unstageable/unspecified stage
- Stage I: non-blanching erythema (a reddened area on the skin).
- Stage II: abrasion, blister, shallow open crater, or other partial thickness skin loss.
- Stage III: full thickness skin loss involving damage or necrosis into subcutaneous soft tissues.
- Stage IV: full thickness skin loss with necrosis of soft tissues through to the muscle, tendons, or tissues around underlying bone.

Undetermined or Unknown: ______________________________

If so, please document the ulcer stage in the progress notes.

Signature ______________________________

Date ______________________________

Thank you!

Cathy Coder

X 5437

Pneumonia Clarification

Dr. Miller:

This patient's final diagnosis is documented as "Pneumonia." Can the pneumonia be further specified to causal organism or type?

Pneumonia due to (Causal type/organism):______________________

The following clinical indicators support this query for further information:

- The 7/5 Gram stain is positive for predominance of Gram negative rods.
- Your 7/5 progress note documents, "sputum culture invalid due to antibiotic therapy, patient unable to produce adequate sample."
- The patient was treated with third generation cephalosporin, which you link in your treatment plan to his immunocompromised status from steroid-dependent chronic obstructive asthma.

If so, please document the type/etiology of the pneumonia in the progress notes.

Undetermined or Unknown: ______________________

Signature ______________________

Date ______________________

Thanks!

CDI Dan

Extension 435

Respiratory Diagnosis Clarification

Dr. Smith:

This patient's final diagnosis is documented as "respiratory distress." Your H&P indicates that the patient was admitted with COPD exacerbation and on admission she had 85 percent oxygen saturation on room air, respiratory rate of 28, and arterial blood gas (ABG) results were: pO_2 47, pCO_2 52, pH 7.34. Admission orders included oxygen and BiPAP.

Can your final diagnosis documentation of respiratory distress be further clarified?:

Acute respiratory failure: ______________________

Acute on chronic respiratory failure: ______________________

Acute respiratory insufficiency: ______________________

Another cause of respiratory distress: ______________________

Other: ______________________

Unable to determine: ______________________

Not Applicable: ______________________

Signature ______________________

Date ______________________

Thank you,

Elaine Record

X7676

Diagnosis Linkage Clarification

Dr. Jones:

The H&P for this patient indicates the presence of diabetes mellitus type 2 and peripheral vascular disease with gangrene.

If possible, can you please clarify whether or not these conditions are believed to be associated?

Please document any associated or unrelated status in the progress notes.

Unable to determine: ______________________________

Not Applicable: ______________________________

Signature ______________________________

Date ______________________________

Thank you,

Mary Med

X9043

Anemia Clarification

Dr. Davis:

This patient was admitted with a duodenal bleed per your admission note. At that time, her hemoglobin was 7.4gm/dl and her hematocrit was 22.6 percent . The H&P states "anemia." After admission, the patient was treated with two units packed red blood cells (PRBC).

Can your diagnosis of anemia be further specified to any of the following?:

Acute blood loss anemia: ______________________________

Chronic blood loss anemia: ______________________________

Other type of anemia: ______________________________

Unable to determine: ______________________________

Please document any clarification in the progress notes or on the discharge summary.

Signature ______________________________

Date ______________________________

Thank you,

John Jay

X349

Intracerebral Bleeding Clarification

Dr. Santos:

In your progress note of October 31, you documented "subarachnoid hemorrhage." Can you please clarify the specific vessel involved?

Anterior Communicating Artery ______________________________

Basilar Artery ______________________________

Carotid Siphon & Bifurcation ______________________________

Middle Cerebral Artery ______________________________

Posterior Communicating Artery ______________________________

Other Intracranial Artery ______________________________

Vertebral Artery ______________________________

Cannot determine ______________________________

Also, please specify the underlying cause and laterality:

Traumatic ______________________________

Non-traumatic ______________________________

Cannot determine ______________________________

Right Brain ______________________________

Left Brain ______________________________

Cannot determine ______________________________

Please document this information in the progress notes.

Signature ______________________________

Date ______________________________

Thanks very much!

Tom Terry, CDI Specialist, 3 North Unit

X6676

Chest Pain Clarification

Dr. Ellis:

The admitting diagnosis in the progress notes for this patient indicates "unspecified chest pain."

Please review the following list of potential diagnoses and clarify the underlying cause, if known.

Note: for hospital admissions, the final diagnosis may be presumptive. Terms such as "probable," "likely," or "suspected" may be used.

Cardiac arrhythmia (please specify type, if known) ________________________________

Coronary artery disease (specify with or w/o unstable angina) ________________________

Costochondritis ________________________________

Gastroesophageal reflux ________________________________

Pleuritic ________________________________

Psychogenic causes ________________________________

Stress and/or anxiety ________________________________

Other cause ________________________________

Chest pain, cause undetermined ________________________________

Please document this information in the progress notes or discharge summary.

Thanks,

Hannah Hospital

X9989

Confirmation Request for Pathology Findings

ATTENTION: THIS FORM IS A PERMANENT PART OF THE MEDICAL RECORD

Dr. Green (attending physician):

This patient had surgery on ________ (date) and the corresponding pathology report indicated an abnormal finding of ______________.

Abnormal findings of this nature are not allowed as reportable conditions unless substantiated by an authorized provider, indicating their clinical significance.

Please specify below:

I concur with this finding/diagnosis ____________________

I do not concur with this finding/diagnosis ____________________

I am unable to concur at this time (unable to determine) ____________________

There is no clinical significance to this finding ____________________

Other diagnosis based on these findings ____________________

____

____

____

____

Attending signature ____________________

Date: ____________________

Appendix 2: HCC and QPP Associated Codes

The following lists include the number and official description of the HCC or QPP measures referenced in the table below. To save space the official descriptions have been provided once in this list. The table includes CPT codes, ICD-10-CM codes, and any applicable HCC and/or QPP measures for **topics covered in this book.** Note that to save space, some ICD-10-CM codes ranges are listed within certain topics in the body of this book. The individual code should be verified in this table.

CMS-HCC Model Category

1	HIV/AIDS
2	Septicemia, Sepsis, Systemic Inflammatory Response Syndrome/Shock
8	Metastatic Cancer and Acute Leukemia
9	Lung and Other Severe Cancers
10	Lymphoma and Other Cancers
12	Breast, Prostate, and Other Cancers and Tumors
17	Diabetes with Acute Complications
18	Diabetes with Chronic Complications
19	Diabetes without Complication
21	Protein-Calorie Malnutrition
22	Morbid Obesity
23	Other Significant Endocrine and Metabolic Disorders
33	Intestinal Obstruction/Perforation
35	Inflammatory Bowel Disease
40	Rheumatoid Arthritis and Inflammatory Connective Tissue Disease
46	Severe Hematological Disorders
54	Drug/Alcohol Psychosis
55	Drug/Alcohol Dependence
79	Seizure Disorders and Convulsions
82	Respirator Dependence/Tracheostomy Status
84	Cardio-Respiratory Failure and Shock
85	Congestive Heart Failure
86	Acute Myocardial Infarction
87	Unstable Angina, Other Acute Ischemic Heart Disease
88	Angina Pectoris
96	Specified Heart Arrhythmias
99	Cerebral Hemorrhage
100	Ischemic or Unspecified Stroke
106	Atherosclerosis of the Extremities with Ulceration or Gangrene
108	Vascular Disease
111	Chronic Obstructive Pulmonary Disease
114	Aspiration and Specified Bacterial Pneumonias
122	Proliferative Diabetic Retinopathy and Vitreous Hemorrhage
136	Chronic Kidney Disease (Stage 5)
157	Pressure Ulcer w/ Necrosis to Muscle, Tendon, Bone
158	Pressure Ulcer with Full Thickness Skin Loss
161	Chronic Ulcer of Skin, Except Pressure
166	Severe Head Injury
167	Major Head Injury
169	Vertebral Fractures without Spinal Cord Injury
170	Hip Fracture/Dislocation
176	Complication of Specified Implanted Device or Graft

QPP Measures Category

1	Diabetes: Hemoglobin A1c (HbA1c) Poor Control (>9%)
12	Primary Open-Angle Glaucoma (POAG): Optic Nerve Evaluation
19	Diabetic Retinopathy: Communication with the Physician Managing Ongoing Diabetes Care
21	Perioperative Care: Selection of Prophylactic Antibiotic – First OR Second Generation Cephalosporin
23	Perioperative Care: Venous Thromboembolism (VTE) Prophylaxis (When Indicated in ALL Patients)
24	Communication with the Physician or Other Clinician Managing On-going Care Post-Fracture for Men and Women Aged 50 Years and Older
32	Stroke and Stroke Rehabilitation: Discharged on Antithrombotic Therapy
39	Screening for Osteoporosis for Women Aged 65-85 years of Age
47	Care Plan
51	Chronic Obstructive Pulmonary Disease (COPD): Spirometry Evaluation
52	Chronic Obstructive Pulmonary Disease (COPD): Inhaled Bronchodilator Therapy
99	Breast Cancer Resection Pathology Reporting: pT Category (Primary Tumor) and pN Category (Regional Lymph Nodes) with Histologic Grade
117	Diabetes: Eye Exam
141	Primary Open-Angle Glaucoma (POAG): Reduction of Intraocular Pressure (IOP) by 15% OR Documentation of a Plan of Care
145	Radiology: Exposure Dose or Time Reported for Procedures Using Fluoroscopy
156	Oncology: Radiation Dose Limits to Normal Tissues
185	Colonoscopy Interval for Patients with a History of Adenomatous Polyps
204	Ischemic Vascular Disease (IVD): Use of Aspirin or Another Antiplatelet
236	Controlling High Blood Pressure
251	Quantitative Immunohistochemical (IHC) Evaluation of Human Epidermal Growth Factor Receptor 2 Testing (HER2) for Breast Cancer Patients
254	Ultrasound Determination of Pregnancy Location for Pregnant Patients with Abdominal Pain
255	Rh Immunoglobulin (RhoGAM) for Rh-Negative Pregnant Women at Risk of Fetal Blood Exposure
268	Epilepsy: Counseling for Women of Childbearing Potential with Epilepsy
320	Appropriate Follow-Up Interval for Normal Colonoscopy in Average Risk Patients
326	Atrial Fibrillation and Atrial Flutter: Chronic Anticoagulation Therapy
407	Appropriate Treatment of Methicillin-Sensitive Staphylococcus Aureus (MSSA) Bacteremia
415	Emergency Medicine: ED Utilization of CT for Minor Blunt Head Trauma for Patients Aged 18 Years and Older
416	Emergency Medicine: ED Utilization of CT for Minor Blunt Head Trauma for Patients Aged 2 Through 17 years
418	Osteoporosis Management in Women Who Had a Fracture
419	Overuse Of Neuroimaging For Patients With Primary Headache And A Normal Neurological Examination
425	Photodocumentation of Cecal Intubation
435	Quality of Life Assessment For Patients With Primary Headache Disorders

Code	Description	CMS-HCC Model Category	QPP Individual Measures–Claims
19300	Mastectomy for gynecomastia		21, 23
19301	Mastectomy, partial (eg, lumpectomy, tylectomy, quadrantectomy, segmentectomy);		21, 23
19302	Mastectomy, partial (eg, lumpectomy, tylectomy, quadrantectomy, segmentectomy); with axillary lymphadenectomy		21, 23
19303	Mastectomy, simple, complete		21, 23
19304	Mastectomy, subcutaneous		21, 23
19305	Mastectomy, radical, including pectoral muscles, axillary lymph nodes		21, 23
19306	Mastectomy, radical, including pectoral muscles, axillary and internal mammary lymph nodes (Urban type operation)		21, 23
19307	Mastectomy, modified radical, including axillary lymph nodes, with or without pectoralis minor muscle, but excluding pectoralis major muscle		21, 23
33250	Operative ablation of supraventricular arrhythmogenic focus or pathway (eg, Wolff-Parkinson-White, atrioventricular node re-entry), tract(s) and/or focus (foci); without cardiopulmonary bypass		21

Code	Description	CMS-HCC Model Category	QPP Individual Measures–Claims
33251	Operative ablation of supraventricular arrhythmogenic focus or pathway (eg, Wolff-Parkinson-White, atrioventricular node re-entry), tract(s) and/or focus (foci); with cardiopulmonary bypass		21
33256	Operative tissue ablation and reconstruction of atria, extensive (eg, maze procedure); with cardiopulmonary bypass		21
33261	Operative ablation of ventricular arrhythmogenic focus with cardiopulmonary bypass		21
33320	Suture repair of aorta or great vessels; without shunt or cardiopulmonary bypass		21, 23
33321	Suture repair of aorta or great vessels; with shunt bypass		21
33322	Suture repair of aorta or great vessels; with cardiopulmonary bypass		21
44120	Enterectomy, resection of small intestine; single resection and anastomosis		21, 23
44140	Colectomy, partial; with anastomosis		21, 23
44150	Colectomy, total, abdominal, without proctectomy; with ileostomy or ileoproctostomy		21
44155	Colectomy, total, abdominal, with proctectomy; with ileostomy		21, 23
44160	Colectomy, total, abdominal, with proctectomy; with ileostomy		21
45378	Colonoscopy, flexible; diagnostic, including collection of specimen(s) by brushing or washing, when performed (separate procedure)		185, 320, 425
45380	Colonoscopy, flexible; with biopsy, single or multiple		185, 425
45381	Colonoscopy, flexible; with directed submucosal injection(s), any substance		185, 425
45384	Colonoscopy, flexible; with removal of tumor(s), polyp(s), or other lesion(s) by hot biopsy forceps		185, 425
45385	Colonoscopy, flexible; with removal of tumor(s), polyp(s), or other lesion(s) by snare technique		185, 425
45395	Laparoscopy, surgical; proctectomy, complete, combined abdominoperineal, with colostomy		21, 23
45397	Laparoscopy, surgical; proctectomy, combined abdominoperineal pull-through procedure (eg, colo-anal anastomosis), with creation of colonic reservoir (eg, J-pouch), with diverting enterostomy, when performed		21, 23
93453	Combined right and left heart catheterization including intraprocedural injection(s) for left ventriculography, imaging supervision and interpretation, when performed		145
44150	Colectomy, total, abdominal, without proctectomy; with ileostomy or ileoproctostomy		23
44160	Colectomy, partial, with removal of terminal ileum with ileocolostomy		23
99291	Critical care, evaluation and management of the critically ill or critically injured patient; first 30-74 minutes		1, 47, 254, 255, 407
A40.0	Sepsis due to streptococcus, group A	2	
A40.1	Sepsis due to streptococcus, group B	2	
A40.3	Sepsis due to Streptococcus pneumoniae	2	
A40.8	Other streptococcal sepsis	2	
A40.9	Streptococcal sepsis, unspecified	2	
A41.01	Sepsis due to Methicillin susceptible Staphylococcus aureus	2	407
A41.02	Sepsis due to Methicillin resistant Staphylococcus aureus	2	407
A41.1	Sepsis due to other specified staphylococcus	2	
A41.2	Sepsis due to unspecified staphylococcus	2	
A41.3	Sepsis due to Hemophilus influenzae	2	
A41.4	Sepsis due to anaerobes	2	
A41.50	Gram-negative sepsis, unspecified	2	

Code	Description	CMS-HCC Model Category	QPP Individual Measures–Claims
A41.51	Sepsis due to Escherichia coli [E. coli]	2	
A41.52	Sepsis due to Pseudomonas	2	
A41.53	Sepsis due to Serratia	2	
A41.59	Other Gram-negative sepsis	2	
A41.81	Sepsis due to Enterococcus	2	
A41.89	Other specified sepsis	2	
B2Ø	Human immunodeficiency virus [HIV] disease	1	
C22.Ø	Liver cell carcinoma	9	
C22.1	Intrahepatic bile duct carcinoma	9	
C22.2	Hepatoblastoma	9	
C22.3	Angiosarcoma of liver	9	
C22.4	Other sarcomas of liver	9	
C22.7	Other specified carcinomas of liver	9	
C22.8	Malignant neoplasm of liver, primary, unspecified as to type	9	
C22.9	Malignant neoplasm of liver, not specified as primary or secondary	9	
C5Ø.Ø11	Malignant neoplasm of nipple and areola, right female breast	12	99, 156, 251
C5Ø.Ø12	Malignant neoplasm of nipple and areola, left female breast	12	99, 156, 251
C5Ø.Ø19	Malignant neoplasm of nipple and areola, unspecified female breast	12	99, 156, 251
C5Ø.Ø21	Malignant neoplasm of nipple and areola, right male breast	12	99, 156, 251
C5Ø.Ø22	Malignant neoplasm of nipple and areola, left male breast	12	99, 156, 251
C5Ø.Ø29	Malignant neoplasm of nipple and areola, unspecified male breast	12	99, 156, 251
C5Ø.111	Malignant neoplasm of central portion of right female breast	12	99, 156, 251
C5Ø.112	Malignant neoplasm of central portion of left female breast	12	99, 156, 251
C5Ø.119	Malignant neoplasm of central portion of unspecified female breast	12	99, 156, 251
C5Ø.121	Malignant neoplasm of central portion of right male breast	12	99, 156, 251
C5Ø.122	Malignant neoplasm of central portion of left male breast	12	99, 156, 251
C5Ø.129	Malignant neoplasm of central portion of unspecified male breast	12	99, 156, 251
C5Ø.211	Malignant neoplasm of upper-inner quadrant of right female breast	12	99, 156, 251
C5Ø.212	Malignant neoplasm of upper-inner quadrant of left female breast	12	99, 156, 251
C5Ø.219	Malignant neoplasm of upper-inner quadrant of unspecified female breast	12	99, 156, 251
C5Ø.221	Malignant neoplasm of upper-inner quadrant of right male breast	12	99, 156, 251
C5Ø.222	Malignant neoplasm of upper-inner quadrant of left male breast	12	99, 156, 251
C5Ø.229	Malignant neoplasm of upper-inner quadrant of unspecified male breast	12	99, 156, 251
C5Ø.311	Malignant neoplasm of lower-inner quadrant of right female breast	12	99, 156, 251
C5Ø.312	Malignant neoplasm of lower-inner quadrant of left female breast	12	99, 156, 251
C5Ø.319	Malignant neoplasm of lower-inner quadrant of unspecified female breast	12	99, 156, 251
C5Ø.321	Malignant neoplasm of lower-inner quadrant of right male breast	12	99, 156, 251
C5Ø.322	Malignant neoplasm of lower-inner quadrant of left male breast	12	99, 156, 251
C5Ø.329	Malignant neoplasm of lower-inner quadrant of unspecified male breast	12	99, 156, 251
C5Ø.411	Malignant neoplasm of upper-outer quadrant of right female breast	12	99, 156, 251
C5Ø.412	Malignant neoplasm of upper-outer quadrant of left female breast	12	99, 156, 251
C5Ø.419	Malignant neoplasm of upper-outer quadrant of unspecified female breast	12	99, 156, 251

Code	Description	CMS-HCC Model Category	QPP Individual Measures–Claims
C5Ø.421	Malignant neoplasm of upper-outer quadrant of right male breast	12	99, 156, 251
C5Ø.422	Malignant neoplasm of upper-outer quadrant of left male breast	12	99, 156, 251
C5Ø.429	Malignant neoplasm of upper-outer quadrant of unspecified male breast	12	99, 156, 251
C5Ø.511	Malignant neoplasm of lower-outer quadrant of right female breast	12	99, 156, 251
C5Ø.512	Malignant neoplasm of lower-outer quadrant of left female breast	12	99, 156, 251
C5Ø.519	Malignant neoplasm of lower-outer quadrant of unspecified female breast	12	99, 156, 251
C5Ø.521	Malignant neoplasm of lower-outer quadrant of right male breast	12	99, 156, 251
C5Ø.522	Malignant neoplasm of lower-outer quadrant of left male breast	12	99, 156, 251
C5Ø.529	Malignant neoplasm of lower-outer quadrant of unspecified male breast	12	99, 156, 251
C5Ø.611	Malignant neoplasm of axillary tail of right female breast	12	99, 156, 251
C5Ø.612	Malignant neoplasm of axillary tail of left female breast	12	99, 156, 251
C5Ø.619	Malignant neoplasm of axillary tail of unspecified female breast	12	99, 156, 251
C5Ø.621	Malignant neoplasm of axillary tail of right male breast	12	99, 156, 251
C5Ø.622	Malignant neoplasm of axillary tail of left male breast	12	99, 156, 251
C5Ø.629	Malignant neoplasm of axillary tail of unspecified male breast	12	99, 156, 251
C5Ø.811	Malignant neoplasm of overlapping sites of right female breast	12	99, 156, 251
C5Ø.812	Malignant neoplasm of overlapping sites of left female breast	12	99, 156, 251
C5Ø.819	Malignant neoplasm of overlapping sites of unspecified female breast	12	99, 156, 251
C5Ø.821	Malignant neoplasm of overlapping sites of right male breast	12	99, 156, 251
C5Ø.822	Malignant neoplasm of overlapping sites of left male breast	12	99, 156, 251
C5Ø.829	Malignant neoplasm of overlapping sites of unspecified male breast	12	99, 156, 251
C5Ø.911	Malignant neoplasm of unspecified site of right female breast	12	99, 156, 251
C5Ø.912	Malignant neoplasm of unspecified site of left female breast	12	99, 156, 251
C5Ø.919	Malignant neoplasm of unspecified site of unspecified female breast	12	99, 156, 251
C5Ø.921	Malignant neoplasm of unspecified site of right male breast	12	99, 156, 251
C5Ø.922	Malignant neoplasm of unspecified site of left male breast	12	99, 156, 251
C5Ø.929	Malignant neoplasm of unspecified site of unspecified male breast	12	99, 156, 251
C79.11	Secondary malignant neoplasm of bladder	8	156
C79.19	Secondary malignant neoplasm of other urinary organs	8	156
C79.2	Secondary malignant neoplasm of skin	1Ø	156
C79.31	Secondary malignant neoplasm of brain	8	156
C79.81	Secondary malignant neoplasm of breast	1Ø	156
C79.82	Secondary malignant neoplasm of genital organs	1Ø	156
C79.89	Secondary malignant neoplasm of other specified sites	8	156
C79.9	Secondary malignant neoplasm of unspecified site	8	156
D59.1	Other autoimmune hemolytic anemias	46	
D59.2	Drug-induced nonautoimmune hemolytic anemia	46	
D59.3	Hemolytic-uremic syndrome	46	
D59.4	Other nonautoimmune hemolytic anemias	46	
D59.5	Paroxysmal nocturnal hemoglobinuria [Marchiafava-Micheli]	46	
D59.6	Hemoglobinuria due to hemolysis from other external causes	46	
D59.8	Other acquired hemolytic anemias	46	

Code	Description	CMS-HCC Model Category	QPP Individual Measures–Claims
D59.9	Acquired hemolytic anemia, unspecified	46	
EØ8.ØØ	Diabetes mellitus due to underlying condition with hyperosmolarity without nonketotic hyperglycemic-hyperosmolar coma (NKHHC)	17	
EØ8.Ø1	Diabetes mellitus due to underlying condition with hyperosmolarity with coma	17	
EØ8.1Ø	Diabetes mellitus due to underlying condition with ketoacidosis without coma	17	
EØ8.11	Diabetes mellitus due to underlying condition with ketoacidosis with coma	17	
EØ8.21	Diabetes mellitus due to underlying condition with diabetic nephropathy	18	
EØ8.22	Diabetes mellitus due to underlying condition with diabetic chronic kidney disease	18	
EØ8.29	Diabetes mellitus due to underlying condition with other diabetic kidney complication	18	
EØ8.311	Diabetes mellitus due to underlying condition with unspecified diabetic retinopathy with macular edema	18	19
EØ8.319	Diabetes mellitus due to underlying condition with unspecified diabetic retinopathy without macular edema	18	19
EØ8.321	Diabetes mellitus due to underlying condition with mild nonproliferative diabetic retinopathy with macular edema	18	
EØ8.3211	Diabetes mellitus due to underlying condition with mild nonproliferative diabetic retinopathy with macular edema, right eye	18	19
EØ8.3212	Diabetes mellitus due to underlying condition with mild nonproliferative diabetic retinopathy with macular edema, left eye	18	19
EØ8.3213	Diabetes mellitus due to underlying condition with mild nonproliferative diabetic retinopathy with macular edema, bilateral	18	19
EØ8.3219	Diabetes mellitus due to underlying condition with mild nonproliferative diabetic retinopathy with macular edema, unspecified eye	18	19
EØ8.329	Diabetes mellitus due to underlying condition with mild nonproliferative diabetic retinopathy without macular edema	18	
EØ8.3291	Diabetes mellitus due to underlying condition with mild nonproliferative diabetic retinopathy without macular edema, right eye	18	19
EØ8.3292	Diabetes mellitus due to underlying condition with mild nonproliferative diabetic retinopathy without macular edema, left eye	18	19
EØ8.3293	Diabetes mellitus due to underlying condition with mild nonproliferative diabetic retinopathy without macular edema, bilateral	18	19
EØ8.3299	Diabetes mellitus due to underlying condition with mild nonproliferative diabetic retinopathy without macular edema, unspecified eye	18	19
EØ8.331	Diabetes mellitus due to underlying condition with moderate nonproliferative diabetic retinopathy with macular edema	18	
EØ8.3311	Diabetes mellitus due to underlying condition with moderate nonproliferative diabetic retinopathy with macular edema, right eye	18	19
EØ8.3312	Diabetes mellitus due to underlying condition with moderate nonproliferative diabetic retinopathy with macular edema, left eye	18	19
EØ8.3313	Diabetes mellitus due to underlying condition with moderate nonproliferative diabetic retinopathy with macular edema, bilateral	18	19
EØ8.3319	Diabetes mellitus due to underlying condition with moderate nonproliferative diabetic retinopathy with macular edema, unspecified eye	18	19
EØ8.339	Diabetes mellitus due to underlying condition with moderate nonproliferative diabetic retinopathy without macular edema	18	
EØ8.3391	Diabetes mellitus due to underlying condition with moderate nonproliferative diabetic retinopathy without macular edema, right eye	18	19

Code	Description	CMS-HCC Model Category	QPP Individual Measures–Claims
EØ8.3392	Diabetes mellitus due to underlying condition with moderate nonproliferative diabetic retinopathy without macular edema, left eye	18	19
EØ8.3393	Diabetes mellitus due to underlying condition with moderate nonproliferative diabetic retinopathy without macular edema, bilateral	18	19
EØ8.3399	Diabetes mellitus due to underlying condition with moderate nonproliferative diabetic retinopathy without macular edema, unspecified eye	18	19
EØ8.341	Diabetes mellitus due to underlying condition with severe nonproliferative diabetic retinopathy with macular edema	18	
EØ8.3411	Diabetes mellitus due to underlying condition with severe nonproliferative diabetic retinopathy with macular edema, right eye	18	19
EØ8.3412	Diabetes mellitus due to underlying condition with severe nonproliferative diabetic retinopathy with macular edema, left eye	18	19
EØ8.3413	Diabetes mellitus due to underlying condition with severe nonproliferative diabetic retinopathy with macular edema, bilateral	18	19
EØ8.3419	Diabetes mellitus due to underlying condition with severe nonproliferative diabetic retinopathy with macular edema, unspecified eye	18	19
EØ8.349	Diabetes mellitus due to underlying condition with severe nonproliferative diabetic retinopathy without macular edema	18	
EØ8.3491	Diabetes mellitus due to underlying condition with severe nonproliferative diabetic retinopathy without macular edema, right eye	18	19
EØ8.3492	Diabetes mellitus due to underlying condition with severe nonproliferative diabetic retinopathy without macular edema, left eye	18	19
EØ8.3493	Diabetes mellitus due to underlying condition with severe nonproliferative diabetic retinopathy without macular edema, bilateral	18	19
EØ8.3499	Diabetes mellitus due to underlying condition with severe nonproliferative diabetic retinopathy without macular edema, unspecified eye	18	19
EØ8.351	Diabetes mellitus due to underlying condition with proliferative diabetic retinopathy with macular edema	18, 122	
EØ8.3511	Diabetes mellitus due to underlying condition with proliferative diabetic retinopathy with macular edema, right eye	18, 122	19
EØ8.3512	Diabetes mellitus due to underlying condition with proliferative diabetic retinopathy with macular edema, left eye	18, 122	19
EØ8.3513	Diabetes mellitus due to underlying condition with proliferative diabetic retinopathy with macular edema, bilateral	18, 122	19
EØ8.3519	Diabetes mellitus due to underlying condition with proliferative diabetic retinopathy with macular edema, unspecified eye	18, 122	19
EØ8.3521	Diabetes mellitus due to underlying condition with proliferative diabetic retinopathy with traction retinal detachment involving the macula, right eye	18, 122	19
EØ8.3522	Diabetes mellitus due to underlying condition with proliferative diabetic retinopathy with traction retinal detachment involving the macula, left eye	18, 122	19
EØ8.3523	Diabetes mellitus due to underlying condition with proliferative diabetic retinopathy with traction retinal detachment involving the macula, bilateral	18, 122	19
EØ8.3529	Diabetes mellitus due to underlying condition with proliferative diabetic retinopathy with traction retinal detachment involving the macula, unspecified eye	18, 122	19
EØ8.3531	Diabetes mellitus due to underlying condition with proliferative diabetic retinopathy with traction retinal detachment not involving the macula, right eye	18, 122	19
EØ8.3532	Diabetes mellitus due to underlying condition with proliferative diabetic retinopathy with traction retinal detachment not involving the macula, left eye	18, 122	19

Code	Description	CMS-HCC Model Category	QPP Individual Measures–Claims
E08.3533	Diabetes mellitus due to underlying condition with proliferative diabetic retinopathy with traction retinal detachment not involving the macula, bilateral	18, 122	19
E08.3539	Diabetes mellitus due to underlying condition with proliferative diabetic retinopathy with traction retinal detachment not involving the macula, unspecified eye	18, 122	19
E08.3541	Diabetes mellitus due to underlying condition with proliferative diabetic retinopathy with combined traction retinal detachment and rhegmatogenous retinal detachment, right eye	18, 122	19
E08.3542	Diabetes mellitus due to underlying condition with proliferative diabetic retinopathy with combined traction retinal detachment and rhegmatogenous retinal detachment, left eye	18, 122	19
E08.3543	Diabetes mellitus due to underlying condition with proliferative diabetic retinopathy with combined traction retinal detachment and rhegmatogenous retinal detachment, bilateral	18, 122	19
E08.3549	Diabetes mellitus due to underlying condition with proliferative diabetic retinopathy with combined traction retinal detachment and rhegmatogenous retinal detachment, unspecified eye	18, 122	19
E08.3551	Diabetes mellitus due to underlying condition with stable proliferative diabetic retinopathy, right eye	18, 122	19
E08.3552	Diabetes mellitus due to underlying condition with stable proliferative diabetic retinopathy, left eye	18, 122	19
E08.3553	Diabetes mellitus due to underlying condition with stable proliferative diabetic retinopathy, bilateral	18, 122	19
E08.3559	Diabetes mellitus due to underlying condition with stable proliferative diabetic retinopathy, unspecified eye	18, 122	19
E08.359	Diabetes mellitus due to underlying condition with proliferative diabetic retinopathy without macular edema	18, 122	
E08.3591	Diabetes mellitus due to underlying condition with proliferative diabetic retinopathy without macular edema, right eye	18, 122	19
E08.3592	Diabetes mellitus due to underlying condition with proliferative diabetic retinopathy without macular edema, left eye	18, 122	19
E08.3593	Diabetes mellitus due to underlying condition with proliferative diabetic retinopathy without macular edema, bilateral	18, 122	19
E08.3599	Diabetes mellitus due to underlying condition with proliferative diabetic retinopathy without macular edema, unspecified eye	18, 122	19
E08.36	Diabetes mellitus due to underlying condition with diabetic cataract	18	
E08.37X1	Diabetes mellitus due to underlying condition with diabetic macular edema, resolved following treatment, right eye	18	
E08.37X2	Diabetes mellitus due to underlying condition with diabetic macular edema, resolved following treatment, left eye	18	
E08.37X3	Diabetes mellitus due to underlying condition with diabetic macular edema, resolved following treatment, bilateral	18	
E08.37X9	Diabetes mellitus due to underlying condition with diabetic macular edema, resolved following treatment, unspecified eye	18	
E08.39	Diabetes mellitus due to underlying condition with other diabetic ophthalmic complication	18	
E08.40	Diabetes mellitus due to underlying condition with diabetic neuropathy, unspecified	18	
E08.41	Diabetes mellitus due to underlying condition with diabetic mononeuropathy	18	
E08.42	Diabetes mellitus due to underlying condition with diabetic polyneuropathy	18	
E08.43	Diabetes mellitus due to underlying condition with diabetic autonomic (poly)neuropathy	18	

Code	Description	CMS-HCC Model Category	QPP Individual Measures–Claims
E08.44	Diabetes mellitus due to underlying condition with diabetic amyotrophy	18	
E08.49	Diabetes mellitus due to underlying condition with other diabetic neurological complication	18	
E08.51	Diabetes mellitus due to underlying condition with diabetic peripheral angiopathy without gangrene	18, 108	
E08.52	Diabetes mellitus due to underlying condition with diabetic peripheral angiopathy with gangrene	18, 106, 108	
E08.59	Diabetes mellitus due to underlying condition with other circulatory complications	18	
E08.610	Diabetes mellitus due to underlying condition with diabetic neuropathic arthropathy	18	
E08.618	Diabetes mellitus due to underlying condition with other diabetic arthropathy	18	
E08.620	Diabetes mellitus due to underlying condition with diabetic dermatitis	18	
E08.621	Diabetes mellitus due to underlying condition with foot ulcer	18	
E08.622	Diabetes mellitus due to underlying condition with other skin ulcer	18	
E08.628	Diabetes mellitus due to underlying condition with other skin complications	18	
E08.630	Diabetes mellitus due to underlying condition with periodontal disease	18	
E08.638	Diabetes mellitus due to underlying condition with other oral complications	18	
E08.641	Diabetes mellitus due to underlying condition with hypoglycemia with coma	17	
E08.649	Diabetes mellitus due to underlying condition with hypoglycemia without coma	18	
E08.65	Diabetes mellitus due to underlying condition with hyperglycemia	18	
E08.69	Diabetes mellitus due to underlying condition with other specified complication	18	
E08.8	Diabetes mellitus due to underlying condition with unspecified complications	18	
E08.9	Diabetes mellitus due to underlying condition without complications	19	
E09.00	Drug or chemical induced diabetes mellitus with hyperosmolarity without nonketotic hyperglycemic-hyperosmolar coma (NKHHC)	17	
E09.01	Drug or chemical induced diabetes mellitus with hyperosmolarity with coma	17	
E09.10	Drug or chemical induced diabetes mellitus with ketoacidosis without coma	17	
E09.11	Drug or chemical induced diabetes mellitus with ketoacidosis with coma	17	
E09.21	Drug or chemical induced diabetes mellitus with diabetic nephropathy	18	
E09.22	Drug or chemical induced diabetes mellitus with diabetic chronic kidney disease	18	
E09.29	Drug or chemical induced diabetes mellitus with other diabetic kidney complication	18	
E09.311	Drug or chemical induced diabetes mellitus with unspecified diabetic retinopathy with macular edema	18	19
E09.319	Drug or chemical induced diabetes mellitus with unspecified diabetic retinopathy without macular edema	18	19
E09.321	Drug or chemical induced diabetes mellitus with mild nonproliferative diabetic retinopathy with macular edema	18	
E09.3211	Drug or chemical induced diabetes mellitus with mild nonproliferative diabetic retinopathy with macular edema, right eye	18	19
E09.3212	Drug or chemical induced diabetes mellitus with mild nonproliferative diabetic retinopathy with macular edema, left eye	18	19
E09.3213	Drug or chemical induced diabetes mellitus with mild nonproliferative diabetic retinopathy with macular edema, bilateral	18	19
E09.3219	Drug or chemical induced diabetes mellitus with mild nonproliferative diabetic retinopathy with macular edema, unspecified eye	18	19
E09.329	Drug or chemical induced diabetes mellitus with mild nonproliferative diabetic retinopathy without macular edema	18	

Code	Description	CMS-HCC Model Category	QPP Individual Measures–Claims
EØ9.3291	Drug or chemical induced diabetes mellitus with mild nonproliferative diabetic retinopathy without macular edema, right eye	18	19
EØ9.3292	Drug or chemical induced diabetes mellitus with mild nonproliferative diabetic retinopathy without macular edema, left eye	18	19
EØ9.3293	Drug or chemical induced diabetes mellitus with mild nonproliferative diabetic retinopathy without macular edema, bilateral	18	19
EØ9.3299	Drug or chemical induced diabetes mellitus with mild nonproliferative diabetic retinopathy without macular edema, unspecified eye	18	19
EØ9.331	Drug or chemical induced diabetes mellitus with moderate nonproliferative diabetic retinopathy with macular edema	18	
EØ9.3311	Drug or chemical induced diabetes mellitus with moderate nonproliferative diabetic retinopathy with macular edema, right eye	18	19
EØ9.3312	Drug or chemical induced diabetes mellitus with moderate nonproliferative diabetic retinopathy with macular edema, left eye	18	19
EØ9.3313	Drug or chemical induced diabetes mellitus with moderate nonproliferative diabetic retinopathy with macular edema, bilateral	18	19
EØ9.3319	Drug or chemical induced diabetes mellitus with moderate nonproliferative diabetic retinopathy with macular edema, unspecified eye	18	19
EØ9.339	Drug or chemical induced diabetes mellitus with moderate nonproliferative diabetic retinopathy without macular edema	18	
EØ9.3391	Drug or chemical induced diabetes mellitus with moderate nonproliferative diabetic retinopathy without macular edema, right eye	18	19
EØ9.3392	Drug or chemical induced diabetes mellitus with moderate nonproliferative diabetic retinopathy without macular edema, left eye	18	19
EØ9.3393	Drug or chemical induced diabetes mellitus with moderate nonproliferative diabetic retinopathy without macular edema, bilateral	18	19
EØ9.3399	Drug or chemical induced diabetes mellitus with moderate nonproliferative diabetic retinopathy without macular edema, unspecified eye	18	19
EØ9.341	Drug or chemical induced diabetes mellitus with severe nonproliferative diabetic retinopathy with macular edema	18	
EØ9.3411	Drug or chemical induced diabetes mellitus with severe nonproliferative diabetic retinopathy with macular edema, right eye	18	19
EØ9.3412	Drug or chemical induced diabetes mellitus with severe nonproliferative diabetic retinopathy with macular edema, left eye	18	19
EØ9.3413	Drug or chemical induced diabetes mellitus with severe nonproliferative diabetic retinopathy with macular edema, bilateral	18	19
EØ9.3419	Drug or chemical induced diabetes mellitus with severe nonproliferative diabetic retinopathy with macular edema, unspecified eye	18	19
EØ9.349	Drug or chemical induced diabetes mellitus with severe nonproliferative diabetic retinopathy without macular edema	18	
EØ9.3491	Drug or chemical induced diabetes mellitus with severe nonproliferative diabetic retinopathy without macular edema, right eye	18	19
EØ9.3492	Drug or chemical induced diabetes mellitus with severe nonproliferative diabetic retinopathy without macular edema, left eye	18	19
EØ9.3493	Drug or chemical induced diabetes mellitus with severe nonproliferative diabetic retinopathy without macular edema, bilateral	18	19
EØ9.3499	Drug or chemical induced diabetes mellitus with severe nonproliferative diabetic retinopathy without macular edema, unspecified eye	18	19

Code	Description	CMS-HCC Model Category	QPP Individual Measures–Claims
EØ9.351	Drug or chemical induced diabetes mellitus with proliferative diabetic retinopathy with macular edema	18, 122	
EØ9.3511	Drug or chemical induced diabetes mellitus with proliferative diabetic retinopathy with macular edema, right eye	18, 122	19
EØ9.3512	Drug or chemical induced diabetes mellitus with proliferative diabetic retinopathy with macular edema, left eye	18, 122	19
EØ9.3513	Drug or chemical induced diabetes mellitus with proliferative diabetic retinopathy with macular edema, bilateral	18, 122	19
EØ9.3519	Drug or chemical induced diabetes mellitus with proliferative diabetic retinopathy with macular edema, unspecified eye	18, 122	19
EØ9.3521	Drug or chemical induced diabetes mellitus with proliferative diabetic retinopathy with traction retinal detachment involving the macula, right eye	18, 122	19
EØ9.3522	Drug or chemical induced diabetes mellitus with proliferative diabetic retinopathy with traction retinal detachment involving the macula, left eye	18, 122	19
EØ9.3523	Drug or chemical induced diabetes mellitus with proliferative diabetic retinopathy with traction retinal detachment involving the macula, bilateral	18, 122	19
EØ9.3529	Drug or chemical induced diabetes mellitus with proliferative diabetic retinopathy with traction retinal detachment involving the macula, unspecified eye	18, 122	19
EØ9.3531	Drug or chemical induced diabetes mellitus with proliferative diabetic retinopathy with traction retinal detachment not involving the macula, right eye	18, 122	19
EØ9.3532	Drug or chemical induced diabetes mellitus with proliferative diabetic retinopathy with traction retinal detachment not involving the macula, left eye	18, 122	19
EØ9.3533	Drug or chemical induced diabetes mellitus with proliferative diabetic retinopathy with traction retinal detachment not involving the macula, bilateral	18, 122	19
EØ9.3539	Drug or chemical induced diabetes mellitus with proliferative diabetic retinopathy with traction retinal detachment not involving the macula, unspecified eye	18, 122	19
EØ9.3541	Drug or chemical induced diabetes mellitus with proliferative diabetic retinopathy with combined traction retinal detachment and rhegmatogenous retinal detachment, right eye	18, 122	19
EØ9.3542	Drug or chemical induced diabetes mellitus with proliferative diabetic retinopathy with combined traction retinal detachment and rhegmatogenous retinal detachment, left eye	18, 122	19
EØ9.3543	Drug or chemical induced diabetes mellitus with proliferative diabetic retinopathy with combined traction retinal detachment and rhegmatogenous retinal detachment, bilateral	18, 122	19
EØ9.3549	Drug or chemical induced diabetes mellitus with proliferative diabetic retinopathy with combined traction retinal detachment and rhegmatogenous retinal detachment, unspecified eye	18, 122	19
EØ9.3551	Drug or chemical induced diabetes mellitus with stable proliferative diabetic retinopathy, right eye	18, 122	19
EØ9.3552	Drug or chemical induced diabetes mellitus with stable proliferative diabetic retinopathy, left eye	18, 122	19
EØ9.3553	Drug or chemical induced diabetes mellitus with stable proliferative diabetic retinopathy, bilateral	18, 122	19
EØ9.3559	Drug or chemical induced diabetes mellitus with stable proliferative diabetic retinopathy, unspecified eye	18, 122	19
EØ9.359	Drug or chemical induced diabetes mellitus with proliferative diabetic retinopathy without macular edema	18, 122	
EØ9.3591	Drug or chemical induced diabetes mellitus with proliferative diabetic retinopathy without macular edema, right eye	18, 122	19

Code	Description	CMS-HCC Model Category	QPP Individual Measures–Claims
EØ9.3592	Drug or chemical induced diabetes mellitus with proliferative diabetic retinopathy without macular edema, left eye	18, 122	19
EØ9.3593	Drug or chemical induced diabetes mellitus with proliferative diabetic retinopathy without macular edema, bilateral	18, 122	19
EØ9.3599	Drug or chemical induced diabetes mellitus with proliferative diabetic retinopathy without macular edema, unspecified eye	18, 122	19
EØ9.36	Drug or chemical induced diabetes mellitus with diabetic cataract	18	
EØ9.37X1	Drug or chemical induced diabetes mellitus with diabetic macular edema, resolved following treatment, right eye	18	
EØ9.37X2	Drug or chemical induced diabetes mellitus with diabetic macular edema, resolved following treatment, left eye	18	
EØ9.37X3	Drug or chemical induced diabetes mellitus with diabetic macular edema, resolved following treatment, bilateral	18	
EØ9.37X9	Drug or chemical induced diabetes mellitus with diabetic macular edema, resolved following treatment, unspecified eye	18	
EØ9.39	Drug or chemical induced diabetes mellitus with other diabetic ophthalmic complication	18	
EØ9.4Ø	Drug or chemical induced diabetes mellitus with neurological complications with diabetic neuropathy, unspecified	18	
EØ9.41	Drug or chemical induced diabetes mellitus with neurological complications with diabetic mononeuropathy	18	
EØ9.42	Drug or chemical induced diabetes mellitus with neurological complications with diabetic polyneuropathy	18	
EØ9.43	Drug or chemical induced diabetes mellitus with neurological complications with diabetic autonomic (poly)neuropathy	18	
EØ9.44	Drug or chemical induced diabetes mellitus with neurological complications with diabetic amyotrophy	18	
EØ9.49	Drug or chemical induced diabetes mellitus with neurological complications with other diabetic neurological complication	18	
EØ9.51	Drug or chemical induced diabetes mellitus with diabetic peripheral angiopathy without gangrene	18, 1Ø8	
EØ9.52	Drug or chemical induced diabetes mellitus with diabetic peripheral angiopathy with gangrene	18, 1Ø6, 1Ø8	
EØ9.59	Drug or chemical induced diabetes mellitus with other circulatory complications	18	
EØ9.61Ø	Drug or chemical induced diabetes mellitus with diabetic neuropathic arthropathy	18	
EØ9.618	Drug or chemical induced diabetes mellitus with other diabetic arthropathy	18	
EØ9.62Ø	Drug or chemical induced diabetes mellitus with diabetic dermatitis	18	
EØ9.621	Drug or chemical induced diabetes mellitus with foot ulcer	18	
EØ9.622	Drug or chemical induced diabetes mellitus with other skin ulcer	18	
EØ9.628	Drug or chemical induced diabetes mellitus with other skin complications	18	
EØ9.63Ø	Drug or chemical induced diabetes mellitus with periodontal disease	18	
EØ9.638	Drug or chemical induced diabetes mellitus with other oral complications	18	
EØ9.641	Drug or chemical induced diabetes mellitus with hypoglycemia with coma	17	
EØ9.649	Drug or chemical induced diabetes mellitus with hypoglycemia without coma	18	
EØ9.65	Drug or chemical induced diabetes mellitus with hyperglycemia	18	
EØ9.69	Drug or chemical induced diabetes mellitus with other specified complication	18	
EØ9.8	Drug or chemical induced diabetes mellitus with unspecified complications	18	

Code	Description	CMS-HCC Model Category	QPP Individual Measures–Claims
E09.9	Drug or chemical induced diabetes mellitus without complications	19	
E10.10	Type 1 diabetes mellitus with ketoacidosis without coma	17	1, 117
E10.11	Type 1 diabetes mellitus with ketoacidosis with coma	17	1, 117
E10.21	Type 1 diabetes mellitus with diabetic nephropathy	18	1, 117
E10.22	Type 1 diabetes mellitus with diabetic chronic kidney disease	18	1, 117
E10.29	Type 1 diabetes mellitus with other diabetic kidney complication	18	1, 117
E10.311	Type 1 diabetes mellitus with unspecified diabetic retinopathy with macular edema	18	1, 19, 117
E10.319	Type 1 diabetes mellitus with unspecified diabetic retinopathy without macular edema	18	1, 19, 117
E10.321	Type 1 diabetes mellitus with mild nonproliferative diabetic retinopathy with macular edema	18	
E10.3211	Type 1 diabetes mellitus with mild nonproliferative diabetic retinopathy with macular edema, right eye	18	1, 19, 117
E10.3212	Type 1 diabetes mellitus with mild nonproliferative diabetic retinopathy with macular edema, left eye	18	1, 19, 117
E10.3213	Type 1 diabetes mellitus with mild nonproliferative diabetic retinopathy with macular edema, bilateral	18	1, 19, 117
E10.3219	Type 1 diabetes mellitus with mild nonproliferative diabetic retinopathy with macular edema, unspecified eye	18	1, 19, 117
E10.329	Type 1 diabetes mellitus with mild nonproliferative diabetic retinopathy without macular edema	18	
E10.3291	Type 1 diabetes mellitus with mild nonproliferative diabetic retinopathy without macular edema, right eye	18	1, 19, 117
E10.3292	Type 1 diabetes mellitus with mild nonproliferative diabetic retinopathy without macular edema, left eye	18	1, 19, 117
E10.3293	Type 1 diabetes mellitus with mild nonproliferative diabetic retinopathy without macular edema, bilateral	18	1, 19, 117
E10.3299	Type 1 diabetes mellitus with mild nonproliferative diabetic retinopathy without macular edema, unspecified eye	18	1, 19, 117
E10.331	Type 1 diabetes mellitus with moderate nonproliferative diabetic retinopathy with macular edema	18	
E10.3311	Type 1 diabetes mellitus with moderate nonproliferative diabetic retinopathy with macular edema, right eye	18	1, 19, 117
E10.3312	Type 1 diabetes mellitus with moderate nonproliferative diabetic retinopathy with macular edema, left eye	18	1, 19, 117
E10.3313	Type 1 diabetes mellitus with moderate nonproliferative diabetic retinopathy with macular edema, bilateral	18	1, 19, 117
E10.3319	Type 1 diabetes mellitus with moderate nonproliferative diabetic retinopathy with macular edema, unspecified eye	18	1, 19, 117
E10.339	Type 1 diabetes mellitus with moderate nonproliferative diabetic retinopathy without macular edema	18	
E10.3391	Type 1 diabetes mellitus with moderate nonproliferative diabetic retinopathy without macular edema, right eye	18	1, 19, 117
E10.3392	Type 1 diabetes mellitus with moderate nonproliferative diabetic retinopathy without macular edema, left eye	18	1, 19, 117
E10.3393	Type 1 diabetes mellitus with moderate nonproliferative diabetic retinopathy without macular edema, bilateral	18	1, 19, 117
E10.3399	Type 1 diabetes mellitus with moderate nonproliferative diabetic retinopathy without macular edema, unspecified eye	18	1, 19, 117

Code	Description	CMS-HCC Model Category	QPP Individual Measures–Claims
E10.341	Type 1 diabetes mellitus with severe nonproliferative diabetic retinopathy with macular edema	18	
E10.3411	Type 1 diabetes mellitus with severe nonproliferative diabetic retinopathy with macular edema, right eye	18	1, 19, 117
E10.3412	Type 1 diabetes mellitus with severe nonproliferative diabetic retinopathy with macular edema, left eye	18	1, 19, 117
E10.3413	Type 1 diabetes mellitus with severe nonproliferative diabetic retinopathy with macular edema, bilateral	18	1, 19, 117
E10.3419	Type 1 diabetes mellitus with severe nonproliferative diabetic retinopathy with macular edema, unspecified eye	18	1, 19, 117
E10.349	Type 1 diabetes mellitus with severe nonproliferative diabetic retinopathy without macular edema	18	
E10.3491	Type 1 diabetes mellitus with severe nonproliferative diabetic retinopathy without macular edema, right eye	18	1, 19, 117
E10.3492	Type 1 diabetes mellitus with severe nonproliferative diabetic retinopathy without macular edema, left eye	18	1, 19, 117
E10.3493	Type 1 diabetes mellitus with severe nonproliferative diabetic retinopathy without macular edema, bilateral	18	1, 19, 117
E10.3499	Type 1 diabetes mellitus with severe nonproliferative diabetic retinopathy without macular edema, unspecified eye	18	1, 19, 117
E10.351	Type 1 diabetes mellitus with proliferative diabetic retinopathy with macular edema	18, 122	
E10.3511	Type 1 diabetes mellitus with proliferative diabetic retinopathy with macular edema, right eye	18, 122	1, 19, 117
E10.3512	Type 1 diabetes mellitus with proliferative diabetic retinopathy with macular edema, left eye	18, 122	1, 19, 117
E10.3513	Type 1 diabetes mellitus with proliferative diabetic retinopathy with macular edema, bilateral	18, 122	1, 19, 117
E10.3519	Type 1 diabetes mellitus with proliferative diabetic retinopathy with macular edema, unspecified eye	18, 122	1, 19, 117
E10.3521	Type 1 diabetes mellitus with proliferative diabetic retinopathy with traction retinal detachment involving the macula, right eye	18, 122	1, 19, 117
E10.3522	Type 1 diabetes mellitus with proliferative diabetic retinopathy with traction retinal detachment involving the macula, left eye	18, 122	1, 19, 117
E10.3523	Type 1 diabetes mellitus with proliferative diabetic retinopathy with traction retinal detachment involving the macula, bilateral	18, 122	1, 19, 117
E10.3529	Type 1 diabetes mellitus with proliferative diabetic retinopathy with traction retinal detachment involving the macula, unspecified eye	18, 122	1, 19, 117
E10.3531	Type 1 diabetes mellitus with proliferative diabetic retinopathy with traction retinal detachment not involving the macula, right eye	18, 122	1, 19, 117
E10.3532	Type 1 diabetes mellitus with proliferative diabetic retinopathy with traction retinal detachment not involving the macula, left eye	18, 122	1, 19, 117
E10.3533	Type 1 diabetes mellitus with proliferative diabetic retinopathy with traction retinal detachment not involving the macula, bilateral	18, 122	1, 19, 117
E10.3539	Type 1 diabetes mellitus with proliferative diabetic retinopathy with traction retinal detachment not involving the macula, unspecified eye	18, 122	1, 19, 117
E10.3541	Type 1 diabetes mellitus with proliferative diabetic retinopathy with combined traction retinal detachment and rhegmatogenous retinal detachment, right eye	18, 122	1, 19, 117
E10.3542	Type 1 diabetes mellitus with proliferative diabetic retinopathy with combined traction retinal detachment and rhegmatogenous retinal detachment, left eye	18, 122	1, 19, 117

Code	Description	CMS-HCC Model Category	QPP Individual Measures–Claims
E10.3543	Type 1 diabetes mellitus with proliferative diabetic retinopathy with combined traction retinal detachment and rhegmatogenous retinal detachment, bilateral	18, 122	1, 19, 117
E10.3549	Type 1 diabetes mellitus with proliferative diabetic retinopathy with combined traction retinal detachment and rhegmatogenous retinal detachment, unspecified eye	18, 122	1, 19, 117
E10.3551	Type 1 diabetes mellitus with stable proliferative diabetic retinopathy, right eye	18, 122	1, 19, 117
E10.3552	Type 1 diabetes mellitus with stable proliferative diabetic retinopathy, left eye	18, 122	1, 19, 117
E10.3553	Type 1 diabetes mellitus with stable proliferative diabetic retinopathy, bilateral	18, 122	1, 19, 117
E10.3559	Type 1 diabetes mellitus with stable proliferative diabetic retinopathy, unspecified eye	18, 122	1, 19, 117
E10.359	Type 1 diabetes mellitus with proliferative diabetic retinopathy without macular edema	18, 122	
E10.3591	Type 1 diabetes mellitus with proliferative diabetic retinopathy without macular edema, right eye	18, 122	1, 19, 117
E10.3592	Type 1 diabetes mellitus with proliferative diabetic retinopathy without macular edema, left eye	18, 122	1, 19, 117
E10.3593	Type 1 diabetes mellitus with proliferative diabetic retinopathy without macular edema, bilateral	18, 122	1, 19, 117
E10.3599	Type 1 diabetes mellitus with proliferative diabetic retinopathy without macular edema, unspecified eye	18, 122	1, 19, 117
E10.36	Type 1 diabetes mellitus with diabetic cataract	18	1, 117
E10.37X1	Type 1 diabetes mellitus with diabetic macular edema, resolved following treatment, right eye	18	1, 117
E10.37X2	Type 1 diabetes mellitus with diabetic macular edema, resolved following treatment, left eye	18	1, 117
E10.37X3	Type 1 diabetes mellitus with diabetic macular edema, resolved following treatment, bilateral	18	1, 117
E10.37X9	Type 1 diabetes mellitus with diabetic macular edema, resolved following treatment, unspecified eye	18	1, 117
E10.39	Type 1 diabetes mellitus with other diabetic ophthalmic complication	18	1, 117
E10.40	Type 1 diabetes mellitus with diabetic neuropathy, unspecified	18	1, 117
E10.41	Type 1 diabetes mellitus with diabetic mononeuropathy	18	1, 117
E10.42	Type 1 diabetes mellitus with diabetic polyneuropathy	18	1, 117
E10.43	Type 1 diabetes mellitus with diabetic autonomic (poly)neuropathy	18	1, 117
E10.44	Type 1 diabetes mellitus with diabetic amyotrophy	18	1, 117
E10.49	Type 1 diabetes mellitus with other diabetic neurological complication	18	1, 117
E10.51	Type 1 diabetes mellitus with diabetic peripheral angiopathy without gangrene	18, 108	1, 117
E10.52	Type 1 diabetes mellitus with diabetic peripheral angiopathy with gangrene	18, 106, 108	1, 117
E10.59	Type 1 diabetes mellitus with other circulatory complications	18	1, 117
E10.610	Type 1 diabetes mellitus with diabetic neuropathic arthropathy	18	1, 117
E10.618	Type 1 diabetes mellitus with other diabetic arthropathy	18	1, 117
E10.620	Type 1 diabetes mellitus with diabetic dermatitis	18	1, 117
E10.621	Type 1 diabetes mellitus with foot ulcer	18	1, 117
E10.622	Type 1 diabetes mellitus with other skin ulcer	18	1, 117
E10.628	Type 1 diabetes mellitus with other skin complications	18	1, 117
E10.630	Type 1 diabetes mellitus with periodontal disease	18	1, 117
E10.638	Type 1 diabetes mellitus with other oral complications	18	1, 117
E10.641	Type 1 diabetes mellitus with hypoglycemia with coma	17	1, 117

Code	Description	CMS-HCC Model Category	QPP Individual Measures–Claims
E10.649	Type 1 diabetes mellitus with hypoglycemia without coma	18	1, 117
E10.65	Type 1 diabetes mellitus with hyperglycemia	18	1, 117
E10.69	Type 1 diabetes mellitus with other specified complication	18	1, 117
E10.8	Type 1 diabetes mellitus with unspecified complications	18	1, 117
E10.9	Type 1 diabetes mellitus without complications	19	1, 117
E11.00	Type 2 diabetes mellitus with hyperosmolarity without nonketotic hyperglycemic-hyperosmolar coma (NKHHC)	17	1, 117
E11.01	Type 2 diabetes mellitus with hyperosmolarity with coma	17	1, 117
E11.21	Type 2 diabetes mellitus with diabetic nephropathy	18	1, 117
E11.22	Type 2 diabetes mellitus with diabetic chronic kidney disease	18	1, 117
E11.29	Type 2 diabetes mellitus with other diabetic kidney complication	18	1, 117
E11.311	Type 2 diabetes mellitus with unspecified diabetic retinopathy with macular edema	18	1, 19, 117
E11.319	Type 2 diabetes mellitus with unspecified diabetic retinopathy without macular edema	18	1, 19, 117
E11.321	Type 2 diabetes mellitus with mild nonproliferative diabetic retinopathy with macular edema	18	
E11.3211	Type 2 diabetes mellitus with mild nonproliferative diabetic retinopathy with macular edema, right eye	18	1, 19, 117
E11.3212	Type 2 diabetes mellitus with mild nonproliferative diabetic retinopathy with macular edema, left eye	18	1, 19, 117
E11.3213	Type 2 diabetes mellitus with mild nonproliferative diabetic retinopathy with macular edema, bilateral	18	1, 19, 117
E11.3219	Type 2 diabetes mellitus with mild nonproliferative diabetic retinopathy with macular edema, unspecified eye	18	1, 19, 117
E11.329	Type 2 diabetes mellitus with mild nonproliferative diabetic retinopathy without macular edema	18	
E11.3291	Type 2 diabetes mellitus with mild nonproliferative diabetic retinopathy without macular edema, right eye	18	1, 19, 117
E11.3292	Type 2 diabetes mellitus with mild nonproliferative diabetic retinopathy without macular edema, left eye	18	1, 19, 117
E11.3293	Type 2 diabetes mellitus with mild nonproliferative diabetic retinopathy without macular edema, bilateral	18	1, 19, 117
E11.3299	Type 2 diabetes mellitus with mild nonproliferative diabetic retinopathy without macular edema, unspecified eye	18	1, 19, 117
E11.331	Type 2 diabetes mellitus with moderate nonproliferative diabetic retinopathy with macular edema	18	
E11.3311	Type 2 diabetes mellitus with moderate nonproliferative diabetic retinopathy with macular edema, right eye	18	1, 19, 117
E11.3312	Type 2 diabetes mellitus with moderate nonproliferative diabetic retinopathy with macular edema, left eye	18	1, 19, 117
E11.3313	Type 2 diabetes mellitus with moderate nonproliferative diabetic retinopathy with macular edema, bilateral	18	1, 19, 117
E11.3319	Type 2 diabetes mellitus with moderate nonproliferative diabetic retinopathy with macular edema, unspecified eye	18	1, 19, 117
E11.339	Type 2 diabetes mellitus with moderate nonproliferative diabetic retinopathy without macular edema	18	
E11.3391	Type 2 diabetes mellitus with moderate nonproliferative diabetic retinopathy without macular edema, right eye	18	1, 19, 117

Code	Description	CMS-HCC Model Category	QPP Individual Measures–Claims
E11.3392	Type 2 diabetes mellitus with moderate nonproliferative diabetic retinopathy without macular edema, left eye	18	1, 19, 117
E11.3393	Type 2 diabetes mellitus with moderate nonproliferative diabetic retinopathy without macular edema, bilateral	18	1, 19, 117
E11.3399	Type 2 diabetes mellitus with moderate nonproliferative diabetic retinopathy without macular edema, unspecified eye	18	1, 19, 117
E11.341	Type 2 diabetes mellitus with severe nonproliferative diabetic retinopathy with macular edema	18	
E11.3411	Type 2 diabetes mellitus with severe nonproliferative diabetic retinopathy with macular edema, right eye	18	1, 19, 117
E11.3412	Type 2 diabetes mellitus with severe nonproliferative diabetic retinopathy with macular edema, left eye	18	1, 19, 117
E11.3413	Type 2 diabetes mellitus with severe nonproliferative diabetic retinopathy with macular edema, bilateral	18	1, 19, 117
E11.3419	Type 2 diabetes mellitus with severe nonproliferative diabetic retinopathy with macular edema, unspecified eye	18	1, 19, 117
E11.349	Type 2 diabetes mellitus with severe nonproliferative diabetic retinopathy without macular edema	18	
E11.3491	Type 2 diabetes mellitus with severe nonproliferative diabetic retinopathy without macular edema, right eye	18	1, 19, 117
E11.3492	Type 2 diabetes mellitus with severe nonproliferative diabetic retinopathy without macular edema, left eye	18	1, 19, 117
E11.3493	Type 2 diabetes mellitus with severe nonproliferative diabetic retinopathy without macular edema, bilateral	18	1, 19, 117
E11.3499	Type 2 diabetes mellitus with severe nonproliferative diabetic retinopathy without macular edema, unspecified eye	18	1, 19, 117
E11.351	Type 2 diabetes mellitus with proliferative diabetic retinopathy with macular edema	18, 122	
E11.3511	Type 2 diabetes mellitus with proliferative diabetic retinopathy with macular edema, right eye	18, 122	1, 19, 117
E11.3512	Type 2 diabetes mellitus with proliferative diabetic retinopathy with macular edema, left eye	18, 122	1, 19, 117
E11.3513	Type 2 diabetes mellitus with proliferative diabetic retinopathy with macular edema, bilateral	18, 122	1, 19, 117
E11.3519	Type 2 diabetes mellitus with proliferative diabetic retinopathy with macular edema, unspecified eye	18, 122	1, 19, 117
E11.3521	Type 2 diabetes mellitus with proliferative diabetic retinopathy with traction retinal detachment involving the macula, right eye	18, 122	1, 19, 117
E11.3522	Type 2 diabetes mellitus with proliferative diabetic retinopathy with traction retinal detachment involving the macula, left eye	18, 122	1, 19, 117
E11.3523	Type 2 diabetes mellitus with proliferative diabetic retinopathy with traction retinal detachment involving the macula, bilateral	18, 122	1, 19, 117
E11.3529	Type 2 diabetes mellitus with proliferative diabetic retinopathy with traction retinal detachment involving the macula, unspecified eye	18, 122	1, 19, 117
E11.3531	Type 2 diabetes mellitus with proliferative diabetic retinopathy with traction retinal detachment not involving the macula, right eye	18, 122	1, 19, 117
E11.3532	Type 2 diabetes mellitus with proliferative diabetic retinopathy with traction retinal detachment not involving the macula, left eye	18, 122	1, 19, 117
E11.3533	Type 2 diabetes mellitus with proliferative diabetic retinopathy with traction retinal detachment not involving the macula, bilateral	18, 122	1, 19, 117

Code	Description	CMS-HCC Model Category	QPP Individual Measures–Claims
E11.3539	Type 2 diabetes mellitus with proliferative diabetic retinopathy with traction retinal detachment not involving the macula, unspecified eye	18, 122	1, 19, 117
E11.3541	Type 2 diabetes mellitus with proliferative diabetic retinopathy with combined traction retinal detachment and rhegmatogenous retinal detachment, right eye	18, 122	1, 19, 117
E11.3542	Type 2 diabetes mellitus with proliferative diabetic retinopathy with combined traction retinal detachment and rhegmatogenous retinal detachment, left eye	18, 122	1, 19, 117
E11.3543	Type 2 diabetes mellitus with proliferative diabetic retinopathy with combined traction retinal detachment and rhegmatogenous retinal detachment, bilateral	18, 122	1, 19, 117
E11.3549	Type 2 diabetes mellitus with proliferative diabetic retinopathy with combined traction retinal detachment and rhegmatogenous retinal detachment, unspecified eye	18, 122	1, 19, 117
E11.3551	Type 2 diabetes mellitus with stable proliferative diabetic retinopathy, right eye	18, 122	1, 19, 117
E11.3552	Type 2 diabetes mellitus with stable proliferative diabetic retinopathy, left eye	18, 122	1, 19, 117
E11.3553	Type 2 diabetes mellitus with stable proliferative diabetic retinopathy, bilateral	18, 122	1, 19, 117
E11.3559	Type 2 diabetes mellitus with stable proliferative diabetic retinopathy, unspecified eye	18, 122	1, 19, 117
E11.359	Type 2 diabetes mellitus with proliferative diabetic retinopathy without macular edema	18, 122	
E11.3591	Type 2 diabetes mellitus with proliferative diabetic retinopathy without macular edema, right eye	18, 122	1, 19, 117
E11.3592	Type 2 diabetes mellitus with proliferative diabetic retinopathy without macular edema, left eye	18, 122	1, 19, 117
E11.3593	Type 2 diabetes mellitus with proliferative diabetic retinopathy without macular edema, bilateral	18, 122	1, 19, 117
E11.3599	Type 2 diabetes mellitus with proliferative diabetic retinopathy without macular edema, unspecified eye	18	1, 19, 117
E11.36	Type 2 diabetes mellitus with diabetic cataract	18	1, 117
E11.37X1	Type 2 diabetes mellitus with diabetic macular edema, resolved following treatment, right eye	18	1, 117
E11.37X2	Type 2 diabetes mellitus with diabetic macular edema, resolved following treatment, left eye	18	1, 117
E11.37X3	Type 2 diabetes mellitus with diabetic macular edema, resolved following treatment, bilateral	18	1, 117
E11.37X9	Type 2 diabetes mellitus with diabetic macular edema, resolved following treatment, unspecified eye	18	1, 117
E11.39	Type 2 diabetes mellitus with other diabetic ophthalmic complication	18	1, 117
E11.4Ø	Type 2 diabetes mellitus with diabetic neuropathy, unspecified	18	1, 117
E11.41	Type 2 diabetes mellitus with diabetic mononeuropathy	18	1, 117
E11.42	Type 2 diabetes mellitus with diabetic polyneuropathy	18	1, 117
E11.43	Type 2 diabetes mellitus with diabetic autonomic (poly)neuropathy	18	1, 117
E11.44	Type 2 diabetes mellitus with diabetic amyotrophy	18	1, 117
E11.49	Type 2 diabetes mellitus with other diabetic neurological complication	18	1, 117
E11.51	Type 2 diabetes mellitus with diabetic peripheral angiopathy without gangrene	18, 1Ø8	1, 117
E11.52	Type 2 diabetes mellitus with diabetic peripheral angiopathy with gangrene	18, 1Ø6, 1Ø8	1, 117
E11.59	Type 2 diabetes mellitus with other circulatory complications	18	1, 117
E11.61Ø	Type 2 diabetes mellitus with diabetic neuropathic arthropathy	18	1, 117
E11.618	Type 2 diabetes mellitus with other diabetic arthropathy	18	1, 117
E11.62Ø	Type 2 diabetes mellitus with diabetic dermatitis	18	1, 117
E11.621	Type 2 diabetes mellitus with foot ulcer	18	1, 117

Code	Description	CMS-HCC Model Category	QPP Individual Measures–Claims
E11.622	Type 2 diabetes mellitus with other skin ulcer	18	1, 117
E11.628	Type 2 diabetes mellitus with other skin complications	18	1, 117
E11.630	Type 2 diabetes mellitus with periodontal disease	18	1, 117
E11.638	Type 2 diabetes mellitus with other oral complications	18	1, 117
E11.641	Type 2 diabetes mellitus with hypoglycemia with coma	17	1, 117
E11.649	Type 2 diabetes mellitus with hypoglycemia without coma	18	1, 117
E11.65	Type 2 diabetes mellitus with hyperglycemia	18	1, 117
E11.69	Type 2 diabetes mellitus with other specified complication	18	1, 117
E11.8	Type 2 diabetes mellitus with unspecified complications	18	1, 117
E11.9	Type 2 diabetes mellitus without complications	19	1, 117
E13.00	Other specified diabetes mellitus with hyperosmolarity without nonketotic hyperglycemic-hyperosmolar coma (NKHHC)	17	1, 117
E13.01	Other specified diabetes mellitus with hyperosmolarity with coma	17	1, 117
E13.10	Other specified diabetes mellitus with ketoacidosis without coma	17	1, 117
E13.11	Other specified diabetes mellitus with ketoacidosis with coma	17	1, 117
E13.21	Other specified diabetes mellitus with diabetic nephropathy	18	1, 117
E13.22	Other specified diabetes mellitus with diabetic chronic kidney disease	18	1, 117
E13.29	Other specified diabetes mellitus with other diabetic kidney complication	18	1, 117
E13.311	Other specified diabetes mellitus with unspecified diabetic retinopathy with macular edema	18	1, 19, 117
E13.319	Other specified diabetes mellitus with unspecified diabetic retinopathy without macular edema	18	1, 19, 117
E13.321	Other specified diabetes mellitus with mild nonproliferative diabetic retinopathy with macular edema	18	
E13.3211	Other specified diabetes mellitus with mild nonproliferative diabetic retinopathy with macular edema, right eye	18	1, 19, 117
E13.3212	Other specified diabetes mellitus with mild nonproliferative diabetic retinopathy with macular edema, left eye	18	1, 19, 117
E13.3213	Other specified diabetes mellitus with mild nonproliferative diabetic retinopathy with macular edema, bilateral	18	1, 19, 117
E13.3219	Other specified diabetes mellitus with mild nonproliferative diabetic retinopathy with macular edema, unspecified eye	18	1, 19, 117
E13.329	Other specified diabetes mellitus with mild nonproliferative diabetic retinopathy without macular edema	18	
E13.3291	Other specified diabetes mellitus with mild nonproliferative diabetic retinopathy without macular edema, right eye	18	1, 19, 117
E13.3292	Other specified diabetes mellitus with mild nonproliferative diabetic retinopathy without macular edema, left eye	18	1, 19, 117
E13.3293	Other specified diabetes mellitus with mild nonproliferative diabetic retinopathy without macular edema, bilateral	18	1, 19, 117
E13.3299	Other specified diabetes mellitus with mild nonproliferative diabetic retinopathy without macular edema, unspecified eye	18	1, 19, 117
E13.331	Other specified diabetes mellitus with moderate nonproliferative diabetic retinopathy with macular edema	18	
E13.3311	Other specified diabetes mellitus with moderate nonproliferative diabetic retinopathy with macular edema, right eye	18	1, 19, 117

Code	Description	CMS-HCC Model Category	QPP Individual Measures—Claims
E13.3312	Other specified diabetes mellitus with moderate nonproliferative diabetic retinopathy with macular edema, left eye	18	1, 19, 117
E13.3313	Other specified diabetes mellitus with moderate nonproliferative diabetic retinopathy with macular edema, bilateral	18	1, 19, 117
E13.3319	Other specified diabetes mellitus with moderate nonproliferative diabetic retinopathy with macular edema, unspecified eye	18	1, 19, 117
E13.339	Other specified diabetes mellitus with moderate nonproliferative diabetic retinopathy without macular edema	18	
E13.3391	Other specified diabetes mellitus with moderate nonproliferative diabetic retinopathy without macular edema, right eye	18	1, 19, 117
E13.3392	Other specified diabetes mellitus with moderate nonproliferative diabetic retinopathy without macular edema, left eye	18	1, 19, 117
E13.3393	Other specified diabetes mellitus with moderate nonproliferative diabetic retinopathy without macular edema, bilateral	18	1, 19, 117
E13.3399	Other specified diabetes mellitus with moderate nonproliferative diabetic retinopathy without macular edema, unspecified eye	18	1, 19, 117
E13.341	Other specified diabetes mellitus with severe nonproliferative diabetic retinopathy with macular edema	18	
E13.3411	Other specified diabetes mellitus with severe nonproliferative diabetic retinopathy with macular edema, right eye	18	1, 19, 117
E13.3412	Other specified diabetes mellitus with severe nonproliferative diabetic retinopathy with macular edema, left eye	18	1, 19, 117
E13.3413	Other specified diabetes mellitus with severe nonproliferative diabetic retinopathy with macular edema, bilateral	18	1, 19, 117
E13.3419	Other specified diabetes mellitus with severe nonproliferative diabetic retinopathy with macular edema, unspecified eye	18	1, 19, 117
E13.349	Other specified diabetes mellitus with severe nonproliferative diabetic retinopathy without macular edema	18	
E13.3491	Other specified diabetes mellitus with severe nonproliferative diabetic retinopathy without macular edema, right eye	18	1, 19, 117
E13.3492	Other specified diabetes mellitus with severe nonproliferative diabetic retinopathy without macular edema, left eye	18	1, 19, 117
E13.3493	Other specified diabetes mellitus with severe nonproliferative diabetic retinopathy without macular edema, bilateral	18	1, 19, 117
E13.3499	Other specified diabetes mellitus with severe nonproliferative diabetic retinopathy without macular edema, unspecified eye	18	1, 19, 117
E13.351	Other specified diabetes mellitus with proliferative diabetic retinopathy with macular edema	18, 122	
E13.3511	Other specified diabetes mellitus with proliferative diabetic retinopathy with macular edema, right eye	18, 122	1, 19, 117
E13.3512	Other specified diabetes mellitus with proliferative diabetic retinopathy with macular edema, left eye	18, 122	1, 19, 117
E13.3513	Other specified diabetes mellitus with proliferative diabetic retinopathy with macular edema, bilateral	18, 122	1, 19, 117
E13.3519	Other specified diabetes mellitus with proliferative diabetic retinopathy with macular edema, unspecified eye	18, 122	1, 19, 117
E13.3521	Other specified diabetes mellitus with proliferative diabetic retinopathy with traction retinal detachment involving the macula, right eye	18, 122	1, 19, 117

Code	Description	CMS-HCC Model Category	QPP Individual Measures–Claims
E13.3522	Other specified diabetes mellitus with proliferative diabetic retinopathy with traction retinal detachment involving the macula, left eye	18, 122	1, 19, 117
E13.3523	Other specified diabetes mellitus with proliferative diabetic retinopathy with traction retinal detachment involving the macula, bilateral	18, 122	1, 19, 117
E13.3529	Other specified diabetes mellitus with proliferative diabetic retinopathy with traction retinal detachment involving the macula, unspecified eye	18, 122	1, 19, 117
E13.3531	Other specified diabetes mellitus with proliferative diabetic retinopathy with traction retinal detachment not involving the macula, right eye	18, 122	1, 19, 117
E13.3532	Other specified diabetes mellitus with proliferative diabetic retinopathy with traction retinal detachment not involving the macula, left eye	18, 122	1, 19, 117
E13.3533	Other specified diabetes mellitus with proliferative diabetic retinopathy with traction retinal detachment not involving the macula, bilateral	18, 122	1, 19, 117
E13.3539	Other specified diabetes mellitus with proliferative diabetic retinopathy with traction retinal detachment not involving the macula, unspecified eye	18, 122	1, 19, 117
E13.3541	Other specified diabetes mellitus with proliferative diabetic retinopathy with combined traction retinal detachment and rhegmatogenous retinal detachment, right eye	18, 122	1, 19, 117
E13.3542	Other specified diabetes mellitus with proliferative diabetic retinopathy with combined traction retinal detachment and rhegmatogenous retinal detachment, left eye	18, 122	1, 19, 117
E13.3543	Other specified diabetes mellitus with proliferative diabetic retinopathy with combined traction retinal detachment and rhegmatogenous retinal detachment, bilateral	18, 122	1, 19, 117
E13.3549	Other specified diabetes mellitus with proliferative diabetic retinopathy with combined traction retinal detachment and rhegmatogenous retinal detachment, unspecified eye	18, 122	1, 19, 117
E13.3551	Other specified diabetes mellitus with stable proliferative diabetic retinopathy, right eye	18, 122	1, 19, 117
E13.3552	Other specified diabetes mellitus with stable proliferative diabetic retinopathy, left eye	18, 122	1, 19, 117
E13.3553	Other specified diabetes mellitus with stable proliferative diabetic retinopathy, bilateral	18, 122	1, 19, 117
E13.3559	Other specified diabetes mellitus with stable proliferative diabetic retinopathy, unspecified eye	18, 122	1, 19, 117
E13.359	Other specified diabetes mellitus with proliferative diabetic retinopathy without macular edema	18, 122	
E13.3591	Other specified diabetes mellitus with proliferative diabetic retinopathy without macular edema, right eye	18, 122	1, 19, 117
E13.3592	Other specified diabetes mellitus with proliferative diabetic retinopathy without macular edema, left eye	18, 122	1, 19, 117
E13.3593	Other specified diabetes mellitus with proliferative diabetic retinopathy without macular edema, bilateral	18, 122	1, 19, 117
E13.3599	Other specified diabetes mellitus with proliferative diabetic retinopathy without macular edema, unspecified eye	18, 122	1, 19, 117
E13.36	Other specified diabetes mellitus with diabetic cataract	18	1, 117
E13.37X1	Other specified diabetes mellitus with diabetic cataract	18	1, 117
E13.37X2	Other specified diabetes mellitus with diabetic macular edema, resolved following treatment, left eye	18	1, 117
E13.37X3	Other specified diabetes mellitus with diabetic macular edema, resolved following treatment, bilateral	18	1, 117
E13.37X9	Other specified diabetes mellitus with diabetic macular edema, resolved following treatment, unspecified eye	18	1, 117
E13.39	Other specified diabetes mellitus with other diabetic ophthalmic complication	18	1, 117
E13.4Ø	Other specified diabetes mellitus with diabetic neuropathy, unspecified	18	1, 117
E13.41	Other specified diabetes mellitus with diabetic mononeuropathy	18	1, 117

Code	Description	CMS-HCC Model Category	QPP Individual Measures–Claims
E13.42	Other specified diabetes mellitus with diabetic polyneuropathy	18	1, 117
E13.43	Other specified diabetes mellitus with diabetic autonomic (poly)neuropathy	18	1, 117
E13.44	Other specified diabetes mellitus with diabetic amyotrophy	18	1, 117
E13.49	Other specified diabetes mellitus with other diabetic neurological complication	18	1, 117
E13.51	Other specified diabetes mellitus with diabetic peripheral angiopathy without gangrene	18, 1Ø8	1, 117
E13.52	Other specified diabetes mellitus with diabetic peripheral angiopathy with gangrene	18, 1Ø6, 1Ø8	1, 117
E13.59	Other specified diabetes mellitus with other circulatory complications	18	1, 117
E13.61Ø	Other specified diabetes mellitus with diabetic neuropathic arthropathy	18	1, 117
E13.618	Other specified diabetes mellitus with other diabetic arthropathy	18	1, 117
E13.62Ø	Other specified diabetes mellitus with diabetic dermatitis	18	1, 117
E13.621	Other specified diabetes mellitus with foot ulcer	18	1, 117
E13.622	Other specified diabetes mellitus with other skin ulcer	18	1, 117
E13.628	Other specified diabetes mellitus with other skin complications	18	1, 117
E13.63Ø	Other specified diabetes mellitus with periodontal disease	18	1, 117
E13.638	Other specified diabetes mellitus with other oral complications	18	1, 117
E13.641	Other specified diabetes mellitus with hypoglycemia with coma	17	1, 117
E13.649	Other specified diabetes mellitus with hypoglycemia without coma	18	1, 117
E13.65	Other specified diabetes mellitus with hyperglycemia	18	1, 117
E13.69	Other specified diabetes mellitus with other specified complication	18	1, 117
E13.8	Other specified diabetes mellitus with unspecified complications	18	1, 117
E13.9	Other specified diabetes mellitus without complications	18	1, 117
E4Ø	Kwashiorkor	21	
E41	Nutritional marasmus	21	
E42	Marasmic kwashiorkor	21	
E43	Unspecified severe protein-calorie malnutrition	21	
E44.Ø	Moderate protein-calorie malnutrition	21	
E44.1	Mild protein-calorie malnutrition	21	
E45	Retarded development following protein-calorie malnutrition	21	
E46	Unspecified protein-calorie malnutrition	21	
E85.Ø	Non-neuropathic heredofamilial amyloidosis	23	
E85.1	Neuropathic heredofamilial amyloidosis	23	
E85.2	Heredofamilial amyloidosis, unspecified	23	
E85.3	Secondary systemic amyloidosis	23	
E85.4	Organ-limited amyloidosis	23	
E85.8	Other amyloidosis	23	
E85.9	Amyloidosis, unspecified	23	
F1Ø.12Ø	Alcohol abuse with intoxication, uncomplicated	55	
F1Ø.121	Alcohol abuse with intoxication delirium	55	
F1Ø.129	Alcohol abuse with intoxication, unspecified	55	
F1Ø.14	Alcohol abuse with alcohol-induced mood disorder	55	
F1Ø.15Ø	Alcohol abuse with alcohol-induced psychotic disorder with delusions	54	
F1Ø.151	Alcohol abuse with alcohol-induced psychotic disorder with hallucinations	54	

Code	Description	CMS-HCC Model Category	QPP Individual Measures–Claims
F10.159	Alcohol abuse with alcohol-induced psychotic disorder, unspecified	54	
F10.180	Alcohol abuse with alcohol-induced anxiety disorder	55	
F10.181	Alcohol abuse with alcohol-induced sexual dysfunction	55	
F10.182	Alcohol abuse with alcohol-induced sleep disorder	55	
F10.188	Alcohol abuse with other alcohol-induced disorder	55	
F10.19	Alcohol abuse with unspecified alcohol-induced disorder	55	
F10.20	Alcohol dependence, uncomplicated	55	
F10.21	Alcohol dependence, in remission	55	
F10.220	Alcohol dependence with intoxication, uncomplicated	55	
F10.221	Alcohol dependence with intoxication delirium	55	
F10.229	Alcohol dependence with intoxication, unspecified	55	
F10.230	Alcohol dependence with withdrawal, uncomplicated	55	
F10.231	Alcohol dependence with withdrawal delirium	54	
F10.232	Alcohol dependence with withdrawal with perceptual disturbance	54	
F10.239	Alcohol dependence with withdrawal, unspecified	55	
F10.24	Alcohol dependence with alcohol-induced mood disorder	55	
F10.250	Alcohol dependence with alcohol-induced psychotic disorder with delusions	54	
F10.251	Alcohol dependence with alcohol-induced psychotic disorder with hallucinations	54	
F10.259	Alcohol dependence with alcohol-induced psychotic disorder, unspecified	54	
F10.26	Alcohol dependence with alcohol-induced persisting amnestic disorder	54	
F10.27	Alcohol dependence with alcohol-induced persisting dementia	54	
F10.280	Alcohol dependence with alcohol-induced anxiety disorder	55	
F10.281	Alcohol dependence with alcohol-induced sexual dysfunction	55	
F10.282	Alcohol dependence with alcohol-induced sleep disorder	55	
F10.288	Alcohol dependence with other alcohol-induced disorder	55	
F10.29	Alcohol dependence with unspecified alcohol-induced disorder	55	
F10.920	Alcohol use, unspecified with intoxication, uncomplicated	55	
F10.921	Alcohol use, unspecified with intoxication delirium	55	
F10.929	Alcohol use, unspecified with intoxication, unspecified	55	
F10.94	Alcohol use, unspecified with alcohol-induced mood disorder	55	
F10.950	Alcohol use, unspecified with alcohol-induced psychotic disorder with delusions	54	
F10.951	Alcohol use, unspecified with alcohol-induced psychotic disorder with hallucinations	54	
F10.959	Alcohol use, unspecified with alcohol-induced psychotic disorder, unspecified	54	
F10.96	Alcohol use, unspecified with alcohol-induced persisting amnestic disorder	54	
F10.97	Alcohol use, unspecified with alcohol-induced persisting dementia	54	
F10.980	Alcohol use, unspecified with alcohol-induced anxiety disorder	55	
F10.981	Alcohol use, unspecified with alcohol-induced sexual dysfunction	55	
F10.982	Alcohol use, unspecified with alcohol-induced sleep disorder	55	
F10.988	Alcohol use, unspecified with other alcohol-induced disorder	55	
F10.99	Alcohol use, unspecified with unspecified alcohol-induced disorder	55	
F11.120	Opioid abuse with intoxication, uncomplicated	55	
F11.121	Opioid abuse with intoxication delirium	55	

Code	Description	CMS-HCC Model Category	QPP Individual Measures–Claims
F11.122	Opioid abuse with intoxication with perceptual disturbance	55	
F11.129	Opioid abuse with intoxication, unspecified	55	
F11.14	Opioid abuse with opioid-induced mood disorder	55	
F11.150	Opioid abuse with opioid-induced psychotic disorder with delusions	54	
F11.151	Opioid abuse with opioid-induced psychotic disorder with hallucinations	54	
F11.159	Opioid abuse with opioid-induced psychotic disorder, unspecified	54	
F11.181	Opioid abuse with opioid-induced sexual dysfunction	55	
F11.182	Opioid abuse with opioid-induced sleep disorder	55	
F11.188	Opioid abuse with other opioid-induced disorder	55	
F11.19	Opioid abuse with unspecified opioid-induced disorder	55	
F11.20	Opioid dependence, uncomplicated	55	
F11.21	Opioid dependence, in remission	55	
F11.220	Opioid dependence with intoxication, uncomplicated	55	
F11.221	Opioid dependence with intoxication delirium	55	
F11.222	Opioid dependence with intoxication with perceptual disturbance	55	
F11.229	Opioid dependence with intoxication, unspecified	55	
F11.23	Opioid dependence with withdrawal	55	
F11.24	Opioid dependence with opioid-induced mood disorder	55	
F11.250	Opioid dependence with opioid-induced psychotic disorder with delusions	54	
F11.251	Opioid dependence with opioid-induced psychotic disorder with hallucinations	54	
F11.259	Opioid dependence with opioid-induced psychotic disorder, unspecified	54	
F11.281	Opioid dependence with opioid-induced sexual dysfunction	55	
F11.282	Opioid dependence with opioid-induced sleep disorder	55	
F11.288	Opioid dependence with other opioid-induced disorder	55	
F11.29	Opioid dependence with unspecified opioid-induced disorder	55	
F11.920	Opioid use, unspecified with intoxication, uncomplicated	55	
F11.921	Opioid use, unspecified with intoxication delirium	55	
F11.922	Opioid use, unspecified with intoxication with perceptual disturbance	55	
F11.929	Opioid use, unspecified with intoxication, unspecified	55	
F11.93	Opioid use, unspecified with withdrawal	55	
F11.94	Opioid use, unspecified with opioid-induced mood disorder	55	
F11.950	Opioid use, unspecified with opioid-induced psychotic disorder with delusions	54	
F11.951	Opioid use, unspecified with opioid-induced psychotic disorder with hallucinations	54	
F11.959	Opioid use, unspecified with opioid-induced psychotic disorder, unspecified	54	
F11.981	Opioid use, unspecified with opioid-induced sexual dysfunction	55	
F11.982	Opioid use, unspecified with opioid-induced sleep disorder	55	
F11.988	Opioid use, unspecified with other opioid-induced disorder	55	
F11.99	Opioid use, unspecified with unspecified opioid-induced disorder	55	
F12.120	Cannabis abuse with intoxication, uncomplicated	55	
F12.121	Cannabis abuse with intoxication delirium	55	
F12.122	Cannabis abuse with intoxication with perceptual disturbance	55	
F12.129	Cannabis abuse with intoxication, unspecified	55	

Code	Description	CMS-HCC Model Category	QPP Individual Measures–Claims
F12.15Ø	Cannabis abuse with psychotic disorder with delusions	54	
F12.151	Cannabis abuse with psychotic disorder with hallucinations	54	
F12.159	Cannabis abuse with psychotic disorder, unspecified	54	
F12.18Ø	Cannabis abuse with cannabis-induced anxiety disorder	55	
F12.188	Cannabis abuse with other cannabis-induced disorder	55	
F12.19	Cannabis abuse with unspecified cannabis-induced disorder	55	
F12.2Ø	Cannabis dependence, uncomplicated	55	
F12.21	Cannabis dependence, in remission	55	
F12.22Ø	Cannabis dependence with intoxication, uncomplicated	55	
F12.221	Cannabis dependence with intoxication delirium	55	
F12.222	Cannabis dependence with intoxication with perceptual disturbance	55	
F12.229	Cannabis dependence with intoxication, unspecified	55	
F12.25Ø	Cannabis dependence with psychotic disorder with delusions	54	
F12.251	Cannabis dependence with psychotic disorder with hallucinations	54	
F12.259	Cannabis dependence with psychotic disorder, unspecified	54	
F12.28Ø	Cannabis dependence with cannabis-induced anxiety disorder	55	
F12.288	Cannabis dependence with other cannabis-induced disorder	55	
F12.29	Cannabis dependence with unspecified cannabis-induced disorder	55	
F12.92Ø	Cannabis use, unspecified with intoxication, uncomplicated	55	
F12.921	Cannabis use, unspecified with intoxication delirium	55	
F12.922	Cannabis use, unspecified with intoxication with perceptual disturbance	55	
F12.929	Cannabis use, unspecified with intoxication, unspecified	55	
F12.95Ø	Cannabis use, unspecified with psychotic disorder with delusions	54	
F12.951	Cannabis use, unspecified with psychotic disorder with hallucinations	54	
F12.959	Cannabis use, unspecified with psychotic disorder, unspecified	54	
F12.98Ø	Cannabis use, unspecified with anxiety disorder	55	
F12.988	Cannabis use, unspecified with other cannabis-induced disorder	55	
F12.99	Cannabis use, unspecified with unspecified cannabis-induced disorder	55	
F13.12Ø	Sedative, hypnotic or anxiolytic abuse with intoxication, uncomplicated	55	
F13.121	Sedative, hypnotic or anxiolytic abuse with intoxication delirium	55	
F13.129	Sedative, hypnotic or anxiolytic abuse with intoxication, unspecified	55	
F13.14	Sedative, hypnotic or anxiolytic abuse with sedative, hypnotic or anxiolytic-induced mood disorder	55	
F13.15Ø	Sedative, hypnotic or anxiolytic abuse with sedative, hypnotic or anxiolytic-induced psychotic disorder with delusions	54	
F13.151	Sedative, hypnotic or anxiolytic abuse with sedative, hypnotic or anxiolytic-induced psychotic disorder with hallucinations	54	
F13.159	Sedative, hypnotic or anxiolytic abuse with sedative, hypnotic or anxiolytic-induced psychotic disorder, unspecified	54	
F13.18Ø	Sedative, hypnotic or anxiolytic abuse with sedative, hypnotic or anxiolytic-induced anxiety disorder	55	
F13.181	Sedative, hypnotic or anxiolytic abuse with sedative, hypnotic or anxiolytic-induced sexual dysfunction	55	

Code	Description	CMS-HCC Model Category	QPP Individual Measures–Claims
F13.182	Sedative, hypnotic or anxiolytic abuse with sedative, hypnotic or anxiolytic-induced sleep disorder	55	
F13.188	Sedative, hypnotic or anxiolytic abuse with other sedative, hypnotic or anxiolytic-induced disorder	55	
F13.19	Sedative, hypnotic or anxiolytic abuse with unspecified sedative, hypnotic or anxiolytic-induced disorder	55	
F13.20	Sedative, hypnotic or anxiolytic dependence, uncomplicated	55	
F13.21	Sedative, hypnotic or anxiolytic dependence, in remission	55	
F13.220	Sedative, hypnotic or anxiolytic dependence with intoxication, uncomplicated	55	
F13.221	Sedative, hypnotic or anxiolytic dependence with intoxication delirium	55	
F13.229	Sedative, hypnotic or anxiolytic dependence with intoxication, unspecified	55	
F13.230	Sedative, hypnotic or anxiolytic dependence with withdrawal, uncomplicated	55	
F13.231	Sedative, hypnotic or anxiolytic dependence with withdrawal delirium	54	
F13.232	Sedative, hypnotic or anxiolytic dependence with withdrawal with perceptual disturbance	54	
F13.239	Sedative, hypnotic or anxiolytic dependence with withdrawal, unspecified	55	
F13.24	Sedative, hypnotic or anxiolytic dependence with sedative, hypnotic or anxiolytic-induced mood disorder	55	
F13.250	Sedative, hypnotic or anxiolytic dependence with sedative, hypnotic or anxiolytic-induced psychotic disorder with delusions	54	
F13.251	Sedative, hypnotic or anxiolytic dependence with sedative, hypnotic or anxiolytic-induced psychotic disorder with hallucinations	54	
F13.259	Sedative, hypnotic or anxiolytic dependence with sedative, hypnotic or anxiolytic-induced psychotic disorder, unspecified	54	
F13.26	Sedative, hypnotic or anxiolytic dependence with sedative, hypnotic or anxiolytic-induced persisting amnestic disorder	54	
F13.27	Sedative, hypnotic or anxiolytic dependence with sedative, hypnotic or anxiolytic-induced persisting dementia	54	
F13.280	Sedative, hypnotic or anxiolytic dependence with sedative, hypnotic or anxiolytic-induced anxiety disorder	55	
F13.281	Sedative, hypnotic or anxiolytic dependence with sedative, hypnotic or anxiolytic-induced sexual dysfunction	55	
F13.282	Sedative, hypnotic or anxiolytic dependence with sedative, hypnotic or anxiolytic-induced sleep disorder	55	
F13.288	Sedative, hypnotic or anxiolytic dependence with other sedative, hypnotic or anxiolytic-induced disorder	55	
F13.29	Sedative, hypnotic or anxiolytic dependence with unspecified sedative, hypnotic or anxiolytic-induced disorder	55	
F13.920	Sedative, hypnotic or anxiolytic use, unspecified with intoxication, uncomplicated	55	
F13.921	Sedative, hypnotic or anxiolytic use, unspecified with intoxication delirium	55	
F13.929	Sedative, hypnotic or anxiolytic use, unspecified with intoxication, unspecified	55	
F13.930	Sedative, hypnotic or anxiolytic use, unspecified with withdrawal, uncomplicated	55	
F13.931	Sedative, hypnotic or anxiolytic use, unspecified with withdrawal delirium	54	
F13.932	Sedative, hypnotic or anxiolytic use, unspecified with withdrawal with perceptual disturbances	54	
F13.939	Sedative, hypnotic or anxiolytic use, unspecified with withdrawal, unspecified	55	

Code	Description	CMS-HCC Model Category	QPP Individual Measures–Claims
F13.94	Sedative, hypnotic or anxiolytic use, unspecified with sedative, hypnotic or anxiolytic-induced mood disorder	55	
F13.950	Sedative, hypnotic or anxiolytic use, unspecified with sedative, hypnotic or anxiolytic-induced psychotic disorder with delusions	54	
F13.951	Sedative, hypnotic or anxiolytic use, unspecified with sedative, hypnotic or anxiolytic-induced psychotic disorder with hallucinations	54	
F13.959	Sedative, hypnotic or anxiolytic use, unspecified with sedative, hypnotic or anxiolytic-induced psychotic disorder, unspecified	54	
F13.96	Sedative, hypnotic or anxiolytic use, unspecified with sedative, hypnotic or anxiolytic-induced persisting amnestic disorder	54	
F13.97	Sedative, hypnotic or anxiolytic use, unspecified with sedative, hypnotic or anxiolytic-induced persisting dementia	54	
F13.980	Sedative, hypnotic or anxiolytic use, unspecified with sedative, hypnotic or anxiolytic-induced anxiety disorder	55	
F13.981	Sedative, hypnotic or anxiolytic use, unspecified with sedative, hypnotic or anxiolytic-induced sexual dysfunction	55	
F13.982	Sedative, hypnotic or anxiolytic use, unspecified with sedative, hypnotic or anxiolytic-induced sleep disorder	55	
F13.988	Sedative, hypnotic or anxiolytic use, unspecified with other sedative, hypnotic or anxiolytic-induced disorder	55	
F13.99	Sedative, hypnotic or anxiolytic use, unspecified with unspecified sedative, hypnotic or anxiolytic-induced disorder	55	
F14.120	Cocaine abuse with intoxication, uncomplicated	55	
F14.121	Cocaine abuse with intoxication with delirium	55	
F14.122	Cocaine abuse with intoxication with perceptual disturbance	55	
F14.129	Cocaine abuse with intoxication, unspecified	55	
F14.14	Cocaine abuse with cocaine-induced mood disorder	55	
F14.150	Cocaine abuse with cocaine-induced psychotic disorder with delusions	54	
F14.151	Cocaine abuse with cocaine-induced psychotic disorder with hallucinations	54	
F14.159	Cocaine abuse with cocaine-induced psychotic disorder, unspecified	54	
F14.180	Cocaine abuse with cocaine-induced anxiety disorder	55	
F14.181	Cocaine abuse with cocaine-induced sexual dysfunction	55	
F14.182	Cocaine abuse with cocaine-induced sleep disorder	55	
F14.188	Cocaine abuse with other cocaine-induced disorder	55	
F14.19	Cocaine abuse with unspecified cocaine-induced disorder	55	
F14.20	Cocaine dependence, uncomplicated	55	
F14.21	Cocaine dependence, in remission	55	
F14.220	Cocaine dependence with intoxication, uncomplicated	55	
F14.221	Cocaine dependence with intoxication delirium	55	
F14.222	Cocaine dependence with intoxication with perceptual disturbance	55	
F14.229	Cocaine dependence with intoxication, unspecified	55	
F14.23	Cocaine dependence with withdrawal	55	
F14.24	Cocaine dependence with cocaine-induced mood disorder	55	
F14.250	Cocaine dependence with cocaine-induced psychotic disorder with delusions	54	
F14.251	Cocaine dependence with cocaine-induced psychotic disorder with hallucinations	54	

Code	Description	CMS-HCC Model Category	QPP Individual Measures—Claims
F14.259	Cocaine dependence with cocaine-induced psychotic disorder, unspecified	54	
F14.280	Cocaine dependence with cocaine-induced anxiety disorder	55	
F14.281	Cocaine dependence with cocaine-induced sexual dysfunction	55	
F14.282	Cocaine dependence with cocaine-induced sleep disorder	55	
F14.288	Cocaine dependence with other cocaine-induced disorder	55	
F14.29	Cocaine dependence with unspecified cocaine-induced disorder	55	
F14.920	Cocaine use, unspecified with intoxication, uncomplicated	55	
F14.921	Cocaine use, unspecified with intoxication delirium	55	
F14.922	Cocaine use, unspecified with intoxication with perceptual disturbance	55	
F14.929	Cocaine use, unspecified with intoxication, unspecified	55	
F14.94	Cocaine use, unspecified with cocaine-induced mood disorder	55	
F14.950	Cocaine use, unspecified with cocaine-induced psychotic disorder with delusions	54	
F14.951	Cocaine use, unspecified with cocaine-induced psychotic disorder with hallucinations	54	
F14.959	Cocaine use, unspecified with cocaine-induced psychotic disorder, unspecified	54	
F14.980	Cocaine use, unspecified with cocaine-induced anxiety disorder	55	
F14.981	Cocaine use, unspecified with cocaine-induced sexual dysfunction	55	
F14.982	Cocaine use, unspecified with cocaine-induced sleep disorder	55	
F14.988	Cocaine use, unspecified with other cocaine-induced disorder	55	
F14.99	Cocaine use, unspecified with unspecified cocaine-induced disorder	55	
F15.120	Other stimulant abuse with intoxication, uncomplicated	55	
F15.121	Other stimulant abuse with intoxication delirium	55	
F15.122	Other stimulant abuse with intoxication with perceptual disturbance	55	
F15.129	Other stimulant abuse with intoxication, unspecified	55	
F15.14	Other stimulant abuse with stimulant-induced mood disorder	55	
F15.150	Other stimulant abuse with stimulant-induced psychotic disorder with delusions	54	
F15.151	Other stimulant abuse with stimulant-induced psychotic disorder with hallucinations	54	
F15.159	Other stimulant abuse with stimulant-induced psychotic disorder, unspecified	54	
F15.180	Other stimulant abuse with stimulant-induced anxiety disorder	55	
F15.181	Other stimulant abuse with stimulant-induced sexual dysfunction	55	
F15.182	Other stimulant abuse with stimulant-induced sleep disorder	55	
F15.188	Other stimulant abuse with other stimulant-induced disorder	55	
F15.19	Other stimulant abuse with unspecified stimulant-induced disorder	55	
F15.20	Other stimulant dependence, uncomplicated	55	
F15.21	Other stimulant dependence, in remission	55	
F15.220	Other stimulant dependence with intoxication, uncomplicated	55	
F15.221	Other stimulant dependence with intoxication delirium	55	
F15.222	Other stimulant dependence with intoxication with perceptual disturbance	55	
F15.229	Other stimulant dependence with intoxication, unspecified	55	
F15.23	Other stimulant dependence with withdrawal	55	
F15.24	Other stimulant dependence with stimulant-induced mood disorder	55	
F15.250	Other stimulant dependence with stimulant-induced psychotic disorder with delusions	54	

Code	Description	CMS-HCC Model Category	QPP Individual Measures–Claims
F15.251	Other stimulant dependence with stimulant-induced psychotic disorder with hallucinations	54	
F15.259	Other stimulant dependence with stimulant-induced psychotic disorder, unspecified	54	
F15.280	Other stimulant dependence with stimulant-induced anxiety disorder	55	
F15.281	Other stimulant dependence with stimulant-induced sexual dysfunction	55	
F15.282	Other stimulant dependence with stimulant-induced sleep disorder	55	
F15.288	Other stimulant dependence with other stimulant-induced disorder	55	
F15.29	Other stimulant dependence with unspecified stimulant-induced disorder	55	
F15.920	Other stimulant use, unspecified with intoxication, uncomplicated	55	
F15.921	Other stimulant use, unspecified with intoxication delirium	55	
F15.922	Other stimulant use, unspecified with intoxication with perceptual disturbance	55	
F15.929	Other stimulant use, unspecified with intoxication, unspecified	55	
F15.93	Other stimulant use, unspecified with withdrawal	55	
F15.94	Other stimulant use, unspecified with stimulant-induced mood disorder	55	
F15.950	Other stimulant use, unspecified with stimulant-induced psychotic disorder with delusions	54	
F15.951	Other stimulant use, unspecified with stimulant-induced psychotic disorder with hallucinations	54	
F15.959	Other stimulant use, unspecified with stimulant-induced psychotic disorder, unspecified	54	
F15.980	Other stimulant use, unspecified with stimulant-induced anxiety disorder	55	
F15.981	Other stimulant use, unspecified with stimulant-induced sexual dysfunction	55	
F15.982	Other stimulant use, unspecified with stimulant-induced sleep disorder	55	
F15.988	Other stimulant use, unspecified with other stimulant-induced disorder	55	
F15.99	Other stimulant use, unspecified with unspecified stimulant-induced disorder	55	
F16.120	Hallucinogen abuse with intoxication, uncomplicated	55	
F16.121	Hallucinogen abuse with intoxication with delirium	55	
F16.122	Hallucinogen abuse with intoxication with perceptual disturbance	55	
F16.129	Hallucinogen abuse with intoxication, unspecified	55	
F16.14	Hallucinogen abuse with hallucinogen-induced mood disorder	55	
F16.150	Hallucinogen abuse with hallucinogen-induced psychotic disorder with delusions	54	
F16.151	Hallucinogen abuse with hallucinogen-induced psychotic disorder with hallucinations	54	
F16.159	Hallucinogen abuse with hallucinogen-induced psychotic disorder, unspecified	54	
F16.180	Hallucinogen abuse with hallucinogen-induced anxiety disorder	55	
F16.183	Hallucinogen abuse with hallucinogen persisting perception disorder (flashbacks)	55	
F16.188	Hallucinogen abuse with other hallucinogen-induced disorder	55	
F16.19	Hallucinogen abuse with unspecified hallucinogen-induced disorder	55	
F16.20	Hallucinogen dependence, uncomplicated	55	
F16.21	Hallucinogen dependence, in remission	55	
F16.220	Hallucinogen dependence with intoxication, uncomplicated	55	
F16.221	Hallucinogen dependence with intoxication with delirium	55	
F16.229	Hallucinogen dependence with intoxication, unspecified	55	
F16.24	Hallucinogen dependence with hallucinogen-induced mood disorder	55	
F16.250	Hallucinogen dependence with hallucinogen-induced psychotic disorder with delusions	54	

Code	Description	CMS-HCC Model Category	QPP Individual Measures–Claims
F16.251	Hallucinogen dependence with hallucinogen-induced psychotic disorder with hallucinations	54	
F16.259	Hallucinogen dependence with hallucinogen-induced psychotic disorder, unspecified	54	
F16.280	Hallucinogen dependence with hallucinogen-induced anxiety disorder	55	
F16.283	Hallucinogen dependence with hallucinogen persisting perception disorder (flashbacks)	55	
F16.288	Hallucinogen dependence with other hallucinogen-induced disorder	55	
F16.29	Hallucinogen dependence with unspecified hallucinogen-induced disorder	55	
F16.920	Hallucinogen use, unspecified with intoxication, uncomplicated	55	
F16.921	Hallucinogen use, unspecified with intoxication with delirium	55	
F16.929	Hallucinogen use, unspecified with intoxication, unspecified	55	
F16.94	Hallucinogen use, unspecified with hallucinogen-induced mood disorder	55	
F16.950	Hallucinogen use, unspecified with hallucinogen-induced psychotic disorder with delusions	54	
F16.951	Hallucinogen use, unspecified with hallucinogen-induced psychotic disorder with hallucinations	54	
F16.959	Hallucinogen use, unspecified with hallucinogen-induced psychotic disorder, unspecified	54	
F16.980	Hallucinogen use, unspecified with hallucinogen-induced anxiety disorder	55	
F16.983	Hallucinogen use, unspecified with hallucinogen persisting perception disorder (flashbacks)	55	
F16.988	Hallucinogen use, unspecified with other hallucinogen-induced disorder	55	
F16.99	Hallucinogen use, unspecified with unspecified hallucinogen-induced disorder	55	
F18.120	Inhalant abuse with intoxication, uncomplicated	55	
F18.121	Inhalant abuse with intoxication delirium	55	
F18.129	Inhalant abuse with intoxication, unspecified	55	
F18.14	Inhalant abuse with inhalant-induced mood disorder	55	
F18.150	Inhalant abuse with inhalant-induced psychotic disorder with delusions	54	
F18.151	Inhalant abuse with inhalant-induced psychotic disorder with hallucinations	54	
F18.159	Inhalant abuse with inhalant-induced psychotic disorder, unspecified	54	
F18.17	Inhalant abuse with inhalant-induced dementia	54	
F18.180	Inhalant abuse with inhalant-induced anxiety disorder	55	
F18.188	Inhalant abuse with other inhalant-induced disorder	55	
F18.19	Inhalant abuse with unspecified inhalant-induced disorder	55	
F18.20	Inhalant dependence, uncomplicated	55	
F18.21	Inhalant dependence, in remission	55	
F18.220	Inhalant dependence with intoxication, uncomplicated	55	
F18.221	Inhalant dependence with intoxication delirium	55	
F18.229	Inhalant dependence with intoxication, unspecified	55	
F18.24	Inhalant dependence with inhalant-induced mood disorder	55	
F18.250	Inhalant dependence with inhalant-induced psychotic disorder with delusions	54	
F18.251	Inhalant dependence with inhalant-induced psychotic disorder with hallucinations	54	
F18.259	Inhalant dependence with inhalant-induced psychotic disorder, unspecified	54	
F18.27	Inhalant dependence with inhalant-induced dementia	54	
F18.280	Inhalant dependence with inhalant-induced anxiety disorder	55	

Code	Description	CMS-HCC Model Category	QPP Individual Measures–Claims
F18.288	Inhalant dependence with other inhalant-induced disorder	55	
F18.29	Inhalant dependence with unspecified inhalant-induced disorder	55	
F18.920	Inhalant use, unspecified with intoxication, uncomplicated	55	
F18.921	Inhalant use, unspecified with intoxication with delirium	55	
F18.929	Inhalant use, unspecified with intoxication, unspecified	55	
F18.94	Inhalant use, unspecified with inhalant-induced mood disorder	55	
F18.950	Inhalant use, unspecified with inhalant-induced psychotic disorder with delusions	54	
F18.951	Inhalant use, unspecified with inhalant-induced psychotic disorder with hallucinations	54	
F18.959	Inhalant use, unspecified with inhalant-induced psychotic disorder, unspecified	54	
F18.97	Inhalant use, unspecified with inhalant-induced persisting dementia	54	
F18.980	Inhalant use, unspecified with inhalant-induced anxiety disorder	55	
F18.988	Inhalant use, unspecified with other inhalant-induced disorder	55	
F18.99	Inhalant use, unspecified with unspecified inhalant-induced disorder	55	
F19.121	Other psychoactive substance abuse with intoxication delirium	55	
F19.122	Other psychoactive substance abuse with intoxication with perceptual disturbances	55	
F19.129	Other psychoactive substance abuse with intoxication, unspecified	55	
F19.14	Other psychoactive substance abuse with psychoactive substance-induced mood disorder	55	
F19.150	Other psychoactive substance abuse with psychoactive substance-induced psychotic disorder with delusions	54	
F19.151	Other psychoactive substance abuse with psychoactive substance-induced psychotic disorder with hallucinations	54	
F19.159	Other psychoactive substance abuse with psychoactive substance-induced psychotic disorder, unspecified	54	
F19.16	Other psychoactive substance abuse with psychoactive substance-induced persisting amnestic disorder	54	
F19.17	Other psychoactive substance abuse with psychoactive substance-induced persisting dementia	54	
F19.180	Other psychoactive substance abuse with psychoactive substance-induced anxiety disorder	55	
F19.181	Other psychoactive substance abuse with psychoactive substance-induced sexual dysfunction	55	
F19.182	Other psychoactive substance abuse with psychoactive substance-induced sleep disorder	55	
F19.188	Other psychoactive substance abuse with other psychoactive substance-induced disorder	55	
F19.19	Other psychoactive substance abuse with unspecified psychoactive substance-induced disorder	55	
F19.20	Other psychoactive substance dependence, uncomplicated	55	
F19.21	Other psychoactive substance dependence, in remission	55	
F19.220	Other psychoactive substance dependence with intoxication, uncomplicated	55	
F19.221	Other psychoactive substance dependence with intoxication delirium	55	
F19.222	Other psychoactive substance dependence with intoxication with perceptual disturbance	55	
F19.229	Other psychoactive substance dependence with intoxication, unspecified	55	
F19.230	Other psychoactive substance dependence with withdrawal, uncomplicated	55	

Code	Description	CMS-HCC Model Category	QPP Individual Measures–Claims
F19.231	Other psychoactive substance dependence with withdrawal delirium	54	
F19.232	Other psychoactive substance dependence with withdrawal with perceptual disturbance	54	
F19.239	Other psychoactive substance dependence with withdrawal, unspecified	55	
F19.24	Other psychoactive substance dependence with psychoactive substance-induced mood disorder	55	
F19.25Ø	Other psychoactive substance dependence with psychoactive substance-induced psychotic disorder with delusions	54	
F19.251	Other psychoactive substance dependence with psychoactive substance-induced psychotic disorder with hallucinations	54	
F19.259	Other psychoactive substance dependence with psychoactive substance-induced psychotic disorder, unspecified	54	
F19.26	Other psychoactive substance dependence with psychoactive substance-induced persisting amnestic disorder	54	
F19.27	Other psychoactive substance dependence with psychoactive substance-induced persisting dementia	54	
F19.28Ø	Other psychoactive substance dependence with psychoactive substance-induced anxiety disorder	55	
F19.281	Other psychoactive substance dependence with psychoactive substance-induced sexual dysfunction	55	
F19.282	Other psychoactive substance dependence with psychoactive substance-induced sleep disorder	55	
F19.288	Other psychoactive substance dependence with other psychoactive substance-induced disorder	55	
F19.29	Other psychoactive substance dependence with unspecified psychoactive substance-induced disorder	55	
F19.92Ø	Other psychoactive substance use, unspecified with intoxication, uncomplicated	55	
F19.921	Other psychoactive substance use, unspecified with intoxication with delirium	55	
F19.922	Other psychoactive substance use, unspecified with intoxication with perceptual disturbance	55	
F19.929	Other psychoactive substance use, unspecified with intoxication, unspecified	55	
F19.93Ø	Other psychoactive substance use, unspecified with withdrawal, uncomplicated	55	
F19.931	Other psychoactive substance use, unspecified with withdrawal delirium	54	
F19.932	Other psychoactive substance use, unspecified with withdrawal with perceptual disturbance	54	
F19.939	Other psychoactive substance use, unspecified with withdrawal, unspecified	55	
F19.94	Other psychoactive substance use, unspecified with psychoactive substance-induced mood disorder	55	
F19.95Ø	Other psychoactive substance use, unspecified with psychoactive substance-induced psychotic disorder with delusions	54	
F19.951	Other psychoactive substance use, unspecified with psychoactive substance-induced psychotic disorder with hallucinations	54	
F19.959	Other psychoactive substance use, unspecified with psychoactive substance-induced psychotic disorder, unspecified	54	
F19.96	Other psychoactive substance use, unspecified with psychoactive substance-induced persisting amnestic disorder	54	
F19.97	Other psychoactive substance use, unspecified with psychoactive substance-induced persisting dementia	54	

Code	Description	CMS-HCC Model Category	QPP Individual Measures–Claims
F19.980	Other psychoactive substance use, unspecified with psychoactive substance-induced anxiety disorder	55	
F19.981	Other psychoactive substance use, unspecified with psychoactive substance-induced sexual dysfunction	55	
F19.982	Other psychoactive substance use, unspecified with psychoactive substance-induced sleep disorder	55	
F19.988	Other psychoactive substance use, unspecified with other psychoactive substance-induced disorder	55	
F19.99	Other psychoactive substance use, unspecified with unspecified psychoactive substance-induced disorder	55	
G40.001	Localization-related (focal) (partial) idiopathic epilepsy and epileptic syndromes with seizures of localized onset, not intractable, with status epilepticus	79	
G40.009	Localization-related (focal) (partial) idiopathic epilepsy and epileptic syndromes with seizures of localized onset, not intractable, without status epilepticus	79	
G40.011	Localization-related (focal) (partial) idiopathic epilepsy and epileptic syndromes with seizures of localized onset, intractable, with status epilepticus	79	
G40.019	Localization-related (focal) (partial) idiopathic epilepsy and epileptic syndromes with seizures of localized onset, intractable, without status epilepticus	79	
G40.101	Localization-related (focal) (partial) symptomatic epilepsy and epileptic syndromes with simple partial seizures, not intractable, with status epilepticus	79	
G40.109	Localization-related (focal) (partial) symptomatic epilepsy and epileptic syndromes with simple partial seizures, not intractable, without status epilepticus	79	268
G40.111	Localization-related (focal) (partial) symptomatic epilepsy and epileptic syndromes with simple partial seizures, intractable, with status epilepticus	79	
G40.119	Localization-related (focal) (partial) symptomatic epilepsy and epileptic syndromes with simple partial seizures, intractable, without status epilepticus	79	268
G40.201	Localization-related (focal) (partial) symptomatic epilepsy and epileptic syndromes with complex partial seizures, not intractable, with status epilepticus	79	
G40.209	Localization-related (focal) (partial) symptomatic epilepsy and epileptic syndromes with complex partial seizures, not intractable, without status epilepticus	79	268
G40.211	Localization-related (focal) (partial) symptomatic epilepsy and epileptic syndromes with complex partial seizures, intractable, with status epilepticus	79	
G40.219	Localization-related (focal) (partial) symptomatic epilepsy and epileptic syndromes with complex partial seizures, intractable, without status epilepticus	79	268
G40.301	Generalized idiopathic epilepsy and epileptic syndromes, not intractable, with status epilepticus	79	
G40.309	Generalized idiopathic epilepsy and epileptic syndromes, not intractable, without status epilepticus	79	268
G40.311	Generalized idiopathic epilepsy and epileptic syndromes, intractable, with status epilepticus	79	
G40.319	Generalized idiopathic epilepsy and epileptic syndromes, intractable, without status epilepticus	79	
G40.401	Other generalized epilepsy and epileptic syndromes, not intractable, with status epilepticus	79	
G40.409	Other generalized epilepsy and epileptic syndromes, not intractable, without status epilepticus	79	268
G40.411	Other generalized epilepsy and epileptic syndromes, intractable, with status epilepticus	79	268
G40.419	Other generalized epilepsy and epileptic syndromes, intractable, without status epilepticus	79	

Code	Description	CMS-HCC Model Category	QPP Individual Measures–Claims
G40.501	Epileptic seizures related to external causes, not intractable, with status epilepticus	79	
G40.509	Epileptic seizures related to external causes, not intractable, without status epilepticus	79	
G40.801	Other epilepsy, not intractable, with status epilepticus	79	
G40.802	Other epilepsy, not intractable, without status epilepticus	79	
G40.803	Other epilepsy, intractable, with status epilepticus	79	
G40.804	Other epilepsy, intractable, without status epilepticus	79	
G40.811	Lennox-Gastaut syndrome, not intractable, with status epilepticus	79	
G40.812	Lennox-Gastaut syndrome, not intractable, without status epilepticus	79	
G40.813	Lennox-Gastaut syndrome, intractable, with status epilepticus	79	
G40.814	Lennox-Gastaut syndrome, intractable, without status epilepticus	79	
G40.821	Epileptic spasms, not intractable, with status epilepticus	79	
G40.822	Epileptic spasms, not intractable, without status epilepticus	79	268
G40.823	Epileptic spasms, intractable, with status epilepticus	79	
G40.824	Epileptic spasms, intractable, without status epilepticus	79	268
G40.89	Other seizures	79	
G40.901	Epilepsy, unspecified, not intractable, with status epilepticus	79	
G40.909	Epilepsy, unspecified, not intractable, without status epilepticus	79	268
G40.911	Epilepsy, unspecified, intractable, with status epilepticus	79	
G40.919	Epilepsy, unspecified, intractable, without status epilepticus	79	
G40.A01	Absence epileptic syndrome, not intractable, with status epilepticus	79	
G40.A09	Absence epileptic syndrome, not intractable, without status epilepticus	79	268
G40.A11	Absence epileptic syndrome, intractable, with status epilepticus	79	
G40.A19	Absence epileptic syndrome, intractable, without status epilepticus	79	268
G40.B01	Juvenile myoclonic epilepsy, not intractable, with status epilepticus	79	
G40.B09	Juvenile myoclonic epilepsy, not intractable, without status epilepticus	79	
G40.B11	Juvenile myoclonic epilepsy, intractable, with status epilepticus	79	
G40.B19	Juvenile myoclonic epilepsy, intractable, without status epilepticus	79	
G43.001	Migraine without aura, not intractable, with status migrainosus		419, 435
G43.009	Migraine without aura, not intractable, without status migrainosus		419, 435
G43.011	Migraine without aura, intractable, with status migrainosus		419, 435
G43.019	Migraine without aura, intractable, without status migrainosus		419, 435
G43.101	Migraine with aura, not intractable, with status migrainosus		419, 435
G43.109	Migraine with aura, not intractable, without status migrainosus		419, 435
G43.111	Migraine with aura, intractable, with status migrainosus		419, 435
G43.119	Migraine with aura, intractable, without status migrainosus		419, 435
G43.401	Hemiplegic migraine, not intractable, with status migrainosus		419, 435
G43.409	Hemiplegic migraine, not intractable, without status migrainosus		419, 435
G43.411	Hemiplegic migraine, intractable, with status migrainosus		419, 435
G43.419	Hemiplegic migraine, intractable, without status migrainosus		419, 435
G43.501	Persistent migraine aura without cerebral infarction, not intractable, with status migrainosus		419, 435
G43.509	Persistent migraine aura without cerebral infarction, not intractable, without status migrainosus		419, 435

Code	Description	CMS-HCC Model Category	QPP Individual Measures–Claims
G43.511	Persistent migraine aura without cerebral infarction, intractable, with status migrainosus		419, 435
G43.519	Persistent migraine aura without cerebral infarction, intractable, without status migrainosus		419, 435
G43.7Ø1	Chronic migraine without aura, not intractable, with status migrainosus		419, 435
G43.7Ø9	Chronic migraine without aura, not intractable, without status migrainosus		419, 435
G43.711	Chronic migraine without aura, intractable, with status migrainosus		419, 435
G43.8Ø1	Other migraine, not intractable, with status migrainosus		419, 435
G43.8Ø9	Other migraine, not intractable, without status migrainosus		419, 435
G43.811	Other migraine, intractable, with status migrainosus		419, 435
G43.819	Other migraine, intractable, without status migrainosus		419, 435
G43.9Ø1	Migraine, unspecified, not intractable, with status migrainosus		419, 435
G43.9Ø9	Migraine, unspecified, not intractable, without status migrainosus		419, 435
G43.911	Migraine, unspecified, intractable, with status migrainosus		419, 435
G43.919	Migraine, unspecified, intractable, without status migrainosus		419, 435
G43.BØ	Ophthalmoplegic migraine, not intractable		419, 435
G43.B1	Ophthalmoplegic migraine, intractable		419, 435
G43.CØ	Periodic headache syndromes in child or adult, not intractable		419, 435
G43.C1	Periodic headache syndromes in child or adult, intractable		419, 435
G45.Ø	Vertebro-basilar artery syndrome		32
G45.1	Carotid artery syndrome (hemispheric)		32
G45.2	Multiple and bilateral precerebral artery syndromes		32
G45.8	Other transient cerebral ischemic attacks and related syndromes		32
G45.9	Transient cerebral ischemic attack, unspecified		32
H4Ø.1ØXØ	Unspecified open-angle glaucoma, stage unspecified		12
H4Ø.1ØX1	Unspecified open-angle glaucoma, mild stage		12
H4Ø.1ØX2	Unspecified open-angle glaucoma, moderate stage		12
H4Ø.1ØX3	Unspecified open-angle glaucoma, severe stage		12
H4Ø.1ØX4	Unspecified open-angle glaucoma, indeterminate stage		12
H4Ø.111Ø	Primary open-angle glaucoma, right eye, stage unspecified		12
H4Ø.1111	Primary open-angle glaucoma, right eye, mild stage		12, 141
H4Ø.1112	Primary open-angle glaucoma, right eye, moderate stage		12, 141
H4Ø.1113	Primary open-angle glaucoma, right eye, severe stage		12, 141
H4Ø.1114	Primary open-angle glaucoma, right eye, indeterminate stage		12, 141
H4Ø.112Ø	Primary open-angle glaucoma, left eye, stage unspecified		12
H4Ø.1121	Primary open-angle glaucoma, left eye, mild stage		12, 141
H4Ø.1122	Primary open-angle glaucoma, left eye, moderate stage		12, 141
H4Ø.1123	Primary open-angle glaucoma, left eye, severe stage		12, 141
H4Ø.1124	Primary open-angle glaucoma, left eye, indeterminate stage		12, 141
H4Ø.113Ø	Primary open-angle glaucoma, bilateral, stage unspecified		12
H4Ø.1131	Primary open-angle glaucoma, bilateral, mild stage		12, 141
H4Ø.1132	Primary open-angle glaucoma, bilateral, moderate stage		12, 141
H4Ø.1133	Primary open-angle glaucoma, bilateral, severe stage		12, 141

Code	Description	CMS-HCC Model Category	QPP Individual Measures–Claims
H40.1134	Primary open-angle glaucoma, bilateral, indeterminate stage		12, 141
H40.1190	Primary open-angle glaucoma, unspecified eye, stage unspecified		12
H40.1191	Primary open-angle glaucoma, unspecified eye, mild stage		12
H40.1192	Primary open-angle glaucoma, unspecified eye, moderate stage		12
H40.1193	Primary open-angle glaucoma, unspecified eye, severe stage		12
H40.1194	Primary open-angle glaucoma, unspecified eye, indeterminate stage		12
H40.1210	Low-tension glaucoma, right eye, stage unspecified		12
H40.1211	Low-tension glaucoma, right eye, mild stage		12, 141
H40.1212	Low-tension glaucoma, right eye, moderate stage		12, 141
H40.1213	Low-tension glaucoma, right eye, severe stage		12, 141
H40.1214	Low-tension glaucoma, right eye, indeterminate stage		12, 141
H40.1220	Low-tension glaucoma, left eye, stage unspecified		12
H40.1221	Low-tension glaucoma, left eye, mild stage		12, 141
H40.1222	Low-tension glaucoma, left eye, moderate stage		12, 141
H40.1223	Low-tension glaucoma, left eye, severe stage		12, 141
H40.1224	Low-tension glaucoma, left eye, indeterminate stage		12, 141
H40.1230	Low-tension glaucoma, bilateral, stage unspecified		12
H40.1231	Low-tension glaucoma, bilateral, mild stage		12, 141
H40.1232	Low-tension glaucoma, bilateral, moderate stage		12, 141
H40.1233	Low-tension glaucoma, bilateral, severe stage		12, 141
H40.1234	Low-tension glaucoma, bilateral, indeterminate stage		12, 141
H40.1290	Low-tension glaucoma, unspecified eye, stage unspecified		12
H40.1291	Low-tension glaucoma, unspecified eye, mild stage		12
H40.1292	Low-tension glaucoma, unspecified eye, moderate stage		12
H40.1293	Low-tension glaucoma, unspecified eye, severe stage		12
H40.1294	Low-tension glaucoma, unspecified eye, indeterminate stage		12
H40.151	Residual stage of open-angle glaucoma, right eye		12, 141
H40.152	Residual stage of open-angle glaucoma, left eye		12, 141
H40.153	Residual stage of open-angle glaucoma, bilateral		12, 141
H40.159	Residual stage of open-angle glaucoma, unspecified eye		12
I09.81	Rheumatic heart failure	85	
I10	Essential (primary) hypertension		236
I11.0	Hypertensive heart disease with heart failure	85	
I12.0	Hypertensive chronic kidney disease with stage 5 chronic kidney disease or end stage renal disease	136	
I13.0	Hypertensive heart and chronic kidney disease with heart failure and stage 1 through stage 4 chronic kidney disease, or unspecified chronic kidney disease	85	
I13.11	Hypertensive heart and chronic kidney disease without heart failure, with stage 5 chronic kidney disease, or end stage renal disease	136	
I13.2	Hypertensive heart and chronic kidney disease with heart failure and with stage 5 chronic kidney disease, or end stage renal disease	85, 136	
I21.01	ST elevation (STEMI) myocardial infarction involving left main coronary artery	86	204

Code	Description	CMS-HCC Model Category	QPP Individual Measures–Claims
I21.Ø2	ST elevation (STEMI) myocardial infarction involving left anterior descending coronary artery	86	2Ø4
I21.Ø9	ST elevation (STEMI) myocardial infarction involving other coronary artery of anterior wall	86	2Ø4
I21.11	ST elevation (STEMI) myocardial infarction involving right coronary artery	86	2Ø4
I21.19	ST elevation (STEMI) myocardial infarction involving other coronary artery of inferior wall	86	2Ø4
I21.21	ST elevation (STEMI) myocardial infarction involving left circumflex coronary artery	86	2Ø4
I21.29	ST elevation (STEMI) myocardial infarction involving other sites	86	2Ø4
I21.3	ST elevation (STEMI) myocardial infarction of unspecified site	86	2Ø4
I21.4	Non-ST elevation (NSTEMI) myocardial infarction	86	2Ø4
I22.Ø	Subsequent ST elevation (STEMI) myocardial infarction of anterior wall	86	
I22.1	Subsequent ST elevation (STEMI) myocardial infarction of inferior wall	86	
I22.2	Subsequent non-ST elevation (NSTEMI) myocardial infarction	86	
I22.8	Subsequent ST elevation (STEMI) myocardial infarction of other sites	86	
I22.9	Subsequent ST elevation (STEMI) myocardial infarction of unspecified site	86	
I25.1Ø	Atherosclerotic heart disease of native coronary artery without angina pectoris		2Ø4
I25.11Ø	Atherosclerotic heart disease of native coronary artery with unstable angina pectoris	87	2Ø4
I25.111	Atherosclerotic heart disease of native coronary artery with angina pectoris with documented spasm	88	2Ø4
I25.118	Atherosclerotic heart disease of native coronary artery with other forms of angina pectoris	88	2Ø4
I25.119	Atherosclerotic heart disease of native coronary artery with unspecified angina pectoris	88	2Ø4
I25.5	Ischemic cardiomyopathy		2Ø4
I25.6	Silent myocardial ischemia		2Ø4
I25.7ØØ	Atherosclerosis of coronary artery bypass graft(s), unspecified, with unstable angina pectoris	87	2Ø4
I25.7Ø1	Atherosclerosis of coronary artery bypass graft(s), unspecified, with angina pectoris with documented spasm	88	2Ø4
I25.7Ø8	Atherosclerosis of coronary artery bypass graft(s), unspecified, with other forms of angina pectoris	88	2Ø4
I25.7Ø9	Atherosclerosis of coronary artery bypass graft(s), unspecified, with unspecified angina pectoris	88	2Ø4
I25.71Ø	Atherosclerosis of autologous vein coronary artery bypass graft(s) with unstable angina pectoris	87	2Ø4
I25.711	Atherosclerosis of autologous vein coronary artery bypass graft(s) with angina pectoris with documented spasm	88	2Ø4
I25.718	Atherosclerosis of autologous vein coronary artery bypass graft(s) with other forms of angina pectoris	88	2Ø4
I25.719	Atherosclerosis of autologous vein coronary artery bypass graft(s) with unspecified angina pectoris	88	2Ø4
I25.72Ø	Atherosclerosis of autologous artery coronary artery bypass graft(s) with unstable angina pectoris	87	2Ø4
I25.721	Atherosclerosis of autologous artery coronary artery bypass graft(s) with angina pectoris with documented spasm	88	2Ø4
I25.728	Atherosclerosis of autologous artery coronary artery bypass graft(s) with other forms of angina pectoris	88	2Ø4

Code	Description	CMS-HCC Model Category	QPP Individual Measures–Claims
I25.729	Atherosclerosis of autologous artery coronary artery bypass graft(s) with unspecified angina pectoris	88	204
I25.730	Atherosclerosis of nonautologous biological coronary artery bypass graft(s) with unstable angina pectoris	87	204
I25.731	Atherosclerosis of nonautologous biological coronary artery bypass graft(s) with angina pectoris with documented spasm	88	204
I25.738	Atherosclerosis of nonautologous biological coronary artery bypass graft(s) with other forms of angina pectoris	88	204
I25.739	Atherosclerosis of nonautologous biological coronary artery bypass graft(s) with unspecified angina pectoris	88	204
I25.750	Atherosclerosis of native coronary artery of transplanted heart with unstable angina	87	204
I25.751	Atherosclerosis of native coronary artery of transplanted heart with angina pectoris with documented spasm	88	204
I25.758	Atherosclerosis of native coronary artery of transplanted heart with other forms of angina pectoris	88	204
I25.759	Atherosclerosis of native coronary artery of transplanted heart with unspecified angina pectoris	88	204
I25.760	Atherosclerosis of bypass graft of coronary artery of transplanted heart with unstable angina	87	204
I25.761	Atherosclerosis of bypass graft of coronary artery of transplanted heart with angina pectoris with documented spasm	88	204
I25.768	Atherosclerosis of bypass graft of coronary artery of transplanted heart with other forms of angina pectoris	88	204
I25.769	Atherosclerosis of bypass graft of coronary artery of transplanted heart with unspecified angina pectoris	88	204
I25.790	Atherosclerosis of other coronary artery bypass graft(s) with unstable angina pectoris	87	204
I25.791	Atherosclerosis of other coronary artery bypass graft(s) with angina pectoris with documented spasm	88	204
I25.798	Atherosclerosis of other coronary artery bypass graft(s) with other forms of angina pectoris	88	204
I25.799	Atherosclerosis of other coronary artery bypass graft(s) with unspecified angina pectoris	88	204
I25.810	Atherosclerosis of coronary artery bypass graft(s) without angina pectoris		204
I25.811	Atherosclerosis of native coronary artery of transplanted heart without angina pectoris		204
I25.812	Atherosclerosis of bypass graft of coronary artery of transplanted heart without angina pectoris		204
I25.82	Chronic total occlusion of coronary artery		204
I25.83	Coronary atherosclerosis due to lipid rich plaque		204
I25.84	Coronary atherosclerosis due to calcified coronary lesion		204
I25.89	Other forms of chronic ischemic heart disease		204
I25.9	Chronic ischemic heart disease, unspecified		204
I44.2	Atrioventricular block, complete	96	
I48.0	Paroxysmal atrial fibrillation	96	326
I48.1	Persistent atrial fibrillation	96	326
I48.2	Chronic atrial fibrillation	96	326
I48.3	Typical atrial flutter	96	326
I48.4	Atypical atrial flutter	96	326

Code	Description	CMS-HCC Model Category	QPP Individual Measures–Claims
I48.91	Unspecified atrial fibrillation	96	326
I48.92	Unspecified atrial flutter	96	326
I49.Ø1	Ventricular fibrillation	84	
I49.Ø2	Ventricular flutter	84	
I49.2	Junctional premature depolarization	96	
I49.5	Sick sinus syndrome	96	
I5Ø.1	Left ventricular failure	85	
I5Ø.2Ø	Unspecified systolic (congestive) heart failure	85	
I5Ø.21	Acute systolic (congestive) heart failure	85	
I5Ø.22	Chronic systolic (congestive) heart failure	85	
I5Ø.23	Acute on chronic systolic (congestive) heart failure	85	
I5Ø.3Ø	Unspecified diastolic (congestive) heart failure	85	
I5Ø.31	Acute diastolic (congestive) heart failure	85	
I5Ø.32	Chronic diastolic (congestive) heart failure	85	
I5Ø.33	Acute on chronic diastolic (congestive) heart failure	85	
I5Ø.4Ø	Unspecified combined systolic (congestive) and diastolic (congestive) heart failure	85	
I5Ø.41	Acute combined systolic (congestive) and diastolic (congestive) heart failure	85	
I5Ø.42	Chronic combined systolic (congestive) and diastolic (congestive) heart failure	85	
I5Ø.43	Acute on chronic combined systolic (congestive) and diastolic (congestive) heart failure	85	
I5Ø.9	Heart failure, unspecified	85	
I6Ø.ØØ	Nontraumatic subarachnoid hemorrhage from unspecified carotid siphon and bifurcation	99	
I6Ø.Ø1	Nontraumatic subarachnoid hemorrhage from right carotid siphon and bifurcation	99	
I6Ø.Ø2	Nontraumatic subarachnoid hemorrhage from left carotid siphon and bifurcation	99	
I6Ø.1Ø	Nontraumatic subarachnoid hemorrhage from unspecified middle cerebral artery	99	
I6Ø.11	Nontraumatic subarachnoid hemorrhage from right middle cerebral artery	99	
I6Ø.12	Nontraumatic subarachnoid hemorrhage from left middle cerebral artery	99	
I6Ø.2	Nontraumatic subarachnoid hemorrhage from anterior communicating artery	99	
I6Ø.2Ø	Nontraumatic subarachnoid hemorrhage from unspecified anterior communicating artery	99	
I6Ø.21	Nontraumatic subarachnoid hemorrhage from right anterior communicating artery	99	
I6Ø.22	Nontraumatic subarachnoid hemorrhage from left anterior communicating artery	99	
I6Ø.3Ø	Nontraumatic subarachnoid hemorrhage from unspecified posterior communicating artery	99	
I6Ø.31	Nontraumatic subarachnoid hemorrhage from right posterior communicating artery	99	
I6Ø.32	Nontraumatic subarachnoid hemorrhage from left posterior communicating artery	99	
I6Ø.4	Nontraumatic subarachnoid hemorrhage from basilar artery	99	
I6Ø.5Ø	Nontraumatic subarachnoid hemorrhage from unspecified vertebral artery	99	
I6Ø.51	Nontraumatic subarachnoid hemorrhage from right vertebral artery	99	
I6Ø.52	Nontraumatic subarachnoid hemorrhage from left vertebral artery	99	
I6Ø.6	Nontraumatic subarachnoid hemorrhage from other intracranial arteries	99	
I6Ø.7	Nontraumatic subarachnoid hemorrhage from unspecified intracranial artery	99	
I6Ø.8	Other nontraumatic subarachnoid hemorrhage	99	
I6Ø.9	Nontraumatic subarachnoid hemorrhage, unspecified	99	

Code	Description	CMS-HCC Model Category	QPP Individual Measures–Claims
I61.Ø	Nontraumatic intracerebral hemorrhage in hemisphere, subcortical	99	
I61.1	Nontraumatic intracerebral hemorrhage in hemisphere, cortical	99	
I61.2	Nontraumatic intracerebral hemorrhage in hemisphere, unspecified	99	
I61.3	Nontraumatic intracerebral hemorrhage in brain stem	99	
I61.4	Nontraumatic intracerebral hemorrhage in cerebellum	99	
I61.5	Nontraumatic intracerebral hemorrhage, intraventricular	99	
I61.6	Nontraumatic intracerebral hemorrhage, multiple localized	99	
I61.8	Other nontraumatic intracerebral hemorrhage	99	
I61.9	Nontraumatic intracerebral hemorrhage, unspecified	99	
I62.ØØ	Nontraumatic subdural hemorrhage, unspecified	99	
I62.Ø1	Nontraumatic acute subdural hemorrhage	99	
I62.Ø2	Nontraumatic subacute subdural hemorrhage	99	
I62.Ø3	Nontraumatic chronic subdural hemorrhage	99	
I62.1	Nontraumatic extradural hemorrhage	99	
I62.9	Nontraumatic intracranial hemorrhage, unspecified	99	
I63.ØØ	Cerebral infarction due to thrombosis of unspecified precerebral artery	1ØØ	32, 2Ø4
I63.Ø11	Cerebral infarction due to thrombosis of right vertebral artery	1ØØ	32, 2Ø4
I63.Ø12	Cerebral infarction due to thrombosis of left vertebral artery	1ØØ	32, 2Ø4
I63.Ø13	Cerebral infarction due to thrombosis of bilateral vertebral arteries	1ØØ	32, 2Ø4
I63.Ø19	Cerebral infarction due to thrombosis of unspecified vertebral artery	1ØØ	32, 2Ø4
I63.Ø2	Cerebral infarction due to thrombosis of basilar artery	1ØØ	32, 2Ø4
I63.Ø31	Cerebral infarction due to thrombosis of right carotid artery	1ØØ	32, 2Ø4
I63.Ø32	Cerebral infarction due to thrombosis of left carotid artery	1ØØ	32, 2Ø4
I63.Ø33	Cerebral infarction due to thrombosis of bilateral carotid arteries	1ØØ	32, 2Ø4
I63.Ø39	Cerebral infarction due to thrombosis of unspecified carotid artery	1ØØ	32, 2Ø4
I63.Ø9	Cerebral infarction due to thrombosis of other precerebral artery	1ØØ	32, 2Ø4
I63.1Ø	Cerebral infarction due to embolism of unspecified precerebral artery	1ØØ	32, 2Ø4
I63.111	Cerebral infarction due to embolism of right vertebral artery	1ØØ	32, 2Ø4
I63.112	Cerebral infarction due to embolism of left vertebral artery	1ØØ	32, 2Ø4
I63.113	Cerebral infarction due to embolism of bilateral vertebral arteries	1ØØ	32, 2Ø4
I63.119	Cerebral infarction due to embolism of unspecified vertebral artery	1ØØ	32, 2Ø4
I63.12	Cerebral infarction due to embolism of basilar artery	1ØØ	32, 2Ø4
I63.131	Cerebral infarction due to embolism of right carotid artery	1ØØ	32, 2Ø4
I63.132	Cerebral infarction due to embolism of left carotid artery	1ØØ	32, 2Ø4
I63.133	Cerebral infarction due to embolism of bilateral carotid arteries	1ØØ	32, 2Ø4
I63.139	Cerebral infarction due to embolism of unspecified carotid artery	1ØØ	32, 2Ø4
I63.19	Cerebral infarction due to embolism of other precerebral artery	1ØØ	32, 2Ø4
I63.2Ø	Cerebral infarction due to unspecified occlusion or stenosis of unspecified precerebral arteries	1ØØ	32, 2Ø4
I63.211	Cerebral infarction due to unspecified occlusion or stenosis of right vertebral arteries	1ØØ	32, 2Ø4
I63.212	Cerebral infarction due to unspecified occlusion or stenosis of left vertebral arteries	1ØØ	32, 2Ø4
I63.213	Cerebral infarction due to unspecified occlusion or stenosis of bilateral vertebral arteries	1ØØ	32, 2Ø4

Code	Description	CMS-HCC Model Category	QPP Individual Measures–Claims
I63.219	Cerebral infarction due to unspecified occlusion or stenosis of unspecified vertebral arteries	1ØØ	32, 2Ø4
I63.22	Cerebral infarction due to unspecified occlusion or stenosis of basilar arteries	1ØØ	32, 2Ø4
I63.231	Cerebral infarction due to unspecified occlusion or stenosis of right carotid arteries	1ØØ	32, 2Ø4
I63.232	Cerebral infarction due to unspecified occlusion or stenosis of left carotid arteries	1ØØ	32, 2Ø4
I63.233	Cerebral infarction due to unspecified occlusion or stenosis of bilateral carotid arteries	1ØØ	32, 2Ø4
I63.239	Cerebral infarction due to unspecified occlusion or stenosis of unspecified carotid arteries	1ØØ	32, 2Ø4
I63.29	Cerebral infarction due to unspecified occlusion or stenosis of other precerebral arteries	1ØØ	32, 2Ø4
I63.3Ø	Cerebral infarction due to thrombosis of unspecified cerebral artery	1ØØ	32, 2Ø4
I63.311	Cerebral infarction due to thrombosis of right middle cerebral artery	1ØØ	32, 2Ø4
I63.312	Cerebral infarction due to thrombosis of left middle cerebral artery	1ØØ	32, 2Ø4
I63.313	Cerebral infarction due to thrombosis of bilateral middle cerebral arteries	1ØØ	32, 2Ø4
I63.319	Cerebral infarction due to thrombosis of unspecified middle cerebral artery	1ØØ	32, 2Ø4
I63.321	Cerebral infarction due to thrombosis of right anterior cerebral artery	1ØØ	32, 2Ø4
I63.322	Cerebral infarction due to thrombosis of left anterior cerebral artery	1ØØ	32, 2Ø4
I63.323	Cerebral infarction due to thrombosis of bilateral anterior arteries	1ØØ	32, 2Ø4
I63.329	Cerebral infarction due to thrombosis of unspecified anterior cerebral artery	1ØØ	32, 2Ø4
I63.331	Cerebral infarction due to thrombosis of right posterior cerebral artery	1ØØ	32, 2Ø4
I63.332	Cerebral infarction due to thrombosis of left posterior cerebral artery	1ØØ	32, 2Ø4
I63.333	Cerebral infarction to thrombosis of bilateral posterior arteries	1ØØ	32, 2Ø4
I63.339	Cerebral infarction due to thrombosis of unspecified posterior cerebral artery	1ØØ	32, 2Ø4
I63.341	Cerebral infarction due to thrombosis of right cerebellar artery	1ØØ	32, 2Ø4
I63.342	Cerebral infarction due to thrombosis of left cerebellar artery	1ØØ	32, 2Ø4
I63.349	Cerebral infarction due to thrombosis of unspecified cerebellar artery	1ØØ	32, 2Ø4
I63.39	Cerebral infarction due to thrombosis of other cerebral artery	1ØØ	32, 2Ø4
I63.4Ø	Cerebral infarction due to embolism of unspecified cerebral artery	1ØØ	32, 2Ø4
I63.411	Cerebral infarction due to embolism of right middle cerebral artery	1ØØ	32, 2Ø4
I63.412	Cerebral infarction due to embolism of left middle cerebral artery	1ØØ	32, 2Ø4
I63.413	Cerebral infarction due to embolism of bilateral middle cerebral arteries	1ØØ	32, 2Ø4
I63.419	Cerebral infarction due to embolism of unspecified middle cerebral artery	1ØØ	32, 2Ø4
I63.421	Cerebral infarction due to embolism of right anterior cerebral artery	1ØØ	32, 2Ø4
I63.422	Cerebral infarction due to embolism of left anterior cerebral artery	1ØØ	32, 2Ø4
I63.423	Cerebral infarction due to embolism of bilateral anterior cerebral arteries	1ØØ	32, 2Ø4
I63.429	Cerebral infarction due to embolism of unspecified anterior cerebral artery	1ØØ	32, 2Ø4
I63.431	Cerebral infarction due to embolism of right posterior cerebral artery	1ØØ	32, 2Ø4
I63.432	Cerebral infarction due to embolism of left posterior cerebral artery	1ØØ	32, 2Ø4
I63.433	Cerebral infarction due to embolism of bilateral posterior cerebral arteries	1ØØ	32, 2Ø4
I63.439	Cerebral infarction due to embolism of unspecified posterior cerebral artery	1ØØ	32, 2Ø4
I63.441	Cerebral infarction due to embolism of right cerebellar artery	1ØØ	32, 2Ø4
I63.442	Cerebral infarction due to embolism of left cerebellar artery	1ØØ	32, 2Ø4
I63.449	Cerebral infarction due to embolism of unspecified cerebellar artery	1ØØ	32, 2Ø4
I63.49	Cerebral infarction due to embolism of other cerebral artery	1ØØ	32, 2Ø4

Code	Description	CMS-HCC Model Category	QPP Individual Measures–Claims
I63.50	Cerebral infarction due to unspecified occlusion or stenosis of unspecified cerebral artery	100	32, 204
I63.511	Cerebral infarction due to unspecified occlusion or stenosis of right middle cerebral artery	100	32, 204
I63.512	Cerebral infarction due to unspecified occlusion or stenosis of left middle cerebral artery	100	32, 204
I63.513	Cerebral infarction due to unspecified occlusion or stenosis of bilateral middle arteries	100	32, 204
I63.519	Cerebral infarction due to unspecified occlusion or stenosis of unspecified middle cerebral artery	100	32, 204
I63.521	Cerebral infarction due to unspecified occlusion or stenosis of right anterior cerebral artery	100	32, 204
I63.522	Cerebral infarction due to unspecified occlusion or stenosis of left anterior cerebral artery	100	204
I63.523	Cerebral infarction due to unspecified occlusion or stenosis of bilateral anterior arteries	100	32, 204
I63.529	Cerebral infarction due to unspecified occlusion or stenosis of unspecified anterior cerebral artery	100	204
I63.531	Cerebral infarction due to unspecified occlusion or stenosis of right posterior cerebral artery	100	32, 204
I63.532	Cerebral infarction due to unspecified occlusion or stenosis of left posterior cerebral artery	100	32, 204
I63.533	Cerebral infarction due to unspecified occlusion or stenosis of bilateral posterior arteries	100	32, 204
I63.539	Cerebral infarction due to unspecified occlusion or stenosis of unspecified posterior cerebral artery	100	32, 204
I63.541	Cerebral infarction due to unspecified occlusion or stenosis of right cerebellar artery	100	32, 204
I63.542	Cerebral infarction due to unspecified occlusion or stenosis of left cerebellar artery	100	32, 204
I63.543	Cerebral infarction due to unspecified occlusion or stenosis of bilateral cerebellar arteries	100	32, 204
I63.549	Cerebral infarction due to unspecified occlusion or stenosis of unspecified cerebellar artery	100	32, 204
I63.59	Cerebral infarction due to unspecified occlusion or stenosis of other cerebral artery	100	32, 204
I63.6	Cerebral infarction due to cerebral venous thrombosis, nonpyogenic	100	32, 204
I63.8	Other cerebral infarction	100	32, 204
I63.9	Cerebral infarction, unspecified	100	32, 204
J43.0	Unilateral pulmonary emphysema [MacLeod's syndrome]	111	51, 52
J43.1	Panlobular emphysema	111	51, 52
J43.2	Centrilobular emphysema	111	51, 52
J43.8	Other emphysema	111	51, 52
J43.9	Emphysema, unspecified	111	51, 52
J44.0	Chronic obstructive pulmonary disease with acute lower respiratory infection	111	51, 52
J44.1	Chronic obstructive pulmonary disease with (acute) exacerbation	111	51, 52
J44.9	Chronic obstructive pulmonary disease, unspecified	111	51, 52
J80	Acute respiratory distress syndrome	84	
J95.821	Acute postprocedural respiratory failure	84	
J95.822	Acute and chronic postprocedural respiratory failure	84	
J95.850	Mechanical complication of respirator	82	
J95.851	Ventilator associated pneumonia	114	
J95.859	Other complication of respirator [ventilator]	82	
J96.00	Acute respiratory failure, unspecified whether with hypoxia or hypercapnia	84	
J96.01	Acute respiratory failure with hypoxia	84	

Code	Description	CMS-HCC Model Category	QPP Individual Measures–Claims
J96.Ø2	Acute respiratory failure with hypercapnia	84	
J96.1Ø	Chronic respiratory failure, unspecified whether with hypoxia or hypercapnia	84	
J96.11	Chronic respiratory failure with hypoxia	84	
J96.12	Chronic respiratory failure with hypercapnia	84	
J96.2Ø	Acute and chronic respiratory failure, unspecified whether with hypoxia or hypercapnia	84	
J96.21	Acute and chronic respiratory failure with hypoxia	84	
J96.22	Acute and chronic respiratory failure with hypercapnia	84	
J96.9Ø	Respiratory failure, unspecified, unspecified whether with hypoxia or hypercapnia	84	
J96.91	Respiratory failure, unspecified with hypoxia	84	
J96.92	Respiratory failure, unspecified with hypercapnia	84	
J98.2	Interstitial emphysema	111	
J98.3	Compensatory emphysema	111	
K5Ø.ØØ	Crohn's disease of small intestine without complications	35	
K5Ø.Ø11	Crohn's disease of small intestine with rectal bleeding	35	
K5Ø.Ø12	Crohn's disease of small intestine with intestinal obstruction	33, 35	
K5Ø.Ø13	Crohn's disease of small intestine with fistula	35	
K5Ø.Ø14	Crohn's disease of small intestine with abscess	35	
K5Ø.Ø18	Crohn's disease of small intestine with other complication	35	
K5Ø.Ø19	Crohn's disease of small intestine with unspecified complications	35	
K5Ø.1Ø	Crohn's disease of large intestine without complications	35	
K5Ø.111	Crohn's disease of large intestine with rectal bleeding	35	
K5Ø.112	Crohn's disease of large intestine with intestinal obstruction	33, 35	
K5Ø.113	Crohn's disease of large intestine with fistula	35	
K5Ø.114	Crohn's disease of large intestine with abscess	35	
K5Ø.118	Crohn's disease of large intestine with other complication	35	
K5Ø.119	Crohn's disease of large intestine with unspecified complications	35	
K5Ø.8Ø	Crohn's disease of both small and large intestine without complications	35	
K5Ø.811	Crohn's disease of both small and large intestine with rectal bleeding	35	
K5Ø.812	Crohn's disease of both small and large intestine with intestinal obstruction	33, 35	
K5Ø.813	Crohn's disease of both small and large intestine with fistula	35	
K5Ø.814	Crohn's disease of both small and large intestine with abscess	35	
K5Ø.818	Crohn's disease of both small and large intestine with other complication	35	
K5Ø.819	Crohn's disease of both small and large intestine with unspecified complications	35	
K5Ø.9Ø	Crohn's disease, unspecified, without complications	35	
K5Ø.911	Crohn's disease, unspecified, with rectal bleeding	35	
K5Ø.912	Crohn's disease, unspecified, with intestinal obstruction	33, 35	
K5Ø.913	Crohn's disease, unspecified, with fistula	35	
K5Ø.914	Crohn's disease, unspecified, with abscess	35	
K5Ø.918	Crohn's disease, unspecified, with other complication	35	
K5Ø.919	Crohn's disease, unspecified, with unspecified complications	35	
K51.ØØ	Ulcerative (chronic) pancolitis without complications	35	
K51.Ø11	Ulcerative (chronic) pancolitis with rectal bleeding	35	

Code	Description	CMS-HCC Model Category	QPP Individual Measures–Claims
K51.Ø12	Ulcerative (chronic) pancolitis with intestinal obstruction	33, 35	
K51.Ø13	Ulcerative (chronic) pancolitis with fistula	35	
K51.Ø14	Ulcerative (chronic) pancolitis with abscess	35	
K51.Ø18	Ulcerative (chronic) pancolitis with other complication	35	
K51.Ø19	Ulcerative (chronic) pancolitis with unspecified complications	35	
K51.2Ø	Ulcerative (chronic) proctitis without complications	35	
K51.211	Ulcerative (chronic) proctitis with rectal bleeding	35	
K51.212	Ulcerative (chronic) proctitis with intestinal obstruction	33, 35	
K51.213	Ulcerative (chronic) proctitis with fistula	35	
K51.214	Ulcerative (chronic) proctitis with abscess	35	
K51.218	Ulcerative (chronic) proctitis with other complication	35	
K51.219	Ulcerative (chronic) proctitis with unspecified complications	35	
K51.3Ø	Ulcerative (chronic) rectosigmoiditis without complications	35	
K51.311	Ulcerative (chronic) rectosigmoiditis with rectal bleeding	35	
K51.312	Ulcerative (chronic) rectosigmoiditis with intestinal obstruction	33, 35	
K51.313	Ulcerative (chronic) rectosigmoiditis with fistula	35	
K51.314	Ulcerative (chronic) rectosigmoiditis with abscess	35	
K51.318	Ulcerative (chronic) rectosigmoiditis with other complication	35	
K51.319	Ulcerative (chronic) rectosigmoiditis with unspecified complications	35	
K51.4Ø	Inflammatory polyps of colon without complications	35	
K51.411	Inflammatory polyps of colon with rectal bleeding	35	
K51.412	Inflammatory polyps of colon with intestinal obstruction	33, 35	
K51.413	Inflammatory polyps of colon with fistula	35	
K51.414	Inflammatory polyps of colon with abscess	35	
K51.418	Inflammatory polyps of colon with other complication	35	
K51.419	Inflammatory polyps of colon with unspecified complications	35	
K51.5Ø	Left sided colitis without complications	35	
K51.511	Left sided colitis with rectal bleeding	35	
K51.512	Left sided colitis with intestinal obstruction	33, 35	
K51.513	Left sided colitis with fistula	35	
K51.514	Left sided colitis with abscess	35	
K51.518	Left sided colitis with other complication	35	
K51.519	Left sided colitis with unspecified complications	35	
K51.8Ø	Other ulcerative colitis without complications	35	
K51.811	Other ulcerative colitis with rectal bleeding	35	
K51.812	Other ulcerative colitis with intestinal obstruction	33, 35	
K51.813	Other ulcerative colitis with fistula	35	
K51.814	Other ulcerative colitis with abscess	35	
K51.818	Other ulcerative colitis with other complication	35	
K51.819	Other ulcerative colitis with unspecified complications	35	
K51.9Ø	Ulcerative colitis, unspecified, without complications	35	
K51.911	Ulcerative colitis, unspecified with rectal bleeding	35	

Code	Description	CMS-HCC Model Category	QPP Individual Measures–Claims
K51.912	Ulcerative colitis, unspecified with intestinal obstruction	33, 35	
K51.913	Ulcerative colitis, unspecified with fistula	35	
K51.914	Ulcerative colitis, unspecified with abscess	35	
K51.918	Ulcerative colitis, unspecified with other complication	35	
K51.919	Ulcerative colitis, unspecified with unspecified complications	35	
L89.43	Pressure ulcer of contiguous site of back, buttock and hip, stage 3	158	
L89.44	Pressure ulcer of contiguous site of back, buttock and hip, stage 4	157	
L89.45	Pressure ulcer of contiguous site of back, buttock and hip, unstageable	158	
L89.500	Pressure ulcer of unspecified ankle, unstageable	158	
L89.503	Pressure ulcer of unspecified ankle, stage 3	158	
L89.504	Pressure ulcer of unspecified ankle, stage 4	157	
L89.510	Pressure ulcer of right ankle, unstageable	158	
L89.513	Pressure ulcer of right ankle, stage 3	158	
L89.514	Pressure ulcer of right ankle, stage 4	157	
L89.520	Pressure ulcer of left ankle, unstageable	158	
L89.523	Pressure ulcer of left ankle, stage 3	158	
L89.524	Pressure ulcer of left ankle, stage 4	157	
L89.600	Pressure ulcer of unspecified heel, unstageable	158	
L89.603	Pressure ulcer of unspecified heel, stage 3	158	
L89.604	Pressure ulcer of unspecified heel, stage 4	157	
L89.610	Pressure ulcer of right heel, unstageable	158	
L89.613	Pressure ulcer of right heel, stage 3	158	
L89.614	Pressure ulcer of right heel, stage 4	157	
L89.620	Pressure ulcer of left heel, unstageable	158	
L89.623	Pressure ulcer of left heel, stage 3	158	
L89.624	Pressure ulcer of left heel, stage 4	157	
L89.810	Pressure ulcer of head, unstageable	158	
L89.813	Pressure ulcer of head, stage 3	158	
L89.814	Pressure ulcer of head, stage 4	157	
L89.890	Pressure ulcer of other site, unstageable	158	
L89.893	Pressure ulcer of other site, stage 3	158	
L89.894	Pressure ulcer of other site, stage 4	157	
L89.93	Pressure ulcer of unspecified site, stage 3	158	
L89.94	Pressure ulcer of unspecified site, stage 4	157	
L89.95	Pressure ulcer of unspecified site, unstageable	158	
L97.101	Non-pressure chronic ulcer of unspecified thigh limited to breakdown of skin	161	
L97.102	Non-pressure chronic ulcer of unspecified thigh with fat layer exposed	161	
L97.103	Non-pressure chronic ulcer of unspecified thigh with necrosis of muscle	161	
L97.104	Non-pressure chronic ulcer of unspecified thigh with necrosis of bone	161	
L97.109	Non-pressure chronic ulcer of unspecified thigh with unspecified severity	161	
L97.111	Non-pressure chronic ulcer of right thigh limited to breakdown of skin	161	
L97.112	Non-pressure chronic ulcer of right thigh with fat layer exposed	161	

Code	Description	CMS-HCC Model Category	QPP Individual Measures–Claims
L97.113	Non-pressure chronic ulcer of right thigh with necrosis of muscle	161	
L97.114	Non-pressure chronic ulcer of right thigh with necrosis of bone	161	
L97.119	Non-pressure chronic ulcer of right thigh with unspecified severity	161	
L97.121	Non-pressure chronic ulcer of left thigh limited to breakdown of skin	161	
L97.122	Non-pressure chronic ulcer of left thigh with fat layer exposed	161	
L97.123	Non-pressure chronic ulcer of left thigh with necrosis of muscle	161	
L97.124	Non-pressure chronic ulcer of left thigh with necrosis of bone	161	
L97.129	Non-pressure chronic ulcer of left thigh with unspecified severity	161	
L97.201	Non-pressure chronic ulcer of unspecified calf limited to breakdown of skin	161	
L97.202	Non-pressure chronic ulcer of unspecified calf with fat layer exposed	161	
L97.203	Non-pressure chronic ulcer of unspecified calf with necrosis of muscle	161	
L97.204	Non-pressure chronic ulcer of unspecified calf with necrosis of bone	161	
L97.209	Non-pressure chronic ulcer of unspecified calf with unspecified severity	161	
L97.211	Non-pressure chronic ulcer of right calf limited to breakdown of skin	161	
L97.212	Non-pressure chronic ulcer of right calf with fat layer exposed	161	
L97.213	Non-pressure chronic ulcer of right calf with necrosis of muscle	161	
L97.214	Non-pressure chronic ulcer of right calf with necrosis of bone	161	
L97.219	Non-pressure chronic ulcer of right calf with unspecified severity	161	
L97.221	Non-pressure chronic ulcer of left calf limited to breakdown of skin	161	
L97.222	Non-pressure chronic ulcer of left calf with fat layer exposed	161	
L97.223	Non-pressure chronic ulcer of left calf with necrosis of muscle	161	
L97.224	Non-pressure chronic ulcer of left calf with necrosis of bone	161	
L97.229	Non-pressure chronic ulcer of left calf with unspecified severity	161	
L97.301	Non-pressure chronic ulcer of unspecified ankle limited to breakdown of skin	161	
L97.302	Non-pressure chronic ulcer of unspecified ankle with fat layer exposed	161	
L97.303	Non-pressure chronic ulcer of unspecified ankle with necrosis of muscle	161	
L97.304	Non-pressure chronic ulcer of unspecified ankle with necrosis of bone	161	
L97.309	Non-pressure chronic ulcer of unspecified ankle with unspecified severity	161	
L97.311	Non-pressure chronic ulcer of right ankle limited to breakdown of skin	161	
L97.312	Non-pressure chronic ulcer of right ankle with fat layer exposed	161	
L97.313	Non-pressure chronic ulcer of right ankle with necrosis of muscle	161	
L97.314	Non-pressure chronic ulcer of right ankle with necrosis of bone	161	
L97.319	Non-pressure chronic ulcer of right ankle with unspecified severity	161	
L97.321	Non-pressure chronic ulcer of left ankle limited to breakdown of skin	161	
L97.322	Non-pressure chronic ulcer of left ankle with fat layer exposed	161	
L97.323	Non-pressure chronic ulcer of left ankle with necrosis of muscle	161	
L97.324	Non-pressure chronic ulcer of left ankle with necrosis of bone	161	
L97.329	Non-pressure chronic ulcer of left ankle with unspecified severity	161	
L97.401	Non-pressure chronic ulcer of unspecified heel and midfoot limited to breakdown of skin	161	
L97.402	Non-pressure chronic ulcer of unspecified heel and midfoot with fat layer exposed	161	
L97.403	Non-pressure chronic ulcer of unspecified heel and midfoot with necrosis of muscle	161	
L97.404	Non-pressure chronic ulcer of unspecified heel and midfoot with necrosis of bone	161	

Code	Description	CMS-HCC Model Category	QPP Individual Measures–Claims
L97.409	Non-pressure chronic ulcer of unspecified heel and midfoot with unspecified severity	161	
L97.411	Non-pressure chronic ulcer of right heel and midfoot limited to breakdown of skin	161	
L97.412	Non-pressure chronic ulcer of right heel and midfoot with fat layer exposed	161	
L97.413	Non-pressure chronic ulcer of right heel and midfoot with necrosis of muscle	161	
L97.414	Non-pressure chronic ulcer of right heel and midfoot with necrosis of bone	161	
L97.419	Non-pressure chronic ulcer of right heel and midfoot with unspecified severity	161	
L97.421	Non-pressure chronic ulcer of left heel and midfoot limited to breakdown of skin	161	
L97.422	Non-pressure chronic ulcer of left heel and midfoot with fat layer exposed	161	
L97.423	Non-pressure chronic ulcer of left heel and midfoot with necrosis of muscle	161	
L97.424	Non-pressure chronic ulcer of left heel and midfoot with necrosis of bone	161	
L97.429	Non-pressure chronic ulcer of left heel and midfoot with unspecified severity	161	
L97.501	Non-pressure chronic ulcer of other part of unspecified foot limited to breakdown of skin	161	
L97.502	Non-pressure chronic ulcer of other part of unspecified foot with fat layer exposed	161	
L97.503	Non-pressure chronic ulcer of other part of unspecified foot with necrosis of muscle	161	
L97.504	Non-pressure chronic ulcer of other part of unspecified foot with necrosis of bone	161	
L97.509	Non-pressure chronic ulcer of other part of unspecified foot with unspecified severity	161	
L97.511	Non-pressure chronic ulcer of other part of right foot limited to breakdown of skin	161	
L97.512	Non-pressure chronic ulcer of other part of right foot with fat layer exposed	161	
L97.513	Non-pressure chronic ulcer of other part of right foot with necrosis of muscle	161	
L97.514	Non-pressure chronic ulcer of other part of right foot with necrosis of bone	161	
L97.519	Non-pressure chronic ulcer of other part of right foot with unspecified severity	161	
L97.521	Non-pressure chronic ulcer of other part of left foot limited to breakdown of skin	161	
L97.522	Non-pressure chronic ulcer of other part of left foot with fat layer exposed	161	
L97.523	Non-pressure chronic ulcer of other part of left foot with necrosis of muscle	161	
L97.524	Non-pressure chronic ulcer of other part of left foot with necrosis of bone	161	
L97.529	Non-pressure chronic ulcer of other part of left foot with unspecified severity	161	
L97.801	Non-pressure chronic ulcer of other part of unspecified lower leg limited to breakdown of skin	161	
L97.802	Non-pressure chronic ulcer of other part of unspecified lower leg with fat layer exposed	161	
L97.803	Non-pressure chronic ulcer of other part of unspecified lower leg with necrosis of muscle	161	
L97.804	Non-pressure chronic ulcer of other part of unspecified lower leg with necrosis of bone	161	
L97.809	Non-pressure chronic ulcer of other part of unspecified lower leg with unspecified severity	161	
L97.811	Non-pressure chronic ulcer of other part of right lower leg limited to breakdown of skin	161	
L97.812	Non-pressure chronic ulcer of other part of right lower leg with fat layer exposed	161	
L97.813	Non-pressure chronic ulcer of other part of right lower leg with necrosis of muscle	161	
L97.814	Non-pressure chronic ulcer of other part of right lower leg with necrosis of bone	161	
L97.819	Non-pressure chronic ulcer of other part of right lower leg with unspecified severity	161	
L97.821	Non-pressure chronic ulcer of other part of left lower leg limited to breakdown of skin	161	
L97.822	Non-pressure chronic ulcer of other part of left lower leg with fat layer exposed	161	
L97.823	Non-pressure chronic ulcer of other part of left lower leg with necrosis of muscle	161	
L97.824	Non-pressure chronic ulcer of other part of left lower leg with necrosis of bone	161	
L97.829	Non-pressure chronic ulcer of other part of left lower leg with unspecified severity	161	

Code	Description	CMS-HCC Model Category	QPP Individual Measures–Claims
L97.901	Non-pressure chronic ulcer of unspecified part of unspecified lower leg limited to breakdown of skin	161	
L97.902	Non-pressure chronic ulcer of unspecified part of unspecified lower leg with fat layer exposed	161	
L97.903	Non-pressure chronic ulcer of unspecified part of unspecified lower leg with necrosis of muscle	161	
L97.904	Non-pressure chronic ulcer of unspecified part of unspecified lower leg with necrosis of bone	161	
L97.909	Non-pressure chronic ulcer of unspecified part of unspecified lower leg with unspecified severity	161	
L97.911	Non-pressure chronic ulcer of unspecified part of right lower leg limited to breakdown of skin	161	
L97.912	Non-pressure chronic ulcer of unspecified part of right lower leg with fat layer exposed	161	
L97.913	Non-pressure chronic ulcer of unspecified part of right lower leg with necrosis of muscle	161	
L97.914	Non-pressure chronic ulcer of unspecified part of right lower leg with necrosis of bone	161	
L97.919	Non-pressure chronic ulcer of unspecified part of right lower leg with unspecified severity	161	
L97.921	Non-pressure chronic ulcer of unspecified part of left lower leg limited to breakdown of skin	161	
L97.922	Non-pressure chronic ulcer of unspecified part of left lower leg with fat layer exposed	161	
L97.923	Non-pressure chronic ulcer of unspecified part of left lower leg with necrosis of muscle	161	
L97.924	Non-pressure chronic ulcer of unspecified part of left lower leg with necrosis of bone	161	
L97.929	Non-pressure chronic ulcer of unspecified part of left lower leg with unspecified severity	161	
L98.411	Non-pressure chronic ulcer of buttock limited to breakdown of skin	161	
L98.412	Non-pressure chronic ulcer of buttock with fat layer exposed	161	
L98.413	Non-pressure chronic ulcer of buttock with necrosis of muscle	161	
L98.414	Non-pressure chronic ulcer of buttock with necrosis of bone	161	
L98.419	Non-pressure chronic ulcer of buttock with unspecified severity	161	
L98.421	Non-pressure chronic ulcer of back limited to breakdown of skin	161	
L98.422	Non-pressure chronic ulcer of back with fat layer exposed	161	
L98.423	Non-pressure chronic ulcer of back with necrosis of muscle	161	
L98.424	Non-pressure chronic ulcer of back with necrosis of bone	161	
L98.429	Non-pressure chronic ulcer of back with unspecified severity	161	
L98.491	Non-pressure chronic ulcer of skin of other sites limited to breakdown of skin	161	
L98.492	Non-pressure chronic ulcer of skin of other sites with fat layer exposed	161	
L98.493	Non-pressure chronic ulcer of skin of other sites with necrosis of muscle	161	
L98.494	Non-pressure chronic ulcer of skin of other sites with necrosis of bone	161	
L98.499	Non-pressure chronic ulcer of skin of other sites with unspecified severity	161	
M08.08	Unspecified juvenile rheumatoid arthritis, vertebrae	40	
M48.40XA	Fatigue fracture of vertebra, site unspecified, initial encounter for fracture		24, 418
M48.41XA	Fatigue fracture of vertebra, occipito-atlanto-axial region, initial encounter for fracture		24, 418
M48.42XA	Fatigue fracture of vertebra, cervical region, initial encounter for fracture		24, 418
M48.43XA	Fatigue fracture of vertebra, cervicothoracic region, initial encounter for fracture		24, 418
M48.44XA	Fatigue fracture of vertebra, cervicothoracic region, initial encounter for fracture		24, 418
M48.45XA	Fatigue fracture of vertebra, cervicothoracic region, initial encounter for fracture		24, 418

Code	Description	CMS-HCC Model Category	QPP Individual Measures–Claims
M48.46XA	Fatigue fracture of vertebra, lumbar region, initial encounter for fracture		24, 418
M48.47XA	Fatigue fracture of vertebra, lumbosacral region, initial encounter for fracture		24, 418
M48.48XA	Fatigue fracture of vertebra, sacral and sacrococcygeal region, initial encounter for fracture		24, 418
M48.5ØXA	Collapsed vertebra, not elsewhere classified, site unspecified, initial encounter for fracture	169	
M48.51XA	Collapsed vertebra, not elsewhere classified, occipito-atlanto-axial region, initial encounter for fracture	169	
M48.52XA	Collapsed vertebra, not elsewhere classified, cervical region, initial encounter for fracture	169	
M48.53XA	Collapsed vertebra, not elsewhere classified, cervicothoracic region, initial encounter for fracture	169	
M48.54XA	Collapsed vertebra, not elsewhere classified, thoracic region, initial encounter for fracture	169	
M48.55XA	Collapsed vertebra, not elsewhere classified, thoracolumbar region, initial encounter for fracture	169	
M48.56XA	Collapsed vertebra, not elsewhere classified, lumbar region, initial encounter for fracture	169	
M48.57XA	Collapsed vertebra, not elsewhere classified, lumbosacral region, initial encounter for fracture	169	
M48.58XA	Collapsed vertebra, not elsewhere classified, sacral and sacrococcygeal region, initial encounter for fracture	169	
M48.8X1	Other specified spondylopathies, occipito-atlanto-axial region	4Ø	
M48.8X2	Other specified spondylopathies, cervical region	4Ø	
M48.8X3	Other specified spondylopathies, cervicothoracic region	4Ø	
M48.8X4	Other specified spondylopathies, thoracic region	4Ø	
M48.8X5	Other specified spondylopathies, thoracolumbar region	4Ø	
M48.8X6	Other specified spondylopathies, lumbar region	4Ø	
M48.8X7	Other specified spondylopathies, lumbosacral region	4Ø	
M48.8X8	Other specified spondylopathies, sacral and sacrococcygeal region	4Ø	
M48.8X9	Other specified spondylopathies, site unspecified	4Ø	
M8Ø.Ø8XA	Age-related osteoporosis with current pathological fracture, vertebra(e), initial encounter for fracture	169	
M8Ø.Ø8XA-S	Age-related osteoporosis with current pathological fracture, vertebra(e)		39
M8Ø.88XA	Other osteoporosis with current pathological fracture, vertebra(e), initial encounter for fracture	169	
M8Ø.88XA-S	Other osteoporosis with current pathological fracture, vertebra(e)		39
N18.4	Chronic kidney disease, stage 4 (severe)	137	
N18.5	Chronic kidney disease, stage 5	136	
N18.6	End stage renal disease	136	
N99.51Ø	Cystostomy hemorrhage	176	
N99.511	Cystostomy infection	176	
N99.512	Cystostomy malfunction	176	
N99.518	Other cystostomy complication	176	
N99.52Ø	Hemorrhage of incontinent external stoma of urinary tract	176	
N99.521	Infection of incontinent external stoma of urinary tract	176	
N99.522	Malfunction of incontinent external stoma of urinary tract	176	
N99.523	Herniation of incontinent stoma of urinary tract	176	

Code	Description	CMS-HCC Model Category	QPP Individual Measures–Claims
N99.524	Stenosis of incontinent stoma of urinary tract	176	
N99.528	Other complication of incontinent external stoma of urinary tract	176	
N99.530	Hemorrhage of continent stoma of urinary tract	176	
N99.531	Infection of continent stoma of urinary tract	176	
N99.532	Malfunction of continent stoma of urinary tract	176	
N99.533	Herniation of continent stoma of urinary tract	176	
N99.534	Stenosis of continent stoma of urinary tract	176	
N99.538	Other complication of continent stoma of urinary tract	176	
S06.0X0A	Concussion without loss of consciousness, initial encounter		415, 416
S06.0X0S	Concussion without loss of consciousness, sequela	167	
S06.0X1A	Concussion with loss of consciousness of 30 minutes or less, initial encounter		415, 416
S06.0X1S	Concussion with loss of consciousness of 30 minutes or less, sequela	167	
S06.0X9A	Concussion with loss of consciousness of unspecified duration, initial encounter		415, 416
S06.0X9S	Concussion with loss of consciousness of unspecified duration, sequela	167	
S06.1X0A	Traumatic cerebral edema without loss of consciousness, initial encounter	167	415, 416
S06.1X0S	Traumatic cerebral edema without loss of consciousness, sequela	167	
S06.1X1A	Traumatic cerebral edema with loss of consciousness of 30 minutes or less, initial encounter	167	415, 416
S06.1X1S	Traumatic cerebral edema with loss of consciousness of 30 minutes or less, sequela	167	
S06.1X2A	Traumatic cerebral edema with loss of consciousness of 31 minutes to 59 minutes, initial encounter	167	415, 416
S06.1X2S	Traumatic cerebral edema with loss of consciousness of 31 minutes to 59 minutes, sequela	167	
S06.1X3A	Traumatic cerebral edema with loss of consciousness of 1 hour to 5 hours 59 minutes, initial encounter	166	415, 416
S06.1X3S	Traumatic cerebral edema with loss of consciousness of 1 hour to 5 hours 59 minutes, sequela	167	
S06.1X4A	Traumatic cerebral edema with loss of consciousness of 6 hours to 24 hours, initial encounter	166	415, 416
S06.1X4S	Traumatic cerebral edema with loss of consciousness of 6 hours to 24 hours, sequela	167	
S06.1X5A	Traumatic cerebral edema with loss of consciousness greater than 24 hours with return to pre-existing conscious level, initial encounter	166	
S06.1X5S	Traumatic cerebral edema with loss of consciousness greater than 24 hours with return to pre-existing conscious level, sequela	167	
S06.1X6A	Traumatic cerebral edema with loss of consciousness greater than 24 hours without return to pre-existing conscious level with patient surviving, initial encounter	166	
S06.1X6S	Traumatic cerebral edema with loss of consciousness greater than 24 hours without return to pre-existing conscious level with patient surviving, sequela	167	
S06.1X9A	Traumatic cerebral edema with loss of consciousness of unspecified duration, initial encounter	167	415, 416
S06.1X9S	Traumatic cerebral edema with loss of consciousness of unspecified duration,sequela	167	
S06.2X0A	Diffuse traumatic brain injury without loss of consciousness, initial encounter	167	415, 416
S06.2X0S	Diffuse traumatic brain injury without loss of consciousness, sequela	167	
S06.2X1A	Diffuse traumatic brain injury with loss of consciousness of 30 minutes or less, initial encounter	167	415, 416
S06.2X1S	Diffuse traumatic brain injury with loss of consciousness of 30 minutes or less, sequela	167	

Code	Description	CMS-HCC Model Category	QPP Individual Measures–Claims
SØ6.2X2A	Diffuse traumatic brain injury with loss of consciousness of 31 minutes to 59 minutes, initial encounter	167	415, 416
SØ6.2X2S	Diffuse traumatic brain injury with loss of consciousness of 31 minutes to 59 minutes, sequela	167	
SØ6.2X3A	Diffuse traumatic brain injury with loss of consciousness of 1 hour to 5 hours 59 minutes, initial encounter	166	415, 416
SØ6.2X3S	Diffuse traumatic brain injury with loss of consciousness of 1 hour to 5 hours 59 minutes, sequela	167	
SØ6.2X4A	Diffuse traumatic brain injury with loss of consciousness of 6 hours to 24 hours, initial encounter	166	415, 416
SØ6.2X4S	Diffuse traumatic brain injury with loss of consciousness of 6 hours to 24 hours, sequela	167	
SØ6.2X5A	Diffuse traumatic brain injury with loss of consciousness greater than 24 hours with return to pre-existing conscious levels, initial encounter	166	
SØ6.2X5S	Diffuse traumatic brain injury with loss of consciousness greater than 24 hours with return to pre-existing conscious levels, sequela	167	
SØ6.2X6A	Diffuse traumatic brain injury with loss of consciousness greater than 24 hours without return to pre-existing conscious level with patient surviving, initial encounter	166	
SØ6.2X6S	Diffuse traumatic brain injury with loss of consciousness greater than 24 hours without return to pre-existing conscious level with patient surviving, sequela	167	
SØ6.2X9A	Diffuse traumatic brain injury with loss of consciousness of unspecified duration, initial encounter	167	415, 416
SØ6.2X9S	Diffuse traumatic brain injury with loss of consciousness of unspecified duration, sequela	167	
SØ6.3ØØA	Unspecified focal traumatic brain injury without loss of consciousness, initial encounter	167	415, 416
SØ6.3ØØS	Unspecified focal traumatic brain injury without loss of consciousness, sequela	167	
SØ6.3Ø1A	Unspecified focal traumatic brain injury with loss of consciousness of 3Ø minutes or less, initial encounter	167	415, 416
SØ6.3Ø1S	Unspecified focal traumatic brain injury with loss of consciousness of 3Ø minutes or less, sequela	167	
SØ6.3Ø2A	Unspecified focal traumatic brain injury with loss of consciousness of 31 minutes to 59 minutes, initial encounter	167	415, 416
SØ6.3Ø2S	Unspecified focal traumatic brain injury with loss of consciousness of 31 minutes to 59 minutes, sequela	167	
SØ6.3Ø3A	Unspecified focal traumatic brain injury with loss of consciousness of 1 hour to 5 hours 59 minutes, initial encounter	166	415, 416
SØ6.3Ø3S	Unspecified focal traumatic brain injury with loss of consciousness of 1 hour to 5 hours 59 minutes, sequela	167	
SØ6.3Ø4A	Unspecified focal traumatic brain injury with loss of consciousness of 6 hours to 24 hours, initial encounter	166	415, 416
SØ6.3Ø4S	Unspecified focal traumatic brain injury with loss of consciousness of 6 hours to 24 hours, sequela	167	
SØ6.3Ø5A	Unspecified focal traumatic brain injury with loss of consciousness greater than 24 hours with return to pre-existing conscious level, initial encounter	166	
SØ6.3Ø5S	Unspecified focal traumatic brain injury with loss of consciousness greater than 24 hours with return to pre-existing conscious level, sequela	167	
SØ6.3Ø6A	Unspecified focal traumatic brain injury with loss of consciousness greater than 24 hours without return to pre-existing conscious level with patient surviving, initial encounter	166	
SØ6.3Ø6S	Unspecified focal traumatic brain injury with loss of consciousness greater than 24 hours without return to pre-existing conscious level with patient surviving, sequela	167	

Code	Description	CMS-HCC Model Category	QPP Individual Measures–Claims
SØ6.3Ø9A	Unspecified focal traumatic brain injury with loss of consciousness of unspecified duration, initial encounter	167	415, 416
SØ6.3Ø9S	Unspecified focal traumatic brain injury with loss of consciousness of unspecified duration, sequela	167	
SØ6.31ØA	Contusion and laceration of right cerebrum without loss of consciousness, initial encounter	167	
SØ6.31ØS	Contusion and laceration of right cerebrum without loss of consciousness, sequela	167	
SØ6.311A	Contusion and laceration of right cerebrum with loss of consciousness of 3Ø minutes or less, initial encounter	167	
SØ6.311S	Contusion and laceration of right cerebrum with loss of consciousness of 3Ø minutes or less, sequela	167	
SØ6.312A	Contusion and laceration of right cerebrum with loss of consciousness of 31 minutes to 59 minutes, initial encounter	167	
SØ6.312S	Contusion and laceration of right cerebrum with loss of consciousness of 31 minutes to 59 minutes, sequela	167	
SØ6.313A	Contusion and laceration of right cerebrum with loss of consciousness of 1 hour to 5 hours 59 minutes, initial encounter	166	
SØ6.313S	Contusion and laceration of right cerebrum with loss of consciousness of 1 hour to 5 hours 59 minutes, sequela	167	
SØ6.314A	Contusion and laceration of right cerebrum with loss of consciousness of 6 hours to 24 hours, initial encounter	166	
SØ6.314S	Contusion and laceration of right cerebrum with loss of consciousness of 6 hours to 24 hours, sequela	167	
SØ6.315A	Contusion and laceration of right cerebrum with loss of consciousness greater than 24 hours with return to pre-existing conscious level, initial encounter	166	
SØ6.315S	Contusion and laceration of right cerebrum with loss of consciousness greater than 24 hours with return to pre-existing conscious level, sequela	167	
SØ6.316A	Contusion and laceration of right cerebrum with loss of consciousness greater than 24 hours without return to pre-existing conscious level with patient surviving, initial encounter	166	
SØ6.316S	Contusion and laceration of right cerebrum with loss of consciousness greater than 24 hours without return to pre-existing conscious level with patient surviving, sequela	167	
SØ6.319A	Contusion and laceration of right cerebrum with loss of consciousness of unspecified duration, initial encounter	167	
SØ6.319S	Contusion and laceration of right cerebrum with loss of consciousness of unspecified duration, sequela	167	
SØ6.32ØA	Contusion and laceration of left cerebrum without loss of consciousness, initial encounter	167	
SØ6.32ØS	Contusion and laceration of left cerebrum without loss of consciousness, sequela	167	
SØ6.321A	Contusion and laceration of left cerebrum with loss of consciousness of 3Ø minutes or less, initial encounter	167	
SØ6.321S	Contusion and laceration of left cerebrum with loss of consciousness of 3Ø minutes or less, sequela	167	
SØ6.322A	Contusion and laceration of left cerebrum with loss of consciousness of 31 minutes to 59 minutes, initial encounter	167	
SØ6.322S	Contusion and laceration of left cerebrum with loss of consciousness of 31 minutes to 59 minutes, sequela	167	
SØ6.323A	Contusion and laceration of left cerebrum with loss of consciousness of 1 hour to 5 hours 59 minutes, initial encounter	166	

Code	Description	CMS-HCC Model Category	QPP Individual Measures–Claims
S06.323S	Contusion and laceration of left cerebrum with loss of consciousness of 1 hour to 5 hours 59 minutes, sequela	167	
S06.324A	Contusion and laceration of left cerebrum with loss of consciousness of 6 hours to 24 hours, initial encounter	166	
S06.324S	Contusion and laceration of left cerebrum with loss of consciousness of 6 hours to 24 hours, sequela	167	
S06.325A	Contusion and laceration of left cerebrum with loss of consciousness greater than 24 hours with return to pre-existing conscious level, initial encounter	166	
S06.325S	Contusion and laceration of left cerebrum with loss of consciousness greater than 24 hours with return to pre-existing conscious level, sequela	167	
S06.326A	Contusion and laceration of left cerebrum with loss of consciousness greater than 24 hours without return to pre-existing conscious level with patient surviving, initial encounter	166	
S06.326S	Contusion and laceration of left cerebrum with loss of consciousness greater than 24 hours without return to pre-existing conscious level with patient surviving, sequela	167	
S06.329A	Contusion and laceration of left cerebrum with loss of consciousness of unspecified duration, initial encounter	167	
S06.329S	Contusion and laceration of left cerebrum with loss of consciousness of unspecified duration, sequela	167	
S06.330A	Contusion and laceration of cerebrum, unspecified, without loss of consciousness, initial encounter	167	
S06.330S	Contusion and laceration of cerebrum, unspecified, without loss of consciousness, sequela	167	
S06.331A	Contusion and laceration of cerebrum, unspecified, with loss of consciousness of 30 minutes or less, initial encounter	167	
S06.331S	Contusion and laceration of cerebrum, unspecified, with loss of consciousness of 30 minutes or less, sequela	167	
S06.332A	Contusion and laceration of cerebrum, unspecified, with loss of consciousness of 31 minutes to 59 minutes, initial encounter	167	
S06.332S	Contusion and laceration of cerebrum, unspecified, with loss of consciousness of 31 minutes to 59 minutes, sequela	167	
S06.333A	Contusion and laceration of cerebrum, unspecified, with loss of consciousness of 1 hour to 5 hours 59 minutes, initial encounter	166	
S06.333S	Contusion and laceration of cerebrum, unspecified, with loss of consciousness of 1 hour to 5 hours 59 minutes, sequela	167	
S06.334A	Contusion and laceration of cerebrum, unspecified, with loss of consciousness of 6 hours to 24 hours, initial encounter	166	
S06.334S	Contusion and laceration of cerebrum, unspecified, with loss of consciousness of 6 hours to 24 hours, sequela	167	
S06.335A	Contusion and laceration of cerebrum, unspecified, with loss of consciousness greater than 24 hours with return to pre-existing conscious level, initial encounter	166	
S06.335S	Contusion and laceration of cerebrum, unspecified, with loss of consciousness greater than 24 hours with return to pre-existing conscious level, sequela	167	
S06.336A	Contusion and laceration of cerebrum, unspecified, with loss of consciousness greater than 24 hours without return to pre-existing conscious level with patient surviving, initial encounter	166	
S06.336S	Contusion and laceration of cerebrum, unspecified, with loss of consciousness greater than 24 hours without return to pre-existing conscious level with patient surviving, sequela	167	

Code	Description	CMS-HCC Model Category	QPP Individual Measures–Claims
S06.339A	Contusion and laceration of cerebrum, unspecified, with loss of consciousness of unspecified duration, initial encounter	167	
S06.339S	Contusion and laceration of cerebrum, unspecified, with loss of consciousness of unspecified duration, sequela	167	
S06.340A	Traumatic hemorrhage of right cerebrum without loss of consciousness, initial encounter	167	415, 416
S06.340S	Traumatic hemorrhage of right cerebrum without loss of consciousness, sequela	167	
S06.341A	Traumatic hemorrhage of right cerebrum with loss of consciousness of 30 minutes or less, initial encounter	167	415, 416
S06.341S	Traumatic hemorrhage of right cerebrum with loss of consciousness of 30 minutes or less, sequela	167	
S06.342A	Traumatic hemorrhage of right cerebrum with loss of consciousness of 31 minutes to 59 minutes, initial encounter	167	415, 416
S06.342S	Traumatic hemorrhage of right cerebrum with loss of consciousness of 31 minutes to 59 minutes, sequela	167	
S06.343A	Traumatic hemorrhage of right cerebrum with loss of consciousness of 1 hours to 5 hours 59 minutes, initial encounter	166	415, 416
S06.343S	Traumatic hemorrhage of right cerebrum with loss of consciousness of 1 hours to 5 hours 59 minutes, sequela	167	
S06.344A	Traumatic hemorrhage of right cerebrum with loss of consciousness of 6 hours to 24 hours, initial encounter	166	415, 416
S06.344S	Traumatic hemorrhage of right cerebrum with loss of consciousness of 6 hours to 24 hours, sequela	167	
S06.345A	Traumatic hemorrhage of right cerebrum with loss of consciousness greater than 24 hours with return to pre-existing conscious level, initial encounter	166	
S06.345S	Traumatic hemorrhage of right cerebrum with loss of consciousness greater than 24 hours with return to pre-existing conscious level, sequela	167	
S06.346A	Traumatic hemorrhage of right cerebrum with loss of consciousness greater than 24 hours without return to pre-existing conscious level with patient surviving, initial encounter	166	
S06.346S	Traumatic hemorrhage of right cerebrum with loss of consciousness greater than 24 hours without return to pre-existing conscious level with patient surviving, sequela	167	
S06.349A	Traumatic hemorrhage of right cerebrum with loss of consciousness of unspecified duration, initial encounter	167	415, 416
S06.349S	Traumatic hemorrhage of right cerebrum with loss of consciousness of unspecified duration, sequela	167	
S06.350A	Traumatic hemorrhage of left cerebrum without loss of consciousness, initial encounter	167	415, 416
S06.350S	Traumatic hemorrhage of left cerebrum without loss of consciousness, sequela	167	
S06.351A	Traumatic hemorrhage of left cerebrum with loss of consciousness of 30 minutes or less, initial encounter	167	415, 416
S06.351S	Traumatic hemorrhage of left cerebrum with loss of consciousness of 30 minutes or less, sequela	167	
S06.352A	Traumatic hemorrhage of left cerebrum with loss of consciousness of 31 minutes to 59 minutes, initial encounter	167	415, 416
S06.352S	Traumatic hemorrhage of left cerebrum with loss of consciousness of 31 minutes to 59 minutes, sequela	167	
S06.353A	Traumatic hemorrhage of left cerebrum with loss of consciousness of 1 hours to 5 hours 59 minutes, initial encounter	166	415, 416
S06.353S	Traumatic hemorrhage of left cerebrum with loss of consciousness of 1 hours to 5 hours 59 minutes, sequela	167	

Code	Description	CMS-HCC Model Category	QPP Individual Measures–Claims
SØ6.354A	Traumatic hemorrhage of left cerebrum with loss of consciousness of 6 hours to 24 hours, initial encounter	166	415, 416
SØ6.354S	Traumatic hemorrhage of left cerebrum with loss of consciousness of 6 hours to 24 hours, sequela	167	
SØ6.355A	Traumatic hemorrhage of left cerebrum with loss of consciousness greater than 24 hours with return to pre-existing conscious level, initial encounter	166	
SØ6.355S	Traumatic hemorrhage of left cerebrum with loss of consciousness greater than 24 hours with return to pre-existing conscious level, sequela	167	
SØ6.356A	Traumatic hemorrhage of left cerebrum with loss of consciousness greater than 24 hours without return to pre-existing conscious level with patient surviving, initial encounter	166	
SØ6.356S	Traumatic hemorrhage of left cerebrum with loss of consciousness greater than 24 hours without return to pre-existing conscious level with patient surviving, sequela	167	
SØ6.359A	Traumatic hemorrhage of left cerebrum with loss of consciousness of unspecified duration, initial encounter	167	415, 416
SØ6.359S	Traumatic hemorrhage of left cerebrum with loss of consciousness of unspecified duration, sequela	167	
SØ6.36ØA	Traumatic hemorrhage of cerebrum, unspecified, without loss of consciousness, initial encounter	167	415, 416
SØ6.36ØS	Traumatic hemorrhage of cerebrum, unspecified, without loss of consciousness, sequela	167	
SØ6.361A	Traumatic hemorrhage of cerebrum, unspecified, with loss of consciousness of 3Ø minutes or less, initial encounter	167	415, 416
SØ6.361S	Traumatic hemorrhage of cerebrum, unspecified, with loss of consciousness of 3Ø minutes or less, sequela	167	
SØ6.362A	Traumatic hemorrhage of cerebrum, unspecified, with loss of consciousness of 31 minutes to 59 minutes, initial encounter	167	415, 416
SØ6.362S	Traumatic hemorrhage of cerebrum, unspecified, with loss of consciousness of 31 minutes to 59 minutes, sequela	167	
SØ6.363A	Traumatic hemorrhage of cerebrum, unspecified, with loss of consciousness of 1 hours to 5 hours 59 minutes, initial encounter	166	415, 416
SØ6.363S	Traumatic hemorrhage of cerebrum, unspecified, with loss of consciousness of 1 hours to 5 hours 59 minutes, sequela	167	
SØ6.364A	Traumatic hemorrhage of cerebrum, unspecified, with loss of consciousness of 6 hours to 24 hours, initial encounter	166	415, 416
SØ6.364S	Traumatic hemorrhage of cerebrum, unspecified, with loss of consciousness of 6 hours to 24 hours, sequela	167	
SØ6.365A	Traumatic hemorrhage of cerebrum, unspecified, with loss of consciousness greater than 24 hours with return to pre-existing conscious level, initial encounter	166	
SØ6.365S	Traumatic hemorrhage of cerebrum, unspecified, with loss of consciousness greater than 24 hours with return to pre-existing conscious level, sequela	167	
SØ6.366A	Traumatic hemorrhage of cerebrum, unspecified, with loss of consciousness greater than 24 hours without return to pre-existing conscious level with patient surviving, initial encounter	166	
SØ6.366S	Traumatic hemorrhage of cerebrum, unspecified, with loss of consciousness greater than 24 hours without return to pre-existing conscious level with patient surviving, sequela	167	
SØ6.369A	Traumatic hemorrhage of cerebrum, unspecified, with loss of consciousness of unspecified duration, initial encounter	167	415, 416
SØ6.369S	Traumatic hemorrhage of cerebrum, unspecified, with loss of consciousness of unspecified duration, sequela	167	

Code	Description	CMS-HCC Model Category	QPP Individual Measures–Claims
S06.370A	Contusion, laceration, and hemorrhage of cerebellum without loss of consciousness, initial encounter	167	
S06.370S	Contusion, laceration, and hemorrhage of cerebellum without loss of consciousness, sequela	167	
S06.371A	Contusion, laceration, and hemorrhage of cerebellum with loss of consciousness of 30 minutes or less, initial encounter	167	
S06.371S	Contusion, laceration, and hemorrhage of cerebellum with loss of consciousness of 30 minutes or less, sequela	167	
S06.372A	Contusion, laceration, and hemorrhage of cerebellum with loss of consciousness of 31 minutes to 59 minutes, initial encounter	167	
S06.372S	Contusion, laceration, and hemorrhage of cerebellum with loss of consciousness of 31 minutes to 59 minutes, sequela	167	
S06.373A	Contusion, laceration, and hemorrhage of cerebellum with loss of consciousness of 1 hour to 5 hours 59 minutes, initial encounter	166	
S06.373S	Contusion, laceration, and hemorrhage of cerebellum with loss of consciousness of 1 hour to 5 hours 59 minutes, sequela	167	
S06.374A	Contusion, laceration, and hemorrhage of cerebellum with loss of consciousness of 6 hours to 24 hours, initial encounter	166	
S06.374S	Contusion, laceration, and hemorrhage of cerebellum with loss of consciousness of 6 hours to 24 hours, sequela	167	
S06.375A	Contusion, laceration, and hemorrhage of cerebellum with loss of consciousness greater than 24 hours with return to pre-existing conscious level, initial encounter	166	
S06.375S	Contusion, laceration, and hemorrhage of cerebellum with loss of consciousness greater than 24 hours with return to pre-existing conscious level, sequela	167	
S06.376A	Contusion, laceration, and hemorrhage of cerebellum with loss of consciousness greater than 24 hours without return to pre-existing conscious level with patient surviving, initial encounter	166	
S06.376S	Contusion, laceration, and hemorrhage of cerebellum with loss of consciousness greater than 24 hours without return to pre-existing conscious level with patient surviving, sequela	167	
S06.379A	Contusion, laceration, and hemorrhage of cerebellum with loss of consciousness of unspecified duration, initial encounter	167	
S06.379S	Contusion, laceration, and hemorrhage of cerebellum with loss of consciousness of unspecified duration, sequela	167	
S06.380A	Contusion, laceration, and hemorrhage of brainstem without loss of consciousness, initial encounter	167	
S06.380S	Contusion, laceration, and hemorrhage of brainstem without loss of consciousness, sequela	167	
S06.381A	Contusion, laceration, and hemorrhage of brainstem with loss of consciousness of 30 minutes or less, initial encounter	167	
S06.381S	Contusion, laceration, and hemorrhage of brainstem with loss of consciousness of 30 minutes or less, sequela	167	
S06.382A	Contusion, laceration, and hemorrhage of brainstem with loss of consciousness of 31 minutes to 59 minutes, initial encounter	167	
S06.382S	Contusion, laceration, and hemorrhage of brainstem with loss of consciousness of 31 minutes to 59 minutes, sequela	167	
S06.383A	Contusion, laceration, and hemorrhage of brainstem with loss of consciousness of 1 hour to 5 hours 59 minutes, initial encounter	166	
S06.383S	Contusion, laceration, and hemorrhage of brainstem with loss of consciousness of 1 hour to 5 hours 59 minutes, sequela	167	

Code	Description	CMS-HCC Model Category	QPP Individual Measures—Claims
SØ6.384A	Contusion, laceration, and hemorrhage of brainstem with loss of consciousness of 6 hours to 24 hours, initial encounter	166	
SØ6.384S	Contusion, laceration, and hemorrhage of brainstem with loss of consciousness of 6 hours to 24 hours, sequela	167	
SØ6.385A	Contusion, laceration, and hemorrhage of brainstem with loss of consciousness greater than 24 hours with return to pre-existing conscious level, initial encounter	166	
SØ6.385S	Contusion, laceration, and hemorrhage of brainstem with loss of consciousness greater than 24 hours with return to pre-existing conscious level, sequela	167	
SØ6.386A	Contusion, laceration, and hemorrhage of brainstem with loss of consciousness greater than 24 hours without return to pre-existing conscious level with patient surviving, initial encounter	166	
SØ6.386S	Contusion, laceration, and hemorrhage of brainstem with loss of consciousness greater than 24 hours without return to pre-existing conscious level with patient surviving, sequela	167	
SØ6.389A	Contusion, laceration, and hemorrhage of brainstem with loss of consciousness of unspecified duration, initial encounter	167	
SØ6.389S	Contusion, laceration, and hemorrhage of brainstem with loss of consciousness of unspecified duration, sequela	167	
SØ6.4XØA	Epidural hemorrhage without loss of consciousness, initial encounter	167	415, 416
SØ6.4XØS	Epidural hemorrhage without loss of consciousness, sequela	167	
SØ6.4X1A	Epidural hemorrhage with loss of consciousness of 3Ø minutes or less, initial encounter	167	415, 416
SØ6.4X1S	Epidural hemorrhage with loss of consciousness of 3Ø minutes or less, sequela	167	
SØ6.4X2A	Epidural hemorrhage with loss of consciousness of 31 minutes to 59 minutes, initial encounter	167	415, 416
SØ6.4X2S	Epidural hemorrhage with loss of consciousness of 31 minutes to 59 minutes, sequela	167	
SØ6.4X3A	Epidural hemorrhage with loss of consciousness of 1 hour to 5 hours 59 minutes, initial encounter	166	415, 416
SØ6.4X3S	Epidural hemorrhage with loss of consciousness of 1 hour to 5 hours 59 minutes, sequela	167	
SØ6.4X4A	Epidural hemorrhage with loss of consciousness of 6 hours to 24 hours, initial encounter	166	415, 416
SØ6.4X4S	Epidural hemorrhage with loss of consciousness of 6 hours to 24 hours, sequela	167	
SØ6.4X5A	Epidural hemorrhage with loss of consciousness greater than 24 hours with return to pre-existing conscious level, initial encounter	166	
SØ6.4X5S	Epidural hemorrhage with loss of consciousness greater than 24 hours with return to pre-existing conscious level, sequela	167	
SØ6.4X6A	Epidural hemorrhage with loss of consciousness greater than 24 hours without return to pre-existing conscious level with patient surviving, initial encounter	166	
SØ6.4X6S	Epidural hemorrhage with loss of consciousness greater than 24 hours without return to pre-existing conscious level with patient surviving, sequela	167	
SØ6.4X9A	Epidural hemorrhage with loss of consciousness of unspecified duration, initial encounter	167	415, 416
SØ6.4X9S	Epidural hemorrhage with loss of consciousness of unspecified duration, sequela	167	
SØ6.5XØA	Traumatic subdural hemorrhage without loss of consciousness, initial encounter	167	415, 416
SØ6.5XØS	Traumatic subdural hemorrhage without loss of consciousness, sequela	167	
SØ6.5X1A	Traumatic subdural hemorrhage with loss of consciousness of 3Ø minutes or less, initial encounter	167	415, 416
SØ6.5X1S	Traumatic subdural hemorrhage with loss of consciousness of 3Ø minutes or less, sequela	167	
SØ6.5X2A	Traumatic subdural hemorrhage with loss of consciousness of 31 minutes to 59 minutes, initial encounter	167	415, 416

Code	Description	CMS-HCC Model Category	QPP Individual Measures–Claims
SØ6.5X2S	Traumatic subdural hemorrhage with loss of consciousness of 31 minutes to 59 minutes, sequela	167	
SØ6.5X3A	Traumatic subdural hemorrhage with loss of consciousness of 1 hour to 5 hours 59 minutes, initial encounter	166	415, 416
SØ6.5X3S	Traumatic subdural hemorrhage with loss of consciousness of 1 hour to 5 hours 59 minutes, sequela	167	
SØ6.5X4A	Traumatic subdural hemorrhage with loss of consciousness of 6 hours to 24 hours, initial encounter	166	415, 416
SØ6.5X4S	Traumatic subdural hemorrhage with loss of consciousness of 6 hours to 24 hours, sequela	167	
SØ6.5X5A	Traumatic subdural hemorrhage with loss of consciousness greater than 24 hours with return to pre-existing conscious level, initial encounter	166	
SØ6.5X5S	Traumatic subdural hemorrhage with loss of consciousness greater than 24 hours with return to pre-existing conscious level, sequela	167	
SØ6.5X6A	Traumatic subdural hemorrhage with loss of consciousness greater than 24 hours without return to pre-existing conscious level with patient surviving, initial encounter	166	
SØ6.5X6S	Traumatic subdural hemorrhage with loss of consciousness greater than 24 hours without return to pre-existing conscious level with patient surviving, sequela	167	
SØ6.5X9A	Traumatic subdural hemorrhage with loss of consciousness of unspecified duration, initial encounter	167	415, 416
SØ6.5X9S	Traumatic subdural hemorrhage with loss of consciousness of unspecified duration, sequela	167	
SØ6.6XØA	Traumatic subarachnoid hemorrhage without loss of consciousness, initial encounter	167	415, 416
SØ6.6XØS	Traumatic subarachnoid hemorrhage without loss of consciousness, sequela	167	
SØ6.6X1A	Traumatic subarachnoid hemorrhage with loss of consciousness of 3Ø minutes or less, initial encounter	167	415, 416
SØ6.6X1S	Traumatic subarachnoid hemorrhage with loss of consciousness of 3Ø minutes or less, sequela	167	
SØ6.6X2A	Traumatic subarachnoid hemorrhage with loss of consciousness of 31 minutes to 59 minutes, initial encounter	167	415, 416
SØ6.6X2S	Traumatic subarachnoid hemorrhage with loss of consciousness of 31 minutes to 59 minutes, sequela	167	
SØ6.6X3A	Traumatic subarachnoid hemorrhage with loss of consciousness of 1 hour to 5 hours 59 minutes, initial encounter	166	415, 416
SØ6.6X3S	Traumatic subarachnoid hemorrhage with loss of consciousness of 1 hour to 5 hours 59 minutes, sequela	167	
SØ6.6X4A	Traumatic subarachnoid hemorrhage with loss of consciousness of 6 hours to 24 hours, initial encounter	166	415, 416
SØ6.6X4S	Traumatic subarachnoid hemorrhage with loss of consciousness of 6 hours to 24 hours, sequela	167	
SØ6.6X5A	Traumatic subarachnoid hemorrhage with loss of consciousness greater than 24 hours with return to pre-existing conscious level, initial encounter	166	
SØ6.6X5S	Traumatic subarachnoid hemorrhage with loss of consciousness greater than 24 hours with return to pre-existing conscious level, sequela	167	
SØ6.6X6A	Traumatic subarachnoid hemorrhage with loss of consciousness greater than 24 hours without return to pre-existing conscious level with patient surviving, initial encounter	166	
SØ6.6X6S	Traumatic subarachnoid hemorrhage with loss of consciousness greater than 24 hours without return to pre-existing conscious level with patient surviving, sequela	167	

Code	Description	CMS-HCC Model Category	QPP Individual Measures–Claims
SØ6.6X9A	Traumatic subarachnoid hemorrhage with loss of consciousness of unspecified duration, initial encounter	167	415, 416
SØ6.6X9S	Traumatic subarachnoid hemorrhage with loss of consciousness of unspecified duration, sequela	167	
SØ6.81ØA	Injury of right internal carotid artery, intracranial portion, not elsewhere classified without loss of consciousness, initial encounter	167	415, 416
SØ6.81ØS	Injury of right internal carotid artery, intracranial portion, not elsewhere classified without loss of consciousness, sequela	167	
SØ6.811A	Injury of right internal carotid artery, intracranial portion, not elsewhere classified with loss of consciousness of 3Ø minutes or less, initial encounter	167	415, 416
SØ6.811S	Injury of right internal carotid artery, intracranial portion, not elsewhere classified with loss of consciousness of 3Ø minutes or less, sequela	167	
SØ6.812A	Injury of right internal carotid artery, intracranial portion, not elsewhere classified with loss of consciousness of 31 minutes to 59 minutes, initial encounter	167	415, 416
SØ6.812S	Injury of right internal carotid artery, intracranial portion, not elsewhere classified with loss of consciousness of 31 minutes to 59 minutes, sequela	167	
SØ6.813A	Injury of right internal carotid artery, intracranial portion, not elsewhere classified with loss of consciousness of 1 hour to 5 hours 59 minutes, initial encounter	166	415, 416
SØ6.813S	Injury of right internal carotid artery, intracranial portion, not elsewhere classified with loss of consciousness of 1 hour to 5 hours 59 minutes, sequela	167	
SØ6.814A	Injury of right internal carotid artery, intracranial portion, not elsewhere classified with loss of consciousness of 6 hours to 24 hours, initial encounter	166	415, 416
SØ6.814S	Injury of right internal carotid artery, intracranial portion, not elsewhere classified with loss of consciousness of 6 hours to 24 hours, sequela	167	
SØ6.815A	Injury of right internal carotid artery, intracranial portion, not elsewhere classified with loss of consciousness greater than 24 hours with return to pre-existing conscious level, initial encounter	166	
SØ6.815S	Injury of right internal carotid artery, intracranial portion, not elsewhere classified with loss of consciousness greater than 24 hours with return to pre-existing conscious level, sequela	167	
SØ6.816A	Injury of right internal carotid artery, intracranial portion, not elsewhere classified with loss of consciousness greater than 24 hours without return to pre-existing conscious level with patient sur	166	
SØ6.816S	Injury of right internal carotid artery, intracranial portion, not elsewhere classified with loss of consciousness greater than 24 hours without return to pre-existing conscious level with patient sur	167	
SØ6.819A	Injury of right internal carotid artery, intracranial portion, not elsewhere classified with loss of consciousness of unspecified duration, initial encounter	167	415, 416
SØ6.819S	Injury of right internal carotid artery, intracranial portion, not elsewhere classified with loss of consciousness of unspecified duration, sequela	167	
SØ6.82ØA	Injury of left internal carotid artery, intracranial portion, not elsewhere classified without loss of consciousness, initial encounter	167	415, 416
SØ6.82ØS	Injury of left internal carotid artery, intracranial portion, not elsewhere classified without loss of consciousness, sequela	167	
SØ6.821A	Injury of left internal carotid artery, intracranial portion, not elsewhere classified with loss of consciousness of 3Ø minutes or less, initial encounter	167	415, 416
SØ6.821S	Injury of left internal carotid artery, intracranial portion, not elsewhere classified with loss of consciousness of 3Ø minutes or less, sequela	167	
SØ6.822A	Injury of left internal carotid artery, intracranial portion, not elsewhere classified with loss of consciousness of 31 minutes to 59 minutes, initial encounter	167	415, 416

Code	Description	CMS-HCC Model Category	QPP Individual Measures–Claims
S06.822S	Injury of left internal carotid artery, intracranial portion, not elsewhere classified with loss of consciousness of 31 minutes to 59 minutes, sequela	167	
S06.823A	Injury of left internal carotid artery, intracranial portion, not elsewhere classified with loss of consciousness of 1 hour to 5 hours 59 minutes, initial encounter	166	415, 416
S06.823S	Injury of left internal carotid artery, intracranial portion, not elsewhere classified with loss of consciousness of 1 hour to 5 hours 59 minutes, sequela	167	
S06.824A	Injury of left internal carotid artery, intracranial portion, not elsewhere classified with loss of consciousness of 6 hours to 24 hours, initial encounter	166	415, 416
S06.824S	Injury of left internal carotid artery, intracranial portion, not elsewhere classified with loss of consciousness of 6 hours to 24 hours, sequela	167	
S06.825A	Injury of left internal carotid artery, intracranial portion, not elsewhere classified with loss of consciousness greater than 24 hours with return to pre-existing conscious level, initial encounter	166	
S06.825S	Injury of left internal carotid artery, intracranial portion, not elsewhere classified with loss of consciousness greater than 24 hours with return to pre-existing conscious level, sequela	167	
S06.826A	Injury of left internal carotid artery, intracranial portion, not elsewhere classified with loss of consciousness greater than 24 hours without return to pre-existing conscious level with patient surv	166	
S06.826S	Injury of left internal carotid artery, intracranial portion, not elsewhere classified with loss of consciousness greater than 24 hours without return to pre-existing conscious level with patient surv	167	
S06.829A	Injury of left internal carotid artery, intracranial portion, not elsewhere classified with loss of consciousness of unspecified duration, initial encounter	167	415, 416
S06.829S	Injury of left internal carotid artery, intracranial portion, not elsewhere classified with loss of consciousness of unspecified duration, sequela	167	
S06.890A	Other specified intracranial injury without loss of consciousness, initial encounter	167	415, 416
S06.890S	Other specified intracranial injury without loss of consciousness, sequela	167	
S06.891A	Other specified intracranial injury with loss of consciousness of 30 minutes or less, initial encounter	167	415, 416
S06.891S	Other specified intracranial injury with loss of consciousness of 30 minutes or less, sequela	167	
S06.892A	Other specified intracranial injury with loss of consciousness of 31 minutes to 59 minutes, initial encounter	167	415, 416
S06.892S	Other specified intracranial injury with loss of consciousness of 31 minutes to 59 minutes, sequela	167	
S06.893A	Other specified intracranial injury with loss of consciousness of 1 hour to 5 hours 59 minutes, initial encounter	166	415, 416
S06.893S	Other specified intracranial injury with loss of consciousness of 1 hour to 5 hours 59 minutes, sequela	167	
S06.894A	Other specified intracranial injury with loss of consciousness of 6 hours to 24 hours, initial encounter	166	415, 416
S06.894S	Other specified intracranial injury with loss of consciousness of 6 hours to 24 hours, sequela	167	
S06.895A	Other specified intracranial injury with loss of consciousness greater than 24 hours with return to pre-existing conscious level, initial encounter	166	
S06.895S	Other specified intracranial injury with loss of consciousness greater than 24 hours with return to pre-existing conscious level, sequela	167	
S06.896A	Other specified intracranial injury with loss of consciousness greater than 24 hours without return to pre-existing conscious level with patient surviving, initial encounter	166	

Code	Description	CMS-HCC Model Category	QPP Individual Measures–Claims
SØ6.896S	Other specified intracranial injury with loss of consciousness greater than 24 hours without return to pre-existing conscious level with patient surviving, sequela	167	
SØ6.899A	Other specified intracranial injury with loss of consciousness of unspecified duration, initial encounter	167	415, 416
SØ6.899S	Other specified intracranial injury with loss of consciousness of unspecified duration, sequela	167	
SØ6.9XØA	Unspecified intracranial injury without loss of consciousness, initial encounter	167	415, 416
SØ6.9XØS	Unspecified intracranial injury without loss of consciousness, sequela	167	
SØ6.9X1A	Unspecified intracranial injury with loss of consciousness of 3Ø minutes or less, initial encounter	167	415, 416
SØ6.9X1S	Unspecified intracranial injury with loss of consciousness of 3Ø minutes or less, sequela	167	
SØ6.9X2A	Unspecified intracranial injury with loss of consciousness of 31 minutes to 59 minutes, initial encounter	167	415, 416
SØ6.9X2S	Unspecified intracranial injury with loss of consciousness of 31 minutes to 59 minutes, sequela	167	
SØ6.9X3A	Unspecified intracranial injury with loss of consciousness of 1 hour to 5 hours 59 minutes, initial encounter	166	415, 416
SØ6.9X3S	Unspecified intracranial injury with loss of consciousness of 1 hour to 5 hours 59 minutes, sequela	167	
SØ6.9X4A	Unspecified intracranial injury with loss of consciousness of 6 hours to 24 hours, initial encounter	166	415, 416
SØ6.9X4S	Unspecified intracranial injury with loss of consciousness of 6 hours to 24 hours, sequela	167	
SØ6.9X5A	Unspecified intracranial injury with loss of consciousness greater than 24 hours with return to pre-existing conscious level, initial encounter	166	
SØ6.9X5S	Unspecified intracranial injury with loss of consciousness greater than 24 hours with return to pre-existing conscious level, sequela	167	
SØ6.9X6A	Unspecified intracranial injury with loss of consciousness greater than 24 hours without return to pre-existing conscious level with patient surviving, initial encounter	166	
SØ6.9X6S	Unspecified intracranial injury with loss of consciousness greater than 24 hours without return to pre-existing conscious level with patient surviving, sequela	167	
SØ6.9X9A	Unspecified intracranial injury with loss of consciousness of unspecified duration, initial encounter	167	415, 416
SØ6.9X9S	Unspecified intracranial injury with loss of consciousness of unspecified duration, sequela	167	
S72.ØØ1A-C	Fracture of unspecified part of neck of right femur	17Ø	24, 418
S72.ØØ2A-C	Fracture of unspecified part of neck of left femur	17Ø	24, 418
S72.ØØ9A-C	Fracture of unspecified part of neck of unspecified femur	17Ø	24, 418
S72.Ø11A-C	Unspecified intracapsular fracture of right femur	17Ø	24, 418
S72.Ø12A-C	Unspecified intracapsular fracture of left femur	17Ø	24, 418
S72.Ø19A-C	Unspecified intracapsular fracture of unspecified femur	17Ø	24, 418
S72.Ø21A-C	Displaced fracture of epiphysis (separation) (upper) of right femur	17Ø	24, 418
S72.Ø22A-C	Displaced fracture of epiphysis (separation) (upper) of left femur	17Ø	24, 418
S72.Ø23A-C	Displaced fracture of epiphysis (separation) (upper) of unspecified femur	17Ø	24, 418
S72.Ø24A-C	Nondisplaced fracture of epiphysis (separation) (upper) of right femur	17Ø	24, 418
S72.Ø25A-C	Nondisplaced fracture of epiphysis (separation) (upper) of left femur	17Ø	24, 418
S72.Ø26A-C	Nondisplaced fracture of epiphysis (separation) (upper) of unspecified femur	17Ø	24, 418
S72.Ø31A-C	Displaced midcervical fracture of right femur	17Ø	24, 418

Code	Description	CMS-HCC Model Category	QPP Individual Measures–Claims
S72.Ø32A-C	Displaced midcervical fracture of left femur	17Ø	24, 418
S72.Ø33A-C	Displaced midcervical fracture of unspecified femur	17Ø	24, 418
S72.Ø34A-C	Nondisplaced midcervical fracture of right femur	17Ø	24, 418
S72.Ø35A-C	Nondisplaced midcervical fracture of left femur	17Ø	24, 418
S72.Ø36A-C	Nondisplaced midcervical fracture of unspecified femur	17Ø	24, 418
S72.Ø41A-C	Displaced fracture of base of neck of right femur	17Ø	24, 418
S72.Ø42A-C	Displaced fracture of base of neck of left femur	17Ø	24, 418
S72.Ø43A-C	Displaced fracture of base of neck of unspecified femur	17Ø	24, 418
S72.Ø44A-C	Nondisplaced fracture of base of neck of right femur	17Ø	24, 418
S72.Ø45A-C	Nondisplaced fracture of base of neck of left femur	17Ø	24, 418
S72.Ø46A-C	Nondisplaced fracture of base of neck of unspecified femur	17Ø	24, 418
S72.Ø51A-C	Unspecified fracture of head of right femur	17Ø	24, 418
S72.Ø52A-C	Unspecified fracture of head of left femur	17Ø	24, 418
S72.Ø59A-C	Unspecified fracture of head of unspecified femur	17Ø	24, 418
S72.Ø61A-C	Displaced articular fracture of head of right femur	17Ø	24, 418
S72.Ø62A-C	Displaced articular fracture of head of left femur	17Ø	24, 418
S72.Ø63A-C	Displaced articular fracture of head of unspecified femur	17Ø	24, 418
S72.Ø64A-C	Nondisplaced articular fracture of head of right femur	17Ø	24, 418
S72.Ø65A-C	Nondisplaced articular fracture of head of left femur	17Ø	24, 418
S72.Ø66A-C	Nondisplaced articular fracture of head of unspecified femur	17Ø	24, 418
S72.Ø91A-C	Other fracture of head and neck of right femur	17Ø	24, 418
S72.Ø92A-C	Other fracture of head and neck of left femur	17Ø	24, 418
S72.Ø99A-C	Other fracture of head and neck of unspecified femur	17Ø	24, 418
S72.1Ø1A-C	Unspecified trochanteric fracture of right femur	17Ø	24, 418
S72.1Ø2A-C	Unspecified trochanteric fracture of left femur	17Ø	24, 418
S72.1Ø9A-C	Unspecified trochanteric fracture of unspecified femur	17Ø	24, 418
S72.111A-C	Displaced fracture of greater trochanter of right femur	17Ø	24, 418
S72.112A-C	Displaced fracture of greater trochanter of left femur	17Ø	24, 418
S72.113A-C	Displaced fracture of greater trochanter of unspecified femur	17Ø	24, 418
S72.114A-C	Nondisplaced fracture of greater trochanter of right femur	17Ø	24, 418
S72.115A-C	Nondisplaced fracture of greater trochanter of left femur	17Ø	24, 418
S72.116A-C	Nondisplaced fracture of greater trochanter of unspecified femur	17Ø	24, 418
S72.121A-C	Displaced fracture of lesser trochanter of right femur	17Ø	24, 418
S72.122A-C	Displaced fracture of lesser trochanter of left femur	17Ø	24, 418
S72.123A-C	Displaced fracture of lesser trochanter of unspecified femur	17Ø	24, 418
S72.124A-C	Nondisplaced fracture of lesser trochanter of right femur	17Ø	24, 418
S72.125A-C	Nondisplaced fracture of lesser trochanter of left femur	17Ø	24, 418
S72.126A-C	Nondisplaced fracture of lesser trochanter of unspecified femur	17Ø	24, 418
S72.131A-C	Displaced apophyseal fracture of right femur	17Ø	24, 418
S72.132A-C	Displaced apophyseal fracture of left femur	17Ø	24, 418
S72.133A-C	Displaced apophyseal fracture of unspecified femur	17Ø	24, 418
S72.134A-C	Nondisplaced apophyseal fracture of right femur	17Ø	24, 418

Code	Description	CMS-HCC Model Category	QPP Individual Measures–Claims
S72.135A-C	Nondisplaced apophyseal fracture of left femur	170	24, 418
S72.136A-C	Nondisplaced apophyseal fracture of unspecified femur	170	24, 418
S72.141A-C	Displaced intertrochanteric fracture of right femur	170	24, 418
S72.142A-C	Displaced intertrochanteric fracture of left femur	170	24, 418
S72.143A-C	Displaced intertrochanteric fracture of unspecified femur	170	24, 418
S72.144A-C	Nondisplaced intertrochanteric fracture of right femur	170	24, 418
S72.145A-C	Nondisplaced intertrochanteric fracture of left femur	170	24, 418
S72.146A-C	Nondisplaced intertrochanteric fracture of unspecified femur	170	24, 418
S72.21XA-C	Displaced subtrochanteric fracture of right femur	170	24, 418
S72.22XA-C	Displaced subtrochanteric fracture of left femur	170	24, 418
S72.23XA-C	Displaced subtrochanteric fracture of unspecified femur	170	24, 418
S72.24XA-C	Nondisplaced subtrochanteric fracture of right femur	170	24, 418
S72.25XA-C	Nondisplaced subtrochanteric fracture of left femur	170	24, 418
S72.26XA-C	Nondisplaced subtrochanteric fracture of unspecified femur	170	24, 418
S72.301A-C	Unspecified fracture of shaft of right femur	170	24, 418
S72.302A-C	Unspecified fracture of shaft of left femur	170	24, 418
S72.309A-C	Unspecified fracture of shaft of unspecified femur	170	24, 418
S72.321A-C	Displaced transverse fracture of shaft of right femur	170	24, 418
S72.322A-C	Displaced transverse fracture of shaft of left femur	170	24, 418
S72.323A-C	Displaced transverse fracture of shaft of unspecified femur	170	24, 418
S72.324A-C	Nondisplaced transverse fracture of shaft of right femur	170	24, 418
S72.325A-C	Nondisplaced transverse fracture of shaft of left femur	170	24, 418
S72.326A-C	Nondisplaced transverse fracture of shaft of unspecified femur	170	24, 418
S72.331A-C	Displaced oblique fracture of shaft of right femur	170	24, 418
S72.332A-C	Displaced oblique fracture of shaft of left femur	170	24, 418
S72.333A-C	Displaced oblique fracture of shaft of unspecified femur	170	24, 418
S72.334A-C	Nondisplaced oblique fracture of shaft of right femur	170	24, 418
S72.335A-C	Nondisplaced oblique fracture of shaft of left femur	170	24, 418
S72.336A-C	Nondisplaced oblique fracture of shaft of unspecified femur	170	24, 418
S72.341A-C	Displaced spiral fracture of shaft of right femur	170	24, 418
S72.342A-C	Displaced spiral fracture of shaft of left femur	170	24, 418
S72.343A-C	Displaced spiral fracture of shaft of unspecified femur	170	24, 418
S72.344A-C	Nondisplaced spiral fracture of shaft of right femur	170	24, 418
S72.345A-C	Nondisplaced spiral fracture of shaft of left femur	170	24, 418
S72.346A-C	Nondisplaced spiral fracture of shaft of unspecified femur	170	24, 418
S72.351A-C	Displaced comminuted fracture of shaft of right femur	170	24, 418
S72.352A-C	Displaced comminuted fracture of shaft of left femur	170	24, 418
S72.353A-C	Displaced comminuted fracture of shaft of unspecified femur	170	24, 418
S72.354A-C	Nondisplaced comminuted fracture of shaft of right femur	170	24, 418
S72.355A-C	Nondisplaced comminuted fracture of shaft of left femur	170	24, 418
S72.356A-C	Nondisplaced comminuted fracture of shaft of unspecified femur	170	24, 418
S72.361A-C	Displaced segmental fracture of shaft of right femur	170	24, 418

Code	Description	CMS-HCC Model Category	QPP Individual Measures–Claims
S72.362A-C	Displaced segmental fracture of shaft of left femur	170	24, 418
S72.363A-C	Displaced segmental fracture of shaft of unspecified femur	170	24, 418
S72.364A-C	Nondisplaced segmental fracture of shaft of right femur	170	24, 418
S72.365A-C	Nondisplaced segmental fracture of shaft of left femur	170	24, 418
S72.366A-C	Nondisplaced segmental fracture of shaft of unspecified femur	170	24, 418
S72.391A-C	Other fracture of shaft of right femur	170	24, 418
S72.392A-C	Other fracture of shaft of left femur	170	24, 418
S72.399A-C	Other fracture of shaft of unspecified femur	170	24, 418
S72.401A-C	Unspecified fracture of lower end of right femur	170	24, 418
S72.402A-C	Unspecified fracture of lower end of left femur	170	24, 418
S72.409A-C	Unspecified fracture of lower end of unspecified femur	170	24, 418
S72.411A-C	Displaced unspecified condyle fracture of lower end of right femur	170	24, 418
S72.412A-C	Displaced unspecified condyle fracture of lower end of left femur	170	24, 418
S72.413A-C	Displaced unspecified condyle fracture of lower end of unspecified femur	170	24, 418
S72.414A-C	Nondisplaced unspecified condyle fracture of lower end of right femur	170	24, 418
S72.415A-C	Nondisplaced unspecified condyle fracture of lower end of left femur	170	24, 418
S72.416A-C	Nondisplaced unspecified condyle fracture of lower end of unspecified femur	170	24, 418
S72.421A-C	Displaced fracture of lateral condyle of right femur	170	24, 418
S72.422A-C	Displaced fracture of lateral condyle of left femur	170	24, 418
S72.423A-C	Displaced fracture of lateral condyle of unspecified femur	170	24, 418
S72.424A-C	Nondisplaced fracture of lateral condyle of right femur	170	24, 418
S72.425A-C	Nondisplaced fracture of lateral condyle of left femur	170	24, 418
S72.426A-C	Nondisplaced fracture of lateral condyle of unspecified femur	170	24, 418
S72.431A-C	Displaced fracture of medial condyle of right femur	170	24, 418
S72.432A-C	Displaced fracture of medial condyle of left femur	170	24, 418
S72.433A-C	Displaced fracture of medial condyle of unspecified femur	170	24, 418
S72.434A-C	Nondisplaced fracture of medial condyle of right femur	170	24, 418
S72.435A-C	Nondisplaced fracture of medial condyle of left femur	170	24, 418
S72.436A-C	Nondisplaced fracture of medial condyle of unspecified femur	170	24, 418
S72.441A-C	Displaced fracture of lower epiphysis (separation) of right femur	170	24, 418
S72.442A-C	Displaced fracture of lower epiphysis (separation) of left femur	170	24, 418
S72.443A-C	Displaced fracture of lower epiphysis (separation) of unspecified femur	170	24, 418
S72.444A-C	Nondisplaced fracture of lower epiphysis (separation) of right femur	170	24, 418
S72.445A-C	Nondisplaced fracture of lower epiphysis (separation) of left femur	170	24, 418
S72.446A-C	Nondisplaced fracture of lower epiphysis (separation) of unspecified femur	170	24, 418
S72.451A-C	Displaced supracondylar fracture without intracondylar extension of lower end of right femur	170	24, 418
S72.452A-C	Displaced supracondylar fracture without intracondylar extension of lower end of left femur	170	24, 418
S72.453A-C	Displaced supracondylar fracture without intracondylar extension of lower end of unspecified femur	170	24, 418
S72.454A-C	Nondisplaced supracondylar fracture without intracondylar extension of lower end of right femur	170	24, 418

Code	Description	CMS-HCC Model Category	QPP Individual Measures–Claims
S72.455A-C	Nondisplaced supracondylar fracture without intracondylar extension of lower end of left femur	170	24, 418
S72.456A-C	Nondisplaced supracondylar fracture without intracondylar extension of lower end of unspecified femur	170	24, 418
S72.461A-C	Displaced supracondylar fracture with intracondylar extension of lower end of right femur	170	24, 418
S72.462A-C	Displaced supracondylar fracture with intracondylar extension of lower end of left femur	170	24, 418
S72.463A-C	Displaced supracondylar fracture with intracondylar extension of lower end of unspecified femur	170	24, 418
S72.464A-C	Nondisplaced supracondylar fracture with intracondylar extension of lower end of right femur	170	24, 418
S72.465A-C	Nondisplaced supracondylar fracture with intracondylar extension of lower end of left femur	170	24, 418
S72.466A-C	Nondisplaced supracondylar fracture with intracondylar extension of lower end of unspecified femur	170	24, 418
S72.471A	Torus fracture of lower end of right femur, initial encounter for closed fracture	170	24, 418
S72.472A	Torus fracture of lower end of left femur, initial encounter for closed fracture	170	24, 418
S72.479A	Torus fracture of lower end of unspecified femur, initial encounter for closed fracture	170	24, 418
S72.491A-C	Other fracture of lower end of right femur	170	24, 418
S72.492A-C	Other fracture of lower end of left femur	170	24, 418
S72.499A-C	Other fracture of lower end of unspecified femur	170	24, 418
S72.8X1A-C	Other fracture of right femur	170	24, 418
S72.8X2A-C	Other fracture of left femur	170	24, 418
S72.8X9A-C	Other fracture of unspecified femur	170	24, 418
S72.90XA-C	Unspecified fracture of unspecified femur	170	24, 418
S72.91XA-C	Unspecified fracture of right femur	170	24, 418
S72.92XA-C	Unspecified fracture of left femur	170	24, 418
Z68.41	Body mass index (BMI) 40.0-44.9, adult	22	
Z68.42	Body mass index (BMI) 45.0-49.9, adult	22	
Z68.43	Body mass index (BMI) 50-59.9 , adult	22	
Z68.44	Body mass index (BMI) 60.0-69.9, adult	22	
Z68.45	Body mass index (BMI) 70 or greater, adult	22	